The Frontier
Nursing Service

CONTRIBUTIONS TO SOUTHERN APPALACHIAN STUDIES

Territory Covered by the
Frontier Nursing Service
1935–1992

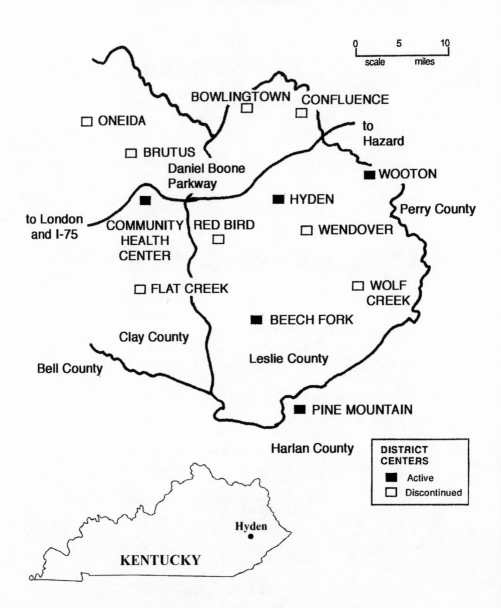

The Frontier Nursing Service

America's First Rural Nurse-Midwife Service and School

MARIE BARTLETT

CONTRIBUTIONS TO SOUTHERN APPALACHIAN STUDIES, 22

McFarland & Company, Inc., Publishers
Jefferson, North Carolina, and London

Library of Congress Cataloguing-in-Publication Data

Maher, Marie Bartlett, 1949–
    The Frontier Nursing Service : America's first rural nurse-
midwife service and school / Marie Bartlett.
       p.   cm.—(Contributions to Southern Appalachian
studies ; 22)
    Includes bibliographical references and index.

    ISBN 978-0-7864-3342-1
    softcover : 50# alkaline paper ∞

    1. Rural nursing—Kentucky.   2. Midwifery—Kentucky.
3. Frontier Nursing Service, Inc.   4. Frontier School of Midwifery and Family Nursing.   5. Breckinridge, Mary, 1881–1965.
I. Title.
RT120.R87M34   2009
610.73'43 — dc22   2008049997

British Library cataloguing data are available

On the cover: A brigade of the Frontier Nursing Service nurse-
midwives in their FNS uniforms, led by Mary Breckinridge
(extreme left), Thanksgiving Day, 1931; *inset* "saddlebag babies"

Manufactured in the United States of America

*McFarland & Company, Inc., Publishers
Box 611, Jefferson, North Carolina 28640
www.mcfarlandpub.com*

To the spirited women
of the Frontier Nursing Service
and to women everywhere
who give freely of themselves
so that others may have a better life.

Acknowledgments

Though writing itself is a lonely business, producing a nonfiction book is never a venture taken alone. The volume of research, time, and commitment necessary to complete it requires extra eyes and helping hands, from content selection to tone and proofing, to finished product.

This book would not have been possible without the assistance of certain people who gave of their time and energies to assist in its completion:

The staff of the Frontier Nursing Service at Wendover, FNS administrator Barb Gibson and Development Coordinator Michael J. Claussen, remained cooperative, kind, and extremely helpful throughout the long process of putting the book together despite numerous requests for materials, facts, photos, and other resources. They were also instrumental in allowing me access to the Big House and providing accommodations for my visits.

Kate Ireland, former head courier of the FNS and FNS board member, provided generous hospitality during a memorable weekend at her plantation home in Tallahassee, Florida. She and former FNS nurse-midwife Anne Cundle also gave me a rare insight into the remarkable type of women who joined the FNS.

My brother Paul Sluder, research assistant extraordinaire, and his wife, Betty Jo, spent untold hours screening files and documents so my debt to them is greater than I can ever repay. So is my gratitude to marketing agent Chuck Werle.

Librarian Shannon Wilson at Berea College Special Collections and University of Kentucky Libraries staff William James Marshall and Gwen Curtis were invaluable sources of information and referral. Dr. Richard A. Carter, of Nashville, Tennessee, offered medical insights and corrections.

And my special thanks to Steve Marks, whose love and support help make *everything* worthwhile.

Table of Contents

Preface

Researching a nonfiction book, in which facts are sacrosanct, can range from joyous to tedious in the extreme. But never did I think it would be a frightening experience ... or at least ghostly. But there I was alone in the deep woods of eastern Kentucky, in the Big House, original site of the rural Frontier Nursing Service and home to its founder, Mary Breckinridge. The cook and housekeeper left the premises at six P.M., telling me to make myself comfortable among Breckinridge's many documents, artifacts, and photos. I could even sleep in her room if I chose.

Around midnight, tired of poring over documents that would help me piece together the story of how midwifery first came to America, I ventured upstairs. The long narrow hallway was dark, seemingly endless, its well-worn plank floors moaning and creaking beneath my feet.

I entered Breckinridge's room, feeling like an intruder in this place she came to love so well. Moonlight peeked through the lacy curtains, shadowed by a huge, lurking elm just outside the window. The room smelled of oilcloth and burnished wood, reminding me of my grandmother's place. Sprawling across the bed fully clothed, I fell fast asleep. It seemed like only minutes passed.

Then I heard a noise: down the hallway the turn of a heavy metal doorknob; the click of a solid door opened and closed; the unmistakable sound of soft footsteps. I awoke suddenly and bolted upright, eyeing the room's entrance. On impulse, I flipped the light switch, by now more afraid of the dark than what was behind the door. I leaned forward, pulled on the handle and peeked down the long, narrow hallway. It was dark and empty. I made the rounds upstairs and down, snapping on every light I could find, searching out every doorway. The place was now lit up like a house on fire. Nothing; no one. All doors were secure, just as I'd left them.

It was only later that I discovered some of the people who worked on the premises—and were much too young to have encountered Mary Breckinridge before her death in 1965 — had seen and heard things throughout the Big House. It was a staple joke among them, and one they shared with very few. After all, jobs and public relations were at stake. A cordial groundskeeper came by as I was sitting outside the next day and asked if I had met Breckinridge yet, chuckling at my expression. I suspected he knew the cook had found me that morning with all the lights on. "I'm not sure," I said. "But I heard someone in the hallway last night. Maybe she didn't like the fact that I was in her room." "Oh, it wouldn't be that," he responded. Then he reached out and patted my shoulder with a steady, reassuring hand. "She took care of everyone," he said. "She probably just wanted to make sure that you were okay."

* * *

There was a time when the average American child-bearing woman was more likely to die from childbirth than from any other condition except tuberculosis. This was especially true in areas where hospitals and quality medical care were scarce or non-existent. But deep in the rolling hills of eastern Kentucky's Cumberland Range, beginning in the 1920s, one woman almost single-handedly changed those dismal figures. Her name was Mary Breckinridge and her goal was to bring rural midwifery to the U.S. for the first time, staffed by trained nurses determined to provide quality maternity care. Opened in 1925 in Leslie County, Kentucky, the Frontier Nursing Service (FNS) set out to lower the local maternal mortality rate from one of the highest in the country to the lowest. Today, the FNS is a National Historic Site, as well as a bed-and-breakfast. And Mary Breckinridge is a local icon, with plays, books, buildings, and children carrying her name. She is referred to as "Mrs. Breckinridge;" it is considered disrespectful to call her "Mary."

Yet she was a most unlikely

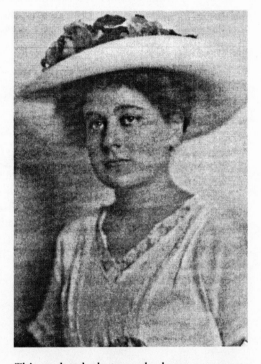

This undated photograph shows a young Mary Breckinridge (probably in her twenties) as she appeared in the early 1900s, prior to establishing the Frontier Nursing Service. A socialite and debutante during this period, Breckinridge once said her aspiration was to become "an explorer." She began the Kentucky Committee for Mothers and Babies in May 1925 at the age of 44. The organization was renamed the Frontier Nursing Service in 1928.

heroine. She would be the first to say so, and the first to emphasize that she could not have achieved this mission alone. She was also extremely complex — highly intelligent yet helpless in some of the minutest ways; generous and warm yet calculating and manipulative; gracious yet condescending; full of self-effacing humor yet deadly serious on those things that mattered most; prim yet raucous and dramatic when it suited her; a forward-thinking progressive yet a social snob; both democratic and autocratic. Demanding, stubborn, endearing, controlling, engaging — in other words a multi-faceted human being with strengths and flaws like the rest of us. As a result, people both loved and feared her, often at the same time. She was also one of the most remarkable women of her time.

While some healthcare professionals have criticized the approach and the data used by Breckinridge which resulted in promoting nurse-midwifery as a noble, romanticized calling rather than a real profession, there is no doubt the FNS provided much-needed comprehensive maternity and general healthcare to a part of the country in which it was desperately needed. There is also no doubt she was a visionary leader and an indelible presence in eastern Kentucky.

Establishing roots in a place she meant only to visit, she knew both success and failure, joy and despair. Her personal life was filled with great loss but in the end was sustained by great satisfaction as well.

This is the story of Breckinridge and the first forty years of the Frontier Nursing Service. It is told in *human terms* as opposed to academic, and in no way is considered a definitive view of the FNS, nor a scholarly attempt at history. That is better left to scholars and historians. It is, instead, the story of an ensemble of strong, dedicated women led by Breckinridge, which changed a community, and allowed a community to change them.

1

In the Beginning

Hyden, Kentucky, lies deep in the arms of the Cumberland Mountains, cradled by rugged, compact hills that shelter it as a mother would encircle and protect her child. As of 2007, slightly fewer than two hundred people called it home. Ninety-eight point five percent of its residents are white. Their ancestry is mostly English, Scotch, and Irish. More than half of adults are married and about one-third have been to college. The median household income is $26,429. The majority of adult males work in construction — truck drivers and sales. Females tend to be teachers, cooks, or service workers. There is no industry to speak of, other than a coal mine twenty-two miles from Hyden.

Unlike a century ago, getting into Hyden today is easy. The well-maintained Hal Rogers Parkway, just off I-75, winds ribbon-like past walls of chiseled granite where small but sturdy homes sit poised on the hillsides as though watching the passers-by. Mobile homes, billboards, a few convenience stores, and an occasional private cemetery dot the landscape. The town of Hyden, the county seat, fifteen miles west of Hazard, sits on a branch of the Middle Fork of the Kentucky River. The town is less than a full square mile in size and its Main Street comes to a T past the public library at a single red light. Going left will take you to the twenty-five-bed Mary Breckinridge Healthcare Center perched at the foot of the old Hyden Hospital. Going right takes you past a popular Dairy Queen, a self-service laundry, a drugstore, and a few small businesses.

As the road begins to snake alongside the Middle Fork creek, the Leslie County High School suddenly looms high and proud on the hillside. It faces the creek bed, fronted by a paved running track, and is topped with a green-tiled roof and an arched exterior that gives it a sleek, sophisticated look. Renovated in 1993 through a multi-million dollar federal project, it startles those who come upon its girth and contemporary beauty. What's also surprising is that there are more students in the high school than in the entire town of Hyden. That's because students come from throughout the entire county to attend school.

Most of the locals are open and friendly despite decades of Appalachian stereotypes that have plagued both them and the region. A few are still sensitive to generalizations of backwoods mountaineers. Some still harbor an understandable reticence to share information with strangers, particularly those who are "brought-on" from the outside.

Near the school, across the concrete bridge that spans the creek, is a single-lane road that twists and turns as it carves its way into the woods. One car must yield to another alongside the creek bed, and in heavy rains the road is often impassable. Deciduous hardwoods form a canopy and in spring and summer, creeping phlox and pink lady slippers add splashes of color. At a sharp bend ahead is a gravel driveway. It is the entrance to Pig Alley, the gateway to Hyden's most renowned tourist attraction, the Frontier Nursing Service (FNS), the first midwife school in rural America. Now a bed-and-breakfast, albeit an isolated one, the rambling two-story log house was also once the home of FNS founder Mary Breckinridge. It is a place that still draws one in.

There is living history that almost seeps from its eighty-year-old walls, a place that epitomizes life-altering sacrifice, dedication to service, intrigue, inspiration, frustration, and more than enough human interest to satisfy even those not interested in long-past events. Within these walls there is even a ghost story or two. Its origins were ambitious; its future uncertain at best. In fact, the concept of professional midwifery was nowhere in the nation's social fabric when Mary Breckinridge set out in 1923 to find the poorest part of America with one of the highest infant mortality rates and reverse that trend. This was god-forsaken country back then, a place few people thought or cared much about. Some even called it the Forgotten Frontier. Thanks to Breckinridge, the brave nurses and staff who helped her build and maintain the Frontier Nursing Service, and a community that seemed strange and foreign at the time, the "god-forsaken" part along with the highest infant mortality rate was about to change.

* * *

Hyden, Kentucky, 1923: A woman with the unlikely name of Lies Pace swore she could tell fortunes just by resting someone's palm inside her calloused hand, for this was how she predicted the future. Often found loitering by the rock wall that guarded the Leslie County courthouse in eastern Kentucky, she made deals with the locals: a reading for a bit of cash, a block of wood to build a fire. The money bought daily food, the wood brought nightly warmth. No one knew where she lived or much about her except her unusual name and her outlandish, prophetic claims.

Near the courthouse was a gristmill, a drugstore set upon a wooden platform reminiscent of a frontier town, a boarding house, a smattering of churches, a general hardware story, a hotel, a bank, and a barber shop. At the post office, locals simply walked in and asked if the mail, delivered by wagon, had arrived. A hitching post for mules and horses formed a centerpiece in the middle of the often muddy morass that passed for Main Street Hyden. The town's population was a meager three hundred souls. One longtime resident said the place was so small you could "fall into one end of town and right out the other."[1] In lieu of sidewalks, two-by-four planks allowed residents to bypass the worst of the puddles. A sweet shop, its exterior walls streaked with an incessant black mud from frequent rains, offered candy and ice cream. To keep the frozen sweets rock-solid, blocks of ice were taken from the creek in winter, placed inside the barns, and buckets of water tossed upon them. Packed tight with sawdust, these blocks would stay cold till nearly mid-summer.

There were no roads other than dirt paths and rocky trails, no railroad as yet, and no phones. Telegraphs and couriers on horseback, many of whom had to guide their trusty animals up and down the steep rocky ridges, kept the flow of information moving. On occasion a wagon-led carnival would pass through town, providing a scant bit of fun. Farmers planted their corn and tobacco by the new moon, as their ancestors had done before them. For a crop of potatoes to do well, they believed it best to plant them deep in the ground by the "old moon." Those who swore by this technique would say "it works because I experienced it out."[2] Everyone grew their own food, mostly corn and potatoes. They raised chickens and hogs which they used to swap for dry goods like flour, a sack of sugar or salt. That could mean a day-long wagon ride to London, the nearest big town, about thirty-five miles away. Industrious children could earn a nickel a day by building a fire for someone or sweeping out the schoolhouse. Attending school was a luxury only a few families could afford, for their offspring were needed worse at home, manning a plow or tending a crop.

A few physicians, or at least those bold enough to call themselves a doctor, operated in and around town. It was hard to tell the licensed from the bogus. One kept his medicines in a jug. Another visited the sick on an old yellow mare. He admitted he had acquired his medical background as an orderly in the Civil War.

When an itinerant doctor arrived in Hyden presenting himself as a foot specialist, he said he could remove corns and bunions "all without a drop of blood, though the other doctors will probably law me for it."[3] A patient, an older woman, finally showed up. The tender corns between her toes were giving her fits, she explained. "You can take these off without drawing blood?" she inquired through narrowed eyes. "I sure can." "I tell you what," she said. "If you draw a drop of blood, I'll kick you right through that wall."[4] He went to work and must have met her expectations for there were no reported injuries.

An ailing youngster was said to "puny around." Children in the decades prior to World War II, particularly in the poverty-stricken Appalachian region, were prone to malnutrition, hookworm, anemia, and typhoid. Young adults were felled by accidents and killer tuberculosis. Pain could be so punishing that patients were often heard to say, "I don't know how I'll live."

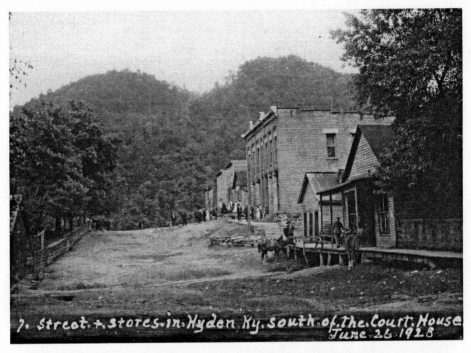

7. Street + stores in Hyden Ky. south of The Court House June 26 1928

Main Street, Hyden, Kentucky, 1928 (courtesy Special Collections and Digital Programs, University of Kentucky Libraries and the Frontier Nursing Service, Inc.).

Though uncommon, there were family feuds that ended in a shootout. One occurred in the middle of Hyden on a day when a large crowd had gathered in front of the courthouse. Some said a man went crazy when his brother was killed and just started shooting up the town. One victim, struck by a .45 bullet between the eyes, kept on running according to a witness. When the melee was over, two men lay dead. The townsfolk quickly scattered, terrified of what might happen next.

High in the hills were a few local, or granny, midwives doing what they thought was best. Often that meant placing an axe under the birthing woman's bed in an effort to cut the pain and facilitate birth or feeding tea made of chimney soot to women in labor.[5] Other natural remedies included black gum bark mixed with sweet apple tree bark, peeled one piece up and one down to ward off miscarriages. Yellow root tea was endorsed by one granny midwife for severe bleeding, while others said roots of the rattleweed, yellow spicewood, peppermint—all made into teas—would assist in childbirth. If herbs were unavailable, quinine and even gunpowder stirred into a drink would suffice.

Among the granny midwives was Aunt Tildy. She grieved the loss of any young mother but a particular case was one she still recalled many years later. "The baby was crossed. I could not reach either head or feet after all day and

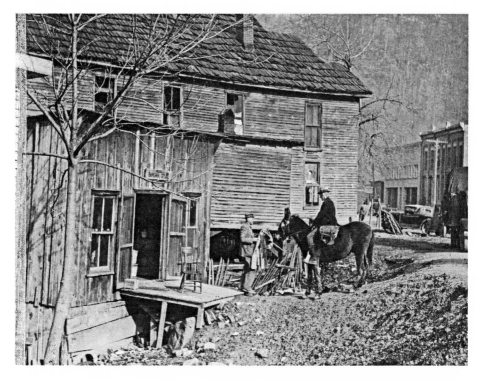

Hyden, Kentucky, in the 1920s was little more than a frontier town. In this photograph, a local resident prepares to dismount his horse at the one of the major retail stores in Hyden (courtesy Special Collections and Digital Programs, University of Kentucky Libraries and the Frontier Nursing Service, Inc.).

all night. Finally, I sent for two doctors. We tried unsuccessfully to deliver the patient. After fifty hours of labor, we sent a fur piece for a real doctor. But before he reached the house, the mother died. And just before that, she called for her sister." "Take keer of my children," was her dying request. "The terrible miseries just kept up until they killed her," recounted Aunt Tildy.[6] A well-respected physician in neighboring Owsley County constantly decried the lack of qualified medical care within the region. "It is impossible for me to reach every hoot-owl hollow in my section in time to be of any use to a woman in childbirth," he complained. "Trained midwives are essential here. I wish they might become nurses as well."[7]

Unbeknownst to him, someone who had the means and the motive to make that wish come true was only a day's horseback ride away, roaming farther into the Appalachian hills than most outsiders ever dared venture. It was late summer in 1923 when she began what she called her investigation. Specifically, she was on a mission to find and interview local granny midwives in order to view their practices, talk with the mothers they served, and attempt to get a handle on medical services needed in three of eastern Kentucky's most isolated counties. This lonely but determined woman was following the heavily forested creek banks on horseback, often stopping to admire a ridgeline or breathe in the woodsy smell of cedar, spruce and hemlock. There was little that her large, intelligent eyes missed. Her name was Mary Breckinridge and she was a most unlikely figure to explore these Kentucky hills.

2

From Socialite to Activist

Born into wealth on February 17, 1881, in Memphis, Tennessee, Breckinridge was the middle child of four children, having an older brother, a younger brother, and a younger sister. Her father, Clifton R. Breckinridge, was born and raised near Lexington, Kentucky; he was a Confederate soldier at fifteen, and in the cotton business as an adult.[1] Her grandfather, John C. Breckinridge, was U.S. vice president under President Buchanan, a major general of the Confederacy, and its last secretary of war.[2] The family was sent to St. Petersburg when Clifton Rodes Breckinridge (who served in the U.S. Congress following Reconstruction) became ambassador to Czar Nicholas II of Russia from 1894 to 1897. It was here that Mary Breckinridge, as an adolescent, learned that her mother was pregnant again. The baby was born assisted by a Russian midwife, an event that planted the first seed for what would eventually become the Frontier Nursing Service.

"If it had been my own, I could not have taken a larger interest in the preparations," she said of her brother's birth. "My mother told me that when the baby was born, two doctors stood by in their white coats while Madame Kourchnova (midwife) did the delivery. It was a normal delivery and there was no reason why they should interfere. I recalled this often. Apparently, there were women called midwives who were trained to do normal deliveries for the doctors."[3] This was unheard of in the States. In fact, during Mrs. Breckinridge's confinements, including her pregnancy with Mary in Tennessee in 1881, there were no trained American nurse-midwives assisting with childbirth.

Worldwide, Europeans were well ahead of the curve on midwifery, assuming that midwives would have an important place in childbirth. Their physicians were, in general, less defensive about their professional status than American doctors. The Midwives Act of 1902 changed things for the better in Britain by creating a central board which examined and supervised midwives, eventually giving them higher status and recognition as opposed to America, where nurse-midwives (when they finally became established in the U.S.) served as stopgaps only until a physician could arrive and attend the birth.[4]

11

Breckinridge was determined to change that in a place that lacked medical attention from healthcare professionals of all types. Her ties to Kentucky were strengthened during summer visits to Hazelwood, a rambling country house near High Bridge, New York. It was the home of a great-aunt whom the Breckinridge children referred to as Grandmother Lees. She was a wealthy, charitable woman born in Kentucky who still contributed money to Southern children for their educations, particularly Kentuckians. Many wrote letters to her, expressing their gratitude. "At Hazelwood," recalled Breckinridge, "I delighted in sitting at her feet and listening to the letters she read aloud from these children. Nearly a lifetime later, when I was living on money that had come from my Grandmother Lees (my share of my mother's share), it seemed altogether right to use this money to start the Frontier Nursing Service in the Kentucky Mountains."

She also learned to horseback ride as a child, often riding bareback behind her brother, and just as often, falling off. Her lifelong love of animals came from having pets as a youngster: a collie she named Shep and a mockingbird she rescued from a nest and called Douce. When the creatures died, she kept a feather and a lock of dog hair in her New Testament Bible. Breckinridge claimed she had no real education, certainly nothing that prepared her for the lifework ahead. But at fifteen, she could write and spell in three languages, though all of them badly, she said. She was extremely poor at math, requiring a tutor to help her understand decimals and fractions in order to get through nursing school. She called them "wretched symbols" and said she "never felt at home with them."[5]

A lonely teen, she found solace in her animals and in books. Among her favorite works: *The Jungle Book* and *Young Marooners.* Writing poetry and creative stories were other pastimes. Attending college was not in the plan for most young women of her day. Families believed that girls should be kept at home and taught domestic skills. Her older brother was sent to first class schools in Washington, D.C., but Breckinridge and her sister Lees had governesses. The children also traveled frequently with their parents where they were exposed to Swiss, German, and French cultures. Despite their wealth (most of which was tied up in heavily taxed land) the family never had a home of their own until Breckinridge was an adult. Her parents preferred to rent after the federal government confiscated a family member's house. It was a sticking point between her parents—Clifton Breckinridge said he would never buy a house; Mrs. Breckinridge always wanted one. That may be why Wendover, which became Mary Breckinridge's permanent home, held so much meaning for her throughout her life.[6]

By the turn of the century, she was a true debutante who attended parties and loved to dance. As a young woman of privilege, she also liked to hunt, mounting the first wild turkey she shot on her uncle's Mississippi plantation. Yet even then, she exhibited a strict code of honor and a deeply engrained set of family rules that she believed were common to Kentucky mountaineers.

Among the Breckinridge family honor code:

- Extend hospitality under all circumstances—"When strangers ride up to your door," she once said, "give them at least a cup of cold water and a bed even if you haven't one."
- Never speak ill of someone who extended hospitality to you.
- Stand by your friends and your people.
- Never hit below the belt, even with your enemies.
- Loyalty to country matters above all else.
- Scandal and slander should be avoided at all costs.[7]

Her sense of decorum was in many respects a product of her times, especially in the upper class South of the early 1900s. Females could travel with a man in the daytime but not at night. Moonlight rides required a chaperone. Men did not use the word "damn" in front of women, nor did they make mention of bulls due to the sexual connotation. Males did not call females by their first names unless they had known them since childhood, and the only gifts a single woman could accept from a single male were books, flowers, and candy.

In her youth Breckinridge was a pretty girl, her soulful face dominated by bright blue eyes round as buttons. She had medium brown hair often topped by a fashionable hat of the day and in stature was small, less than five feet four, with a curvaceous figure. But though she was physically demure, there was little about her spirit and demeanor anyone could call coy. In fact, even in her youth, she was a force to be reckoned with. Her loud laugh could stop a conversation in mid-sentence and she was opinionated to the point of arrogance at times, seldom letting the other person get a word in edgewise. As a young woman, she did not particularly want to be a nurse. She wanted to be an explorer. Later, a member of the national FNS committee, and Breckinridge's peer, said that when Breckinridge eventually traveled overseas to study midwifery in England, she was "more tolerated than welcomed" by the British Mothers and Nurses Committee. "She was very definite about what she thought she knew. So if someone was teaching her something, she would be a rather difficult student. And she was an older person by then, probably set in her ways. The matron told me that if they had known what they were up against, they wouldn't have taken her."[8]

Fashion, make-up, and other forms of vanity would hold less appeal for her as time passed. An acquaintance who once fussed at Breckinridge about wearing the same hat to a public engagement was met with this practical reply: "I only need one hat. I only have one head."[9] Yet in her prime, within her social circles, she was considered quite the catch. She caught the attention of several males, among them Henry Ruffner Morrison, an attorney who became her first husband and one of the few men many believed she truly loved. The couple married in 1904 when Breckinridge was twenty-three, but he died after only a year from what was speculated to be appendicitis. It was a loss so painful to

Breckinridge that she would not speak of it for decades. Instead, she wrote letters to him in her personal journal, making reference to "the darkness of my inner soul."[10]

The question now was what to do next with her restless life. "To stay with my parents, the subject of their endless solicitude was impossible. I wanted to give care, not to receive it."[11] She visited a family friend in New York who suggested she enter nursing school. In February 1907 she was accepted at St. Luke's Hospital School of Nursing. In her third year she was made head of a twenty-four-bed men's surgical ward. By her senior year she was looking for opportunities to work with babies. She found it at the nearby New York Lying-In Hospital where student nurses were sent for obstetrical training. She soon discovered that conditions for the helpless newborns were often dismal. "There were never fewer than twenty babies," Breckinridge recalled, "and sometimes as many as thirty. The heat was turned down at night and the east wind from the river penetrated through the cracks of the windows. Only one thin cotton blanket was allowed to each bassinet. I never had the heart to wear my sweater, for it could provide an extra covering for at least one baby. There weren't anything like enough diapers to keep the babies dry. They were used for other things; face towels for the mothers; dust rags for the ward maids. Most babies were breast-fed and sometimes I despaired over the bottle-fed babies. One had spina bifida and was paralyzed in both legs. Her mother did not want her. More than once the head nurse went off duty leaving no formula, not even milk in the refrigerator. So a young doctor went out on the street to buy milk and brought it back."[12]

After a few months Breckinridge could take it no longer. She approached the hospital board about adopting the handicapped baby, named Margaret. She could well afford to, she told the board. When they refused her request she asked a physician to medically discharge Margaret so Breckinridge could take her home. For her efforts, she was temporarily suspended along with the physician and another nurse. A few days later she received a call that Margaret was dead. Breckinridge was told she could have the body if she wanted it. It would save the child from a pauper's grave. "I arranged with an under-taking firm to buy a grave and we held a brief service. For that crippled baby with the luminous eyes and wisdom beyond her weeks, I have kept affection. I hope, and expect to see her, with my own two children when I have crossed to the other side of death."[13]

After graduation from St. Luke's, Breckinridge took another break to spend time with her family. Her mother was ill and needed attention. She spent a year looking after her in Fort Smith, Arkansas, where she met her second husband, Richard Thompson, president of Crescent College in Eureka Springs. They married in 1912 and lived on the college campus. Breckinridge even taught on occasion, conducting classes in child welfare. Like Breckinridge, Thompson had a sense of humor, evidenced by a ploy to catch his female students sneaking boys onto campus. The girls had commandeered the school's laundry services so their boyfriends could climb into a wicker basket and be hoisted up through a window. When Thompson discovered what the students were doing, he planted himself at the site where the basket was lowered, stepped inside, gave the signal, and had himself delivered to the waiting girls.[14]

But the couple's home life was no laughing matter. Neighbors and friends said they were seldom seen places together and didn't appear harmonious.[15] Of this second marriage, which ended in divorce, Breckinridge divulges very little. Among her social class it was considered poor taste to discuss broken marriages even among friends. Something good did come of the union, however: her two children Breckie and Polly. A precocious tow-headed toddler, Breckie learned French and English simultaneously, could ride a horse by the age of three, and according to his doting mother, distributed toys to the children who came to his house. Breckinridge would make up stories and read to him while he cuddled his favorite toy, Teddy Bear. A chronic climber, he would scamper outside his crib, gather loot and return to his bed. She once found him upright in his crib with an umbrella, an American flag, a dish of prunes, and an innocent grin. Frustrated by his willful nature, she had chicken wire installed over the bed. The climbing stopped.

Tragedy soon followed. On January 23, 1918, her beloved four-year-old Breckie died from peritonitis, an infection of the intestines that a local doctor mistook for appendicitis. By the time surgeons intervened, it was too late. Two years later she was pregnant again. However, Polly was born premature and died within six hours of her birth.[16] Breckinridge and her husband separated soon after, some said because of the loss of their children, while others maintained they were always on divergent paths. Those who knew Thompson said that despite their many differences, he never spoke ill of his ex-wife, telling others she had "a brilliant brain, and was tied down too much in Eureka. She could do more in a life of service."[17]

To the end of her life, Breckinridge would cherish the memories and mourn the deaths of her two children. Whenever she traveled, the first thing she did was pull their pictures from her suitcase and place them on a bureau. A photo of Breckie remained on her dresser till the day she died.[18] In fact, many who knew her said that losing her children was the single most important driving force that led her to establish the Frontier Nursing Service so that other mothers would not suffer the same fate. In the meantime, reaching out to others helped counter her mind-numbing grief. Her first move was to head to Europe, where the First World War had just ended.

By 1920, she was in France assisting villagers through the American Committee for Devastated France. Her role was to serve as director of child hygiene and educate villagers on public health issues. After a year, she announced she was taking a leave of absence to return to America and get a divorce. "I've made up my mind," she told her district nurses. "When I get divorced I want my dear father's name back because the Thompson name doesn't mean anything to me. My son is gone. So when I come back from America, I'll change my name."[19] And that's exactly what she did. A few weeks later she returned to France as promised. Picking up her duties where she left off, she was assigned a woman driver who chauffeured her around in a hand-cranked Model T Ford. Arriving at one small village where she was scheduled to speak, Breckinridge found an audience of mostly peasants. These were French farmers more interested in getting back to their plots of land than listening to this foreign woman lecture them on subjects for which they had little knowledge or interest. To her driver's bemusement, Breckinridge stood up and opened her speech with a personal announcement:

"I am no longer Mrs. Thompson. I'm divorced. And I'm now Mary Breckinridge." The crowd was "quite startled," the driver recalled, "because that was a sophisticated life they did not understand."[20] Yet it was classic Breckinridge, setting the tone for a lifelong talent of capturing an audience's attention. More important was what Breckinridge learned during her years in France that would assist her in establishing the FNS. The village districts, for example, were designed in a manner upon which she would later model the FNS outposts. The field work of the FNS would be set up on a decentralized basis with each nursing center owned by the service, but managed by the nurses. It was the only feasible method in isolated regions like the Scottish Highlands, the rural villages of England and France, and in rural eastern Kentucky. The nursing centers would each have a local committee composed of leading citizens who would meet regularly with the nurses and provide reports. Therefore, the FNS could work *through* the people rather than *for* them, Breckinridge surmised.

She also met numerous French and British midwives, which reinforced her high opinion of their role as health providers. (Ironically, she found that French midwife training was considered of high quality but general nurses' training was not). Perhaps this was due to the stronger emphasis placed on midwife training in Europe. "I also learned it is best to begin small, take root, and then grow. I formed an indispensable habit of learning all I could about native customs so that new things could be grafted onto the old. Finally, I gained a respect for facts—old and new—with the knowledge that change is not brought about by theories."[21]

Upon her return to New York City, it began to dawn upon her that nurse-midwifery was the logical response to the needs of young children, especially in remote areas. She enrolled in Columbia's Teachers College to study public health nursing. There, she had contact with nurses from the Maternity Center Association (MCA), an organization that had attempted and failed in 1923 to open a midwifery program for nurses in conjunction with Bellevue Hospital. MCA was unable to attract interest in a midwifery course among state health administrators. There was also speculation that physicians feared well-educated nurse-midwives as competition.[22] So Breckinridge made plans to become a certified midwife at a school in England with help from Carolyn Conant van Blarcom, best known as the author of an early obstetric textbook, who had midwifery contacts there. Maybe, thought Breckinridge, while in England she could also persuade well-trained British nurses to help in her endeavor to open America's first rural midwifery service. About this time, she learned her mother had died and so she detoured to Arkansas in order to be with the family. She would also need to find and explore one of the poorest parts of the country with the reputation for having one of the highest infant mortality rates, a place in which she could set her plan in motion.

3

Laying the Groundwork

In the spring of 1922, after closing her mother's estate in Fort Smith, Arkansas, Breckinridge made one of several trips to see her father, staying with relatives in Kentucky after his wife's death, and discussed her plan with him. She also began a long series of correspondence to people both in and outside her social circle, doctors, bankers, college administrators, and other public officials, explaining the need for a "child-saving investigation" into health care services. Her plan was to create a free health-care program provided by public health care nurses with advanced education in midwifery based on the British model. Promising physician support, Breckinridge approached the American Child Health Association for funding. But the agency responded by stating it required state support.

Not everyone was convinced Breckinridge had a good idea. Nor was every organization cooperative. Dr. Annie S. Veech, director of Kentucky's Bureau of Maternal and Child Health and the state's project evaluator, vetoed the plan. She believed that Breckinridge was too independent for one thing, unwilling to take her or her staff's advice. For another, Veech thought the plan impractical. She disagreed with the idea of nurse-midwives—they should stick to being midwives rather than public health nurses—and furthermore, she contended, it was more cost effective to train granny midwives than hire professional nurse-midwives.[1]

Undaunted, Breckinridge acquired permission and cooperation from the State Board of Health to complete a house-to-house survey regarding births and deaths of the more than sixteen hundred families living in Leslie County. The state statistician supplemented the records by examining records that dated back to 1911. Bertram Ireland, a certified nurse-midwife who had completed a similar study in the Scottish Highlands, conducted the actual survey along with six people working under her supervision. Though she came from similar geographic terrain, Ireland and her crew encountered difficulties in Leslie County even she did not anticipate. A drought caused a failure of crops, making feed for the horses scarce; that was soon followed by flooding. Corn bread and apples were often the only form of sustenance for residents and animals. One survey worker hitched her horse to a tree near a steep cliff, and turned to see the tree and the horse disappear over the precipice. Another, dismounting at a gap on a mountain ridge, stepped on a rattler, not once but three times, barely avoiding a potentially fatal bite.

"It was an unusual day that did not present a special problem," said Ireland. "And we often heard this was no work for a woman. A few times someone went off with our horse blankets, even our horses. The rains made routes impassable. The mail wagon couldn't bring our anxiously-expected equipment. In my first week there was a 'tide' due to flooding that confined me to a small plot of land for four days. Owing to a shortage of oats, my horse was given a 'green feed' which, together with him being out in a severe hail storm, gave him colic so badly that he could not be ridden for two days."[2] Yet despite the many hardships, Ireland found the mountain residents exhibited a neighborly bond and a strong sense of fair play. Like the Scottish Highlanders, they at least had the good fortune of a natural supply of timber, coal, fruit, and other natural resources. She often shared stories from her native land, convincing them theirs was not the poor country they perceived it to be. "When it became known there was the probability of an increase in the number of nurses in the county," said Ireland, "we were almost embarrassed with offers of land and timber and workers 'if only we would establish a nursing center right here on this creek.'"[3]

In her concluding report to Breckinridge, she wrote that the people of Leslie County were anxious to cooperate with the Kentucky Committee for Mothers and Babies, the new organization Breckinridge had formed with committee members chosen from leading citizens throughout the state. "They are more than willing to help ensure themselves a healthy, happy progeny that will perpetuate their deep love for home and country and equip them for the coming encounter with the industrial competition," Ireland wrote.[4]

Following the report, Breckinridge decided it might be worthwhile to determine the intelligence level of local children compared to those outside the region. She contacted Dr. Ella Woodyard, whom she considered a "brilliant psychologist" and an expert in mental testing. Woodyard tested 66 children, ages six to ten, chosen at random. She used the Stanford Revision of the Binet-Simon test to determine their average I.Q. The result was that with proper education the eastern Kentucky children were just as bright as any child in America. What they lacked were good schools and opportunities for enrichment. The study's outcome would form the justification for working with "this good American stock," as Breckinridge said, and serve her well in her efforts to promote the fledgling organization.[5]

Breckinridge had yet another agenda, and that was to complete an *informal* survey to determine medical availability in the seven-hundred-mile region she wanted her organization to serve. None of the three counties she chose, including Leslie, had decent roads or were on a railroad line. Customary travel was by horseback. Nor did the counties have coal mines as yet, so there was little employment. Subsistence farming and logging were the primary forms of making a living. The steep terrain created geographic obstacles, from high narrow valleys to level land so scarce it was said you couldn't find room for a tennis court. With her was a copy of the 1920 census showing only two foreign-born people in Leslie County, and about one hundred fifty blacks in neighboring Knott County, many of whom were descendants of slaves. The rest, she noted, were "homogenous American stock."[6]

From July through September 1923, she traveled daily, mostly alone, covering more than 650 miles on 13 different horses and 3 mules. She carried her own food, water, and a leather satchel with a notebook and a pen. Occasionally a colleague or a medical student who heard about her work accompanied her either to assist, or to keep her company. Breckinridge calculated her speed at three miles to the hour. The horses' bridles were often pieced with rope; the girths tied with wire or string. A meal sack substituted for a blanket. To her chagrin, the trusty animals suffered sores, ringbone, kidney disorders, and other equine complaints. Since blacksmiths and forges were few and far between, she took her own horseshoes and learned to fit them herself.

There were 17 granny midwives in Leslie County that Breckinridge visited, among them, she noted, "old and young, clean and dirty, capable and shiftless." Of the 53 total midwives throughout the region surveyed, all were mountain natives and all were white except one. They ranged in age from 30 to 90, mostly married with children. Many were widows. One was a county jailer, elected on an independent ticket. Fees for birthing varied from two to five dollars and were charged at random — one fee for a close neighbor, another for someone living farther away.

In most cases, the role of midwife was thrust upon them since there was no medical help nearby. They were neighbors in a lonely country where, as women, they were expected to help others. Their training came from other midwives, older women they accompanied on birthing cases. One had "ketched" her last baby the year before at the age of 90, breaking her own mother's record as a granny midwife. Another was 78 and on crutches, yet her services were still sought. A relatively young midwife told Breckinridge she had trained herself, practicing on cows and pigs as a child. Their homes ran the gamut from windowless one-room log cabins to contemporary frame houses. Breckinridge described a few of these remote residences as "tidy and gay with flowers." She would sit for hours on their front steps, or in a splint-bottomed chair, pen in hand, listening to their obstetrical stories, probing for answers to her questions.

What surprised her most was the native intelligence of these untrained women. "One seventy year-old who could not read or write confided to me that she always wanted to be a doctor. She had no children, but two of her nephews are doctors, graduates of the Medical School at Louisville. It cannot be too strongly emphasized that the question of literacy, especially with the older women, has no bearing whatever upon their relative intelligence. A remarkable old woman of eighty-six was the daughter of a schoolmaster. I found her reading her grandchildren's schoolbooks without spectacles. Another, seventy years old, claimed she had been a 'pure scholar' in her day and 'knew all the words in the blue-backed speller.'"[7]

But it was their medical skills, or lack of, that captured Breckinridge's attention. "The origin of their obstetrical practices lies in unrecorded time," she wrote. "As to one thing I am certain. None give any post-natal care whatever. When the delivery is over and the mother is 'fixed up' and the baby dressed, they go away. And unless something goes wrong and they are sent for again, they do not return."[8] Nor was there anything resembling prenatal care or official documentation of births within the granny midwife ranks. State and county records were spotty at best. (Even the U.S. Census Bureau was not a permanent institution until 1902.) One granny midwife kept marks in a day book and had a neighbor count them — a total of 337 births over 27 years. Another had one thousand marks to her credit. And one, unable to count, kept a ball of string, adding a knot each time she birthed a baby.[9]

All of the midwives performed exams, Breckinridge noted, using hands greased with lard for easier access to the uterus. They were checking "if the womb was open," "if the baby was coming straight," and as one said, "to see if the baby's head was even with the world." A few scrubbed their hands first with homemade potash soap. The umbilical cord was cut with unsterilized scissors and tied with twisted strands of thread. The baby's navel was greased with lard or castor oil and a scorched rag placed over it, though some granny midwives considered that an "ole timey" technique. Care provided to the newborn involved doses of castor oil with a dash of catnip tea. Sugared milk or the milk of another woman was often given. If the child wasn't breathing, its arms and legs were manipulated then the body placed in cold water or dipped in camphor.[10]

As no post-natal visits were provided, nearly all the new mothers were up and about within three to four days of delivery (compared to the modern 1920s world where hospitalized women stayed an average of ten days to two weeks in easy confinement). One midwife said she was convinced the forced reentry into daily chores was why six of her own babies had died within the first month — that and working in the fields until the day of delivery. Breckinridge found the almost universal complaint among multi-pare women (multiple pregnancies) was a prolapsed uterus, or "fallin' womb," as the granny midwives termed it. Again, this was attributed to premature activity following the baby's birth. It was reported with a certain amount of disapproval that the sister of one midwife had risen from her bed "within two to three hours after delivery and didn't retire again until night."

Since books of any type were rare and expensive, there were few medical texts available for reference. One midwife did have a pamphlet a doctor had given her from the State Board of Health. A young midwife, "clean and intelligent" noted Breckinridge, had great potential but was also one of the more "dangerous" practitioners. "She is married to a man who practices as a physician without any justification whatever," Breckinridge explained in her survey. "From him she has learned many bad habits. I found a hypodermic syringe in her rubberized bag and a box of pituitrin which she claimed to use in order to speed labor, without any conception of the gravity of her act. She said her husband authorized its use."[11] (Pituitrin was marketed in 1910 and used to induce or speed up labor but was also *misused* to induce labor, according to contemporary physicians.) Breckinridge went on to say that there were many unlicensed physicians in the area (five in Leslie County alone) and the granny midwives often did not distinguish between them and qualified doctors. As a result, she noted, lives were lost.

Despite the appalling lack of medical standards Breckinridge encountered in her study, there were some positive findings. For example, a few of the mountain midwives had been informally trained by physicians who took them on home visits. "One physician in Owlsey County unquestionably saved many lives he never personally reached," Breckinridge noted. "I found three midwives who described how they scrubbed their hands, trimmed and scraped their nails, held the fundus and used a 'cheap tin container' for a bedpan as this doctor showed her to do."[12] These "real" doctors, said Breckinridge, were all emphatic in the need for local midwives, trained or untrained. Simply put, the granny midwives were often the only medical resources available. Cost was another factor. Sending for a trained physician was prohibitive because of the distance and expense. Even then, few could afford the 30 to 35 dollar fee a doctor would charge. "The midwife is a necessity here," one physician was quoted. "We cannot do without them."[13]

The granny midwives, who could have easily viewed Breckinridge with suspicious alarm, proved surprisingly forthcoming and more often than not opened their homes to this unfamiliar face. "From a few," she said, "I learned nothing for they were frightened, or extraordinarily reticent. Others poured out their experiences. Several talked of the other midwives and their mistakes, especially if a mother or baby died at the hands of the midwife. Among the older midwives, it was common for their patients to deliver sitting on someone's knees, usually the husband, or in a chair with no seat." The term "cotching the baby" may have originated from this custom, Breckinridge surmised. But since no formal records were kept, this tidbit of information, along with more pertinent facts regarding midwifery in eastern Kentucky, raised as many questions as it answered.

When her survey was complete, she carefully pondered the results. While some might argue with her reporting techniques (since they were not considered scientific), no one could deny the maternal death and infant mortality rates within the U.S. Between 1900 and 1930, maternal mortality ranged from 67 to 85 per 10,000 live births, compared to rates of 44 to 48 per 10,000 in England and Wales where midwives were commonly used. (As of 2004, the U.S. maternal mortality rate was 13 deaths per 100,000.)[14] Between 1915 and 1933, neonatal mortality in the U.S. ranged from 34 to 44 for every 1000 live births. Infant mortality (dying within the first year) ranged from 58 to 99 for every 1000 live births. (By contrast, the U.S. infant mortality rate in 2004 was 7 out of every 1000 children dying within their first year, about double the rate found in Hong Kong and Japan.)[15]

Breckinridge cited her statistics to support the dire need for trained midwives and family practitioners in rural regions of America, and emphasized that "of the fifteen nations with lower death rates than the United States; they train and supervise their midwives." "We lose in America every year approximately 100,000 infants in the first month of life from causes to childbirth," she wrote, "with perhaps as many stillbirths over and above that. A newborn baby of the old stock in America has less chance of life than a man ninety years old. There is no more hazardous occupation than just being born an American citizen."[16]

Dr. Annie Veech, whom Breckinridge derisively called "Ready-to-Halt" in her private correspondence, objected to the data Breckinridge had collected in her informal survey, even accusing Breckinridge in a letter of "exploiting" the mountain people of eastern Kentucky. Breckinridge fired back in a letter. "The problem of midwifery in America is not peculiar to the Kentucky Mountains," she replied, "or even to the similar sections of the Appalachian range with its five million people. Never fear that I shall exploit any section of my country, much less the South, and least of all Kentucky. It is not usual, I know, for public interests to take the initiative in pushing forward with new ideas. Private initiative nearly always blazes the trail."[17] She then summarized her survey by focusing on solutions. "It is not the purpose of this report to 'point the moral' regarding the data collected," Breckinridge concluded. "Finding and applying [the solution] will undoubtedly be the work of many people and much time. None the less, the story of my fifty-three midwives will not have ended until that solution has been reached and applied."[18]

To that end, a committee was formed and its first meeting held at the Hyden courthouse in August 1923. Thirty-five people attended as potential committee members, while numerous onlookers jammed the building just to see what was going on. The goals and objectives were explained: Leslie County would serve as a laboratory, or field of research in addition to becoming the first nursing center. The maternal and infant death rate in rural sections of Kentucky would be lowered. A pre-determined area and population would be served by each nurse, combining midwifery and generalized public health nursing. Among the unanswered questions were fees for services (about 20 percent of fees were paid by patients in the Scotland Highland region with the remainder subsidized), how much time would be devoted to midwifery, and most important — would the local population *accept* the new nursing services?

Walter Hoskins, of Hyden, proposed a resolution that active support, both "moral and financial," be forthcoming. Dr. Scott Breckinridge, of Lexington, stood up and said he felt sure the medical profession as a whole would welcome the assistance of trained midwives. "About sixty percent of all maternal deaths come from two causes," he cited, "infections and toxemia, both preventable except in rare instances; one by cleanliness at delivery and the other by simple prenatal precautions."[19] These could easily fall under the scope of the nurse-midwife, he added, and furthermore: What other preventable cause of death could be reduced 60 percent? Numerous other meetings followed and by 1925, the first nursing center was established at Hyden. Edna Rockstroh and Freda "Freddy" Caffin served as the pioneer nurse-midwives, both public health nurses and former members of the Maternity Center Association (MCA) of New York. Rockstroh was the first trained midwife to deliver a Leslie County baby under the auspices of the Kentucky Committee for Mothers and Babies, governed by a medical director and an advisory board. At the time, within Leslie County, there was no licensed physician, no railway station, no paved roads within twenty miles, and less than half a dozen bathtubs listed in households.[20]

Rockstoh recalls that when she and Caffin arrived at Krypton at 4:30 one morning in 1925, there were two men with horses waiting. The foursome went across the street to get breakfast at a small cabin that served as a local eatery. "We had fried cornbread, fried potatoes, and fried eggs with something that looked like raisins. Then we discovered we'd eaten the flies. But we were very hungry." The ride to Hyden was 22 miles. Neither nurse had ever been on a horse. "The men stopped about every five miles and made us get off and walk so we wouldn't get too stiff. When we arrived at Wooten (a local mission and stopover for travelers) someone pulled up well water and filled a metal tub so we could relax in a bath. That was our bathtub for many years. You sat in it, bathed, then stood up and washed your feet."[21]

The temporary facility in Hyden to which the women were assigned was a dilapidated, two-story structure with each room featuring a door that opened one way which you had to exit in order to enter the adjoining room. The veranda lay level with the ground and there was no stable, so horses often trod across the porch, causing the entire building to vibrate. Breckinridge referred to it as "of a sorrowful nature." In short order, they moved to their permanent clinic, just up the hill, and attempted to make it as comfortable as they could with their limited supplies. "It was a cabin, made from plain boards," said Rockstroh, "but it had windows and a little coal and wood heating stove. Somehow, we got it furnished with a cot so people could lie down if they needed to. We had a table and chairs. And I made posters from pictures of food that people ought to eat which I cut from magazines and pasted on the walls."[22]

Patients were hesitant to attend the clinic at first. Some were not certain if the women were missionaries, had ulterior motives, or were just too foreign. One woman came with her twin teenage daughters, about fourteen years old, complaining to the nurses that she couldn't marry them off because "they hadn't had their health yet," meaning they had not begun menstruating. Rockstroh assured her it would happen soon enough, that nothing was wrong, and sent her away "a little happier." A father brought in his son with a severely infected hand. The nurses treated him by lancing it, giving the boy immediate relief. Another parent rushed in telling Rockstroh that his boy was "dying from diphtheria," and to hurry to his place. When she arrived, she found the child had swallowed a wooden splinter through chewing on a piece of stick. She fished out the object, made the boy gargle, and soon had him laughing. Before long, word spread that the nurses were doing good work and the clinic began to fill up. But when the first outside reporters arrived, curious about the new Kentucky Committee for Mothers and Babies and ready to report its outcome, trouble ensued.

In a highly negative article that appeared in *The New York Times* in 1926 titled "Primitive America" *on Screen,* two New York filmmakers, both women, described the region and the people in condescending terms, ranging from a one-sided description of Hyden to the preponderance of young boys named Pearl. Even local wood-cutting techniques were criticized as "haphazard and unscientific, resulting in "whole mountainsides being shorn of any vestige of growth."[23] A Leslie County resident took time to respond in a letter to the county newspaper editor, praising the nurses, honoring Breckinridge for her innovative work, but expressing frustration at their fundraising methods (appealing to the wealthy and more socially connected citizenry). He said he felt it allowed the benefactors to look down their noses at the recipients of their charitable donations. "We feel that we pay in the sacrifice of our honor," he explained. "It seems to me that any organization would find a higher plane upon which to raise funds than to come down to the worn out plan of exaggerating conditions."[24]

Making matters worse was a letter one of the nurses received from a Louisville, Kentucky, committee member following the article's publication. She had arrived for an overnight stay at Wendover and left convinced the nurses exhibited "ridicule" toward the locals, while expressing no interest in community affairs. Furthermore, the woman said, the nurses did not understand the mountain people. Breckinridge and her small staff took great offense and in a blunt rebuttal, responded that nothing could be further from the truth. "This is a totally mistaken view," Breckinridge wrote, "and your brief stay of one night at Hyden would hardly qualify you to form a correct one." She went on to point out that she and her father had lived for months in Hyden, followed the nurses on duty, and watched them perform admirably. If any joking or "ridicule" was done, it was simply a way to minimize the isolation, hardship, and often tragic circumstances the women encountered almost daily.

"Fun among us," stated Breckinridge, "is not ridicule among the people. And as for your statement that the nurses do not understand the mountain people — do you? Mountain people, like lowlanders, are just people, men, women, and children, not so different the world over. I have lived in Russia, Finland, Switzerland, France, and England, as well as many parts of our own land. And I quite honestly can say that I do not understand people. Did I understand them better, I would be writing you today more wisely and tenderly, my dear."[25] It was Breckinridge on the defense — straight-shooting, barbed, and designed to drive her point home. Yet the criticism would not slow her down, or her newly formed brigade of nurses and growing number of supporters. In fact, those who knew Mary Breckinridge well were convinced that once she set her mind to reaching and applying a solution to any problem, large or small, there was no turning back, especially if she believed in what she was doing. More to the point, they also knew this was one determined woman who *never* took no for an answer.

4

The British Connection

More than four thousand miles away in London, at the British Hospital for Mothers and Babies, a young nurse named Betty Lester was mulling over a decision to join the newly formed Kentucky Committee for Mothers and Babies in America's Appalachian Mountains. Breckinridge herself had studied midwifery at the British Hospital since Great Britain was a world leader in midwifery training.

After she graduated as a certified nurse-midwife and conducted her survey, Breckinridge returned to the London-based hospital, mesmerizing the audience of nurses with her tales of critical health care needs in the Kentucky hills. She sent other nurses to recruit as well, one of whom spoke to a group that included Lester. They left behind a photo album with pictures and descriptions of the fledging organization. The pay scale wasn't great — a hundred fifty dollars a month plus your own horse and its upkeep. But it was all so foreign and romantic, Lester recalled. "I had my nursing diploma and went to the General Lying-In Hospital on York Road to take my midwifery training. An American nurse was in the same school. We became good friends and she told me about the horses and the dogs and the people (in eastern Kentucky) and I thought 'what a nice life to be a nurse and midwife, have a horse and a dog, and go riding around the country. What could be better?'"[1]

With both of her parents deceased and her boyfriend, Billy, killed in World War I, Lester was free to travel. She asked her American friend if Breckinridge needed any new midwives. "Why, do you want to come?" the friend responded. "I'd like to very much," Lester said. "I think it's the kind of life that appeals to me, and since I've lived in the country, riding on horseback wouldn't bother me."[2]

But there was one major obstacle to overcome. As Lester was finishing up her midwifery training and word spread that she might leave for the hills of Kentucky, neither her supervisor at the Lying-In Hospital, nor her colleagues, thought it was a good idea. In fact, Lester says the rumors created a "furor" in the hospital. Some who had met Breckinridge on her earlier visits heard her describe the difficult conditions under which the nurse-midwives worked and lived, and many shook their heads at Lester's pending decision.

One day Lester was summoned to her supervisor's office. She recalled the conversation that ensued and her response. "You think you're going to Kentucky?" the nursing supervisor asked Lester. "Yes." "Do you know what you're doing? You've only just got your training. You don't know a thing." *Well, I do too*, Lester thought. "I want to go very badly," she replied.[3]

The supervisor and the hospital medical director both tried to persuade Lester to change her mind by explaining that not only was she inexperienced, but she had advantages staying in England. "Here, you have day sister on day duty to help you," the director pointed out. "You've got night sister on night duty. You've got the doctor within five minutes and you have only twenty cases with supervision. Out there you won't have anybody but yourself."[4] "Well, you can't do this," Lester's supervisor added. "You simply cannot. For one thing, you aren't even properly trained to work without supervision. Yes, you have your diploma but you wouldn't be any good to Mrs. Breckinridge at this point." "But I want to go so badly," said Lester. "Well, for now *stay*," said the director. Lester knew it was not a request. "We want you here for six months for a post-graduate course."[5]

In the meantime, Lester received a letter from Breckinridge telling her that once her post-graduate work was completed, she was welcome to apply to the Kentucky Committee for Mothers and Babies. In addition, the *Glasgow Times* in Scotland and major newspapers London ran advertisements that captured the attention of many English, Welsh, and Scottish nurses, including Lester:

ATTENTION! NURSE GRADUATES
WITH A SENSE OF ADVENTURE!
YOUR OWN HORSE, YOUR OWN DOG, AND A THOUSAND MILES
OF KENTUCKY MOUNTAINS TO SERVE.
JOIN MY NURSES BRIGADE AND HELP SAVE CHILDREN'S LIVES.
WRITE TO: M. BRECKINRIDGE, HYDEN, KENTUCKY USA

In fact, Lester was not the first new Frontier Nurse to cross the Atlantic and travel deep into the Appalachian Mountains. Four others had arrived before her, including one American girl, Dorothy Farrar Buck, from Foxboro, Massachusetts. And like the British nurses, Buck underwent a bout of culture shock once she got past Lexington, Kentucky, in January 1928. "I peered from the train station eager to see something of my new home country, but made out little other than large dark flakes of snow thick between me and the lights of the stations. When it stopped snowing I didn't want to miss any of the beauty of snow-laden trees and rocky mountain slopes."[6]

She struggled into the winter uniform Breckinridge provided—Confederate gray no less—and a bit too snug even for her petite frame. Once in uniform, she was escorted to breakfast by "a kind gentlemen" sent to greet her. "He pointed out small cabins with unchinked walls, propped against the mountain by stilts, their window spaces boarded up for the winter. I was seated before a loaded breakfast table and shown the mark, halfway up the walls, left by the Big Flood of the previous year."[7] Like nearly everything and everyone at the Frontier Nursing Service, Buck would soon acquire a nickname. Hers was "Bucket." Lester would eventually become "The General."

Edna Rockstroh would be gone from the nursing service before Lester's arrival, released from duty by Breckinridge — due in part to a chronic bronchial condition from which Rockstroh suffered — and in part to personality differences between her and Breckinridge. "She was a very strait-laced person." said Rockstroh. "There was no give to her. Black was black and white was white and nothing in-between. It made her a difficult person to work for."[8] Lester described her overseas trip from Southampton to New York as long and arduous. For eight days on the open Atlantic she was seasick most of the way. Ironically for the young Brit, she landed in New York City on the 4th of July. The Stars and Stripes were everywhere that warm holiday, and to Lester this relatively young raw country must have seemed unduly enthusiastic over its release from Great Britain.

The climate was also more than she expected. With temperatures hovering at eighty-five degrees it would have felt like a virtual heat wave after sailing the cool ocean. Ahead was a hot, stuffy train ride from New York down to Lexington, then a transfer to another Pullman train that would take her close to Hyden. A little after five in the morning she was awakened by a porter and informed her stop was next. It was a lonely way station near Hazard, and she was unceremoniously left at the railroad platform. Tired and now hungry, Lester watched the train disappear round the bend. She scanned the horizon. This certainly was a god-forsaken place. Maybe the hospital staff was right all along. Maybe this *was* a crazy idea. "There were mountains on either side of me," she recalled, "the railroad, a valley, and not a soul in sight. It was then I began to wonder what I had done and what to do?"[9]

Suddenly, a man in worn overalls appeared. Lester recounts the exchanges that took place and her first impressions of eastern Kentucky hospitality. "Howdy," the man said, sweeping up her bags. Without introductions Lester had no idea who he was. Not that it mattered for now, for she was famished. "Any idea where I can get some breakfast?" she asked in her lilting British voice. He pointed to a nearby gate and a path leading up to a house. Lester headed in that direction.

As she approached, a matronly woman appeared on the porch, hands on her hips. She seemed kind. Her name was Mrs. Eversole, she told Lester, and she ran the boarding house. "Are you one of Mrs. Breckinridge's nurses?" she asked. "No, but I hope I will be." "Breakfast will be ready in a little while. Come sit a spell on the porch and I'll call you when it's ready."

Lester said she had never seen cornbread, fried potatoes, or hot biscuits (called scones in England) but that she "enjoyed them very much." At the table were several men, all boarders on their way to work. "They came in, sat down at the table, and never said a word," Lester recalled, perplexed. "Then they got up and left."[10] After breakfast Lester returned to the front porch to wait for a nurse who was scheduled to meet her for the horseback ride to Confluence, a community with an FNS nursing center north of Hyden. She sat, resting. And sat, and sat. Maybe they had forgotten all about her. At one point Mrs. Eversole came to the door. "They'll be along shortly," she assured her worried guest.

Peering into the morning mountain mist, Lester spotted a woman on horseback leading a Tennessee Walker. She rose from the porch and gathered her bags. The female nurse, whom they called "Billy" Williams, took one look at the delicate young English woman and said, "Can you *ride?*" "Well, I used to, quite a lot," Lester said. "I grew up in the country." In truth, it had been years since she'd been on a horse. "Have you got any riding clothes?" "Well, no." Williams tossed a pair of riding pants toward her. "Here, put these on and come on. And leave your stuff here. All you got now is a saddlebag." It would be a month before Lester's luggage caught up with her.

Nothing had prepared her for the rough terrain. Her first reaction was "oh my." "We rode straight up a mountain and the rocks looked so big and the trail so bad that I wondered if I would topple over the horse's head. We went straight down the other side and came to the river. I thought, now what do we do? Billy splashed right into the water so I did the same. Confluence Center was just ahead."[11]

The next morning two teenage male couriers arrived for Lester. "Their job was to come to Confluence and meet all the nurses," she said. "Since I was the fifth one, they were getting a bit tired of us. We got on the horses to leave and I was poking along. So they'd ride up behind me, lickety-split, trying to hurry me." She decided she would show them a thing or two about riding. "I gave my horse a light touch, took off, and before long I was right alongside them. We had a lovely ride from there."[12] They rode the dozen or so miles to Hyden, crossing the river four separate times. Their destination was the hospital, a two-story stone building that stood guard above the small town on the side of Thousandsticks Mountain. This was Hyden Hospital, dedicated only two weeks earlier by Mary Breckinridge and a cortège of local and international officials. "Well, you've made it," came the cheery greeting from chief nurse Alice "Al" Logan. An American, she had been sent to England on a scholarship by Breckinridge to become a certified nurse-midwife and help recruit other nurses.[13]

Lester had studied with her the year before, enthralled by Logan's photographs of the region, particularly the nurses on horseback. Logan toured her around and pointed out a small, sparsely furnished room in the hospital that would serve as her quarters. Lester still found the July heat oppressive, noting the hospital had a generator for electricity but no fan in sight. Electrical power was reserved for patient use, she was told. "Are you ready to start work in the morning?" Logan asked. "You'll be assigned to the hospital and Thousandsticks district. We've not had a nurse starting out of here so this will be new work."[14] She had one week to learn the routine. Each nurse at the district outpost centers covered a five mile radius from her designated center. Lester's center was Thousandsticks Mountain at Bull Creek clinic. The mountain gained its name from a Cherokee Indian legend. A former hunting ground for the Cherokees, they supposedly used a thousand sticks to build a signal fire so that other tribesmen would know their location. That was one of several versions she would hear through the years.

For a few days another nurse showed her around. But she was soon left on her own to ride up and down the maze of steep trails. She often got lost, claiming she had no sense of direction. It became a running joke among the nurses that the new girl was out there somewhere wandering around again. It was easy to understand how she could take a wrong turn. Most of her initial duties involved riding into the pitch black night to deliver babies at secluded cabins in the middle of nowhere. Usually the fathers-to-be came for her at whichever clinic she was stationed. "Our slogan," said Lester, "was that regardless of the weather if a man could come for the nurse, the nurse could come to the patient."[15] To her pleasant surprise, these mountaineer men and their grateful families took great care of her in all types of weather conditions. But just getting around would prove extremely difficult at times.

"If a tree fell across the trail, they cleared it right away. The roads were in the creek bed and in the winter travel was often hard. Hyden itself was no more than a village with rutted paths for streets. The courthouse was old and there was an iron bridge which divided the two sides of town. Condemned for years, it shook and rattled as we went across on our horses. We had stores, a post office, and a bank. We could not go out very often as the railroad was twenty-two miles away over four different mountains. I did not see a car for months and months. However, we were all quite happy and everybody helped everyone. We were like old friends together. If a house burned down, or a new barn was needed, people showed up to help. They called these events 'workings.' Whenever I was there at dinner time I was invited to eat, so I never even had to take sandwiches."[16]

Despite her first few busy days, Lester was anxious for one more thing to happen and that was to meet the woman that she had heard so much about, the person without whom none of this adventure would have come about — Mary Breckinridge. She got her chance shortly after arriving at the Hyden Hospital Clinic, when Breckinridge showed up on rounds one day. Lester's first impression was of a petite woman, pleasant, but totally in charge, with a "commander-in-chief" presence. "This little lady walked in dressed in her uniform and she was very hospitable. She said she was glad I was here, how was I getting on, that kind of thing. She was the type of person that when she came into the room you felt as though you had to stand up. I also felt that she was the kind of person who expected the best from you because she was that way herself. I immediately knew that she was someone you looked up to."[17]

Lester, as did all the new nurses, had a scheduled meeting with Breckinridge at the "Big House" in Wendover (headquarters for the FNS and Breckinridge's home) but not before she familiarized herself with required FNS procedures: Once a woman thought she was pregnant, she registered at the hospital. A nurse was assigned and the woman's temperature, blood pressure, urinalysis, and pulse recorded. An external abdominal examination was performed and nutritional advice provided. For the first two trimesters of the pregnancy, home visits were made once a month, followed by every two weeks during the next two months, and every week for the last month. After delivery, the patient was carefully watched for two hours by the nurse who checked for signs of hemorrhage or other abnormalities. Then the nurse returned for post-partum checks every day for the next ten days and every week for the first month. Children were medically monitored as well for malnutrition or what would be known today as "failure to thrive."

One of the first cases handled by Lester was a pregnant mother with six young boys, living on Bad Creek, thirty-two miles from the nearest railway. The woman sent word through her husband to the district nurse that she was bleeding slightly and the nurse, in turn, reported the case direct to Breckinridge. The midwives suspected a case of placenta praevia and began to search for a doctor. "The only Leslie County doctor," said Breckinridge, "was a fine one, but the only one for ten-thousand people over three-hundred seventy-three square miles. Away on holiday, he could not be found. The nearest doctor in Harlan was another day's ride, but he couldn't come. So we tried a fourth. This doctor rode seven hours on horseback to reach Wendover, our nearest center. There we gave him a fresh horse, some sandwiches, and a guide, and he rode through the night three hours longer. He reached the patient and in the end, saved her life."[18]

Ten days later another prenatal patient began bleeding. The nearest physician from her home was twenty-four miles away. But the mother was bleeding so profusely that the nurse-midwife had to give her chloroform and reach in to extract the baby. The doctor later wrote Mary Breckinridge, "If that nurse had not the courage to plunge in and take hold, there would have been a dead patient before I got there."[19] Total cost for midwifery services was five dollars per family, an investment which Breckinridge believed ensured a measure of dignity. It was often paid in fodder for the horses, a cow, a flock of chickens, or a husband's handiwork. One father re-paid a sixty dollar debt for his son by delivering hay to the nurses' headquarters. Another family offered their nurse-midwife a gun, plus lessons in how to use it. She took him up on it until she realized she was such a poor shot she might prove an even greater hazard.[20]

All in all, maintaining the work and the word about the growing FNS was becoming a community endeavor, with one family talking to another about "those fine nurses" and eventually stories getting out to the press in other towns. In addition, Breckinridge, who had a special affinity for public relations, had numerous well-connected friends who not only gave donations, but spoke favorably of the organization and its staff, leading to statewide and national recognition and support. For example, a local chairman of the Kentucky Committee for Mothers and Babies managed to raise funds of over five hundred dollars counting labor and supplies from neighbors to construct a new nursing center. The Louisville and Nashville Railroad furnished passes for patients and nurses needing transport. Lexington doctors gave of their services at reduced or no cost.[21] And due to Breckinridge's tireless fundraising and networking efforts, money began to trickle in from friends and acquaintances throughout the nation.

Within a month after her arrival, Lester was set to visit Breckinridge at Wendover where she first became familiar with the gracious side of her boss' personality. It was a four mile trip from the Hyden hospital across a swinging bridge that spanned the Middle Fork River. As she approached the two-story log cabin poised high on the hillside, windows gleaming in the sunlight, she perceived it as a calm haven in the woods. Not only was it Breckinridge's home, it also served as a well-equipped dispensary and later, a Wendover post office. Lester recalled that Breckinridge met her at the door. "Come in, my child," she greeted Lester. She led her guest through the parlor, past the dining room with its shiny walnut table, and toward a comfortable, oversized chair in the main living area. A window seat with plump print pillows hugged the wall and across the room a hand-hewn banister, polished to a warm glow, led to the upstairs quarters.

Breckinridge summoned the cook and asked her to bring them both some hot tea. "So what was it that brought you here?" Breckinridge asked. "It was the challenge of what you were trying to do," Lester said. "I've always loved people, and these people sounded like they might need me." "You seem well prepared for this work," replied Breckinridge, getting right to the point. "We need nurses who can work on their own, with a physician as backup only for the most difficult cases." She went on to describe the lonely life of a frontier nurse, especially in the outpost centers. "And you must have a dog," added Breckinridge. She excused herself and returned a moment later carrying a collie pup with a tawny-colored coat. "She's the runt of the litter," explained Breckinridge, "which is all we had left since the other new nurses got one." She handed the pup to Lester who quickly found a name for her. "I think I'll call her Ginger."[22]

Now in her late forties, Breckinridge was, to Lester's surprise, a chainsmoker, perhaps influenced by the British nurses who arrived prior to Lester, many of whom smoked incessantly. After dinner, she also liked a glass of sherry or a sip of brandy, maintaining that unlike the hard stuff, sherry did not make

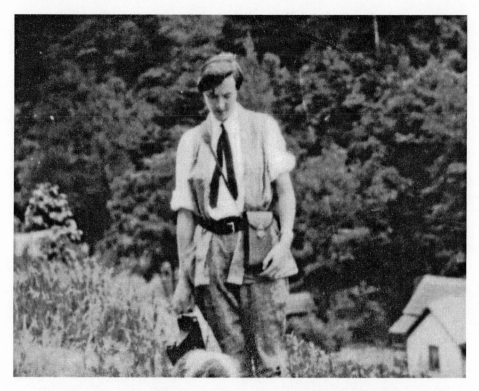

An early 1930s photo of Betty Lester and her dog. One of the many British FNS nurse-midwives who traveled to eastern Kentucky to work with the FNS, Lester arrived in 1928 and said her first reaction to the area was, "*Now* what have I done?" (courtesy Frontier Nursing Service, Inc.)

you drunk. What Lester didn't see that day was the formidable side of Breckinridge in which she liked to hold court and make her opinions known regardless, or perhaps in spite, of others' point of view.

Perched on a cushion in an overstuffed chair near the fireplace in the log house at Wendover, Breckinridge would argue with her employees and guests about current events, government control, and — to the consternation of her staff — who *really* won the Civil War. A lively argument was good for the soul, she believed. However, when family history was involved, especially her own, there was no room for anything but the utmost respect. Carlyle Carter was just ten years old when she came to visit Breckinridge at Wendover. Her grandmother and Breckinridge were first cousins. It was summertime and Carter had spent the day reading books about the Kentucky mountains. Tea time rolled around and Breckinridge told her young charge to come listen to a story about her grandfather, John Breckinridge, who was secretary of war during the Confederacy.

"It was this long recital about her grandfather," said Carter, "and how he escaped to Cuba. I remember it was a very hot day and I went to sleep while she was reading. I didn't think she would notice, but when it was all over she asked me a lot of questions and I didn't know any of the answers." Breckinridge was not amused by the child's disinterest. "She took family history very seriously and expected me to do the same, but I was bored by the whole thing."[23] The two made their peace and Carter accompanied her elder relative to feed the chickens, collect eggs, and work on the flower beds outside the Big House.

When truly aggravated, Breckinridge was known to use colorful language, causing her dignified father to dress her down. Agnes Lewis, her longtime secretary and an occasional recipient of Breckinridge's wrath, recalls overhearing an argument between father and daughter. Throughout his life, he was an important influence on Breckinridge and they shared a close bond. (He also served as secretary to the Kentucky Committee for Mothers and Babies). "She was usually very patient with her father but she was upset that day and said something like, 'I don't give a damn,'" Lewis related. "He shook his finger at her and told her that is not a word that ladies use, and that he didn't want to hear it again."[24]

Clifton Rodes Breckinridge, affectionately known as "Major," was already elderly when Breckinridge began the Frontier Nursing Service. In fact, he would celebrate his eightieth birthday in 1926 with what Breckinridge called a "stag dinner" at the newly constructed Big House at Wendover. To surprise him, she invited several of his cronies who brought him handkerchiefs, cigarettes, and other small gifts. The cook baked a birthday cake and carried it in topped with eighty bright red candles. Later, the Major thanked his daughter for her efforts by telling her it was "an undreamed of birthday."[25]

A white-haired gentleman with a thick, handle-bar mustache, he could be seen striding the Wendover property dressed in a dark wool sports coat, left hand tucked into his pocket, white pants, white shirt and tie, carrying his broad-brimmed hat. One of the dogs usually accompanied him as he pondered over what needing doing and how he could best make it happen. Animals and equipment were his expertise. He wrote a lengthy but informative article published in the FNS *Quarterly Bulletin* about how the nurses should go about selecting the proper horse — "not less than four years old and not older than eight, head flat and eyes full" — and the proper type of saddle, blanket, bridle, halter, girth, and straps to use, as well as how to care for each. He compared treating a horse to that of caring for a child and offered the following advice: "You cannot be too good to him; but you must not spoil him. One must be kind, considerate, and just. Avoid passion; avoid heat; be prudent; but avoid every appearance of fear; be firm if need be; but avoid even a shade of bravado. A horse knows his master, not instantly but soon. Let it be that he shall love, respect, and trust you."[26]

An imposing figure like his daughter, he was one of the few people who could put Breckinridge in her place. Once, while assisting with landscaping and other outdoor projects at Wendover, he approved a concrete foundation for a chicken coop. When Breckinridge found out what he had done in her absence, she didn't like it and told him so. "Mary," he countered, "you know all there is to know about midwifery. But you don't know a damn thing about chicken lots!"[27]

Most of the nurse-midwives, including Betty Lester, had a favorite horse. Hers was known as 'The Old Gray Mare.' Having already served a moonshiner, it had a reputation for steadfast dependability despite the presence of a bullet in its right hip. "This horse knew every trail, every creek, and nearly every boulder in Leslie County," Lester later said. "She was a fine friend to have on the dark nights I was out delivering babies."[28] But first, Lester and her proper English accent had to adapt to the locals and they to her. A month into her arrival she was convinced she would fail miserably as a Frontier nurse-midwife. "They couldn't understand me, and I couldn't understand them. And some of the expressions they used, I simply *didn't* understand."

When she would invite someone to attend the clinic, the response was, "I wouldn't care to." Then they would show up. She eventually realized what they meant was, "It was no bother to come." The twilight hour just before sunset was called "edge of dark," and a woman in labor was "punishing awful bad." Once she learned the dialect things got only slightly better. "I can't get them to talk to me," she complained. "They won't say anything." She took to dropping by unexpectedly and sitting on the patient's front porch in an effort to make friends. Finally, after a few weeks, Lester learned through a third party that she did make an impact. One day at the Hyden Hospital nurse Alice "Al" Logan motioned Betty to her side. "I've got something to tell you," she said. "One of your men from Bull Creek came over here today. He knows all the people in the area. I asked him how they liked the new nurse." Logan paused for effect. Then she repeated what the man said. "Well, we like her fine. But she sure is the *talkingest* woman I ever heard!"[29]

One of the first cases soon after Lester's arrival would seal her acceptance among the locals. On a cold windy night in a torrent of rain, she was summoned by a man named Lem, whose wife was having their first baby. He had come on horseback to the nurses' quarters at the hospital, calling out the familiar "Hallo-oo-oo" as his signal for help. Lester was already in bed, certain that no one would be out on a night like this. "Need you in a hurry!" Lem called out when he saw her. Lester dressed quickly in her blue-gray uniform, donned a rain cape, and grabbed her midwifery bag. Each nurse had two saddle bags, one for midwifery and one for general nursing. The delivery pack held, among numerous other things, an enamel basin, scissors, rectal pads, a cord clamp, a catheter, and a good supply of newspapers for wrapping discards. There were also birth certificate forms, medical directives, and a metal emergency box that included a small suture set.

Lem's face, streaked with rain, cast an eerie shadow from the lantern he carried as they headed for the barn. "She's punishing awful bad," he said in the dark. Together, he and Lester headed over Thousandsticks Mountain as the rain pounded the rocky trail and shifted boulders the size of a cabin. Lem's horse pressed ahead and Lester feared she would lose her way in the darkness. The water was rising and now covered the trail. Thank goodness for Old Gray Mare, her trusty horse. She reached out and gave him a reassuring pat. *Dear Lord, help me*, she prayed silently. *I'll never make it on my own.* As they reached the front porch of the family's home, Lester heard a baby's cry. She rushed inside to find the infant lying between the woman's legs, cord intact. She reached inside her bag for supplies and carefully snipped the cord. Then she laid the infant near its unconscious mother, wrapping it in the bedcovers for warmth. She checked the woman's pulse. It was rapid and thready.

Lester did a vaginal exam on her patient. She could see the placenta coming next and with it, a heavy rush of blood. The woman appeared to be hemorrhaging. From the corner of the room she spotted someone standing in the doorway. "I'm her sister," the woman said. The husband had remained outside. Frontier nurses would find that few men were willing or able to assist in the delivery process. "Then come here and help me lift the foot of the bed onto this chair," Lester instructed. She could use an extra pair of hands. "And get me a couple of extra blankets." Though the room was chilly from the damp mountain air, Lester was perspiring. She tried to stay focused on her midwife training: Massage the abdomen. Control shock. Check the flow of hemorrhage. She positioned a rubber sheet under the patient to capture the troubling loss of blood.

Finally, the young mother stirred, a faint hint of color returning to her lips. The woman's pulse steadied and slowed. Lester glanced up at the woman's sister. Did she realize they had just witnessed a potentially dangerous delivery? It was difficult to tell. She stayed near her patient until dawn, monitoring her vital signs and checking for abnormal bleeding. Everything now appeared under control. She would return daily for the next ten days to determine the woman's progress. Exhausted, she mounted Old Gray Mare and began the trek back to Hyden Hospital. The rain had ceased and the rushing creeks were now receding. She breathed in the musty morning air and brushed past the heavy water-laden trees. She was hungry for breakfast and a steaming cup of tea.

Later in the day she sat at her hospital desk documenting the delivery. She recorded an estimated forty-eight ounces of blood loss, or nearly three pints, with a live healthy baby as the outcome. And she pondered her role and that of the Kentucky Committee for Mothers and Babies. She knew that not everyone was enamored of the upstart organization. "Some people questioned us, or didn't know what we were talking about," she recalled. "Some of the midwives who were already here didn't like us because we were taking work from them. So if someone wanted their own granny midwife and we had all the prenatals, we left people to please themselves. Eventually the local midwives began to help us so it all worked out."[30]

On occasion, a trained midwife would pass a cabin door that was shut tight and knew that meant do not knock or enter. But when they *were* welcomed, there was no denying the good work they performed. "Did I save this woman's life?" she wondered as she concluded her report. It was a question she would ask again and again. Yet, even in her short time as a frontier nurse-midwife, she was beginning to realize that she and the new service as a whole was making a difference. On her next home visit, she overheard one of the local women remark, "If it waren't for these nurses, I declare, I don't know what the women in this part of the country would do."[31]

5

Growing Pains

At the nursing headquarters in Wendover in May 1926, Mary Breckinridge was marking the first anniversary of the Kentucky Committee for Mothers and Babies. Established a year earlier on May 28, 1925, it was the forerunner to what would soon become the Frontier Nursing Service. The organization now covered two hundred and fifty square miles of rugged highlands with ten trained midwives. In her public relations she used concrete examples to emphasize the remoteness of Leslie County, telling readers that "when a letter arrives from Lexington, about a hundred and forty miles away, it has been on the road by mule wagon thirty-six to forty hours."[1] To enlist the support of the locals and get to know them, she had also invited dozens of families with their children to the Big House for the organization's first Christmas that prior December. It had rained the day before and the grounds were muddy as the neighbors drove up in their wagons or arrived on horseback.

Construction on the Wendover site began in the summer and fall of 1925, two years after Breckinridge had conducted her survey and fallen in love with the rolling, wooded site. The land belonged to a local farmer who couldn't decide whether to part with it or not, causing Breckinridge to almost pull out of the deal. In fact, she was ready to leave Hyden and look elsewhere when word came that a price was forthcoming. Thirteen acres were sold to Breckinridge "real cheap," according to Walter Morgan, whose father owned the land.[2] A log barn was constructed first using local help ("A fine crew of men" according to Breckinridge), followed by the first-floor of the house. The work was grueling, and as always, contingent upon good weather. "Men felled the logs on the mountainsides and snaked them down by means of mules hitched with chains," she said. "As the weeks passed, I realized I couldn't expect them to construct a large two-story log house plus an attic and plumbing unless they had expert direction."[3]

So she rode to Hazard looking for a contractor. She found experienced stone masons for the great stone chimneys in the Big House and the nurses' cabin, and laborers for the remainder of the house. Logs for the second story

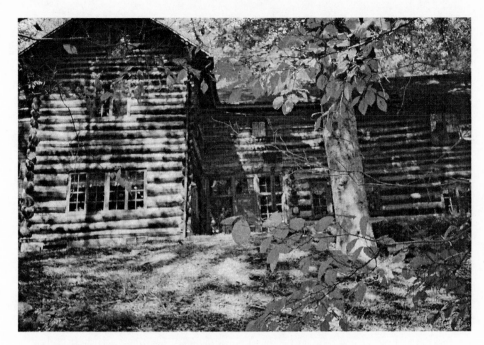

Exterior view of Big House, FNS Headquarters and home of Mary Breckinridge (photograph by Marie Bartlett, courtesy Frontier Nursing Service, Inc.).

were raised by a contraption called a crab in which a pulley was attached to branches on the nearby giant beech trees. Once completed, Breckinridge's home and headquarters for the service was the only two-story log house in the Hyden district and one of few that had a furnace, asphalt shingles on the roof, and two baths.[4] Most of the delays and complications were caused by the weather. To get supplies from the railroad in winter, it often took a team of mules nearly three days for each load of wood, stone, and other materials. Storms arrived to destroy what was put into place. The steep mountainside on which the house was built, soaked with rain and snow, slid onto the house at one point, causing further problems.

On Christmas Day 1925, with parts of the roof still missing and no chinking between the logs, the Big House was opened to the community for a party. Donated presents — dolls and toy trucks — were wrapped and placed under the tall sycamore that served as a Christmas tree in the living room. Major Breckinridge bought the hams for dinner. Each child who arrived was instructed to come forward and choose his own gift but the youngsters were so overwhelmed, they could not decide what they wanted. These were children accustomed to no more than an apple, a bag of nuts, or an orange from Santa. And that was in a good year. The tree was colorfully decorated with paper bows cut from old catalogues and secured with bright wool thread. Paraffin candles set at inter-

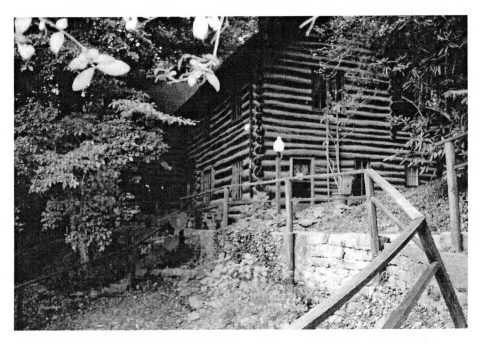

Side view of the Big House (photograph by Marie Bartlett, courtesy Frontier Nursing Service, Inc.).

vals along the stairwell winked their soft lights, and a roaring fire warmed the room. A faint scent of cinnamon, citrus, and clove drifted through the rooms. Platters of turkey, dressing, and ham were prepared along with fruit and custard pies, steamed and boiled vegetables, baked cookies, and homemade candies. The cook had prepared sandwiches but having never seen them, most of the guests bypassed the heaping plates. Cornbread and potatoes were their standard fare. "We called it the Christmas tree party," said Jessie Sheppard, then a child who lived two miles away. "It was awful pretty, all decorated. There were all kinds of things most of us had never seen before. We thought it was most wonderful."[5] Sheppard would eventually grow up and have five healthy babies, all of them delivered by the Frontier Nurses.

After the holidays, ever-changing weather conditions turned the skies dreary again, bringing more challenges to the work and to Breckinridge. Guests, employees, even the occasional patient drifted in and out of Wendover throughout the construction process. At one point, Breckinridge moved out of her upstairs room and into a tent on the grounds just to have some time to herself. "There is a limit to the capacity of even the most elastic house," she explained.[6] She opened an account at Hyden Citizens Bank for weekly payroll and other expenses. Following a vote by the trustees of the Kentucky Committee for Mothers and Babies, the organization officially changed its name to the

Frontier Nursing Service (FNS) in March 1928. Finally, with its name approved, the headquarters built, and her first few nurses in place, she was ready to begin the work of strengthening the FNS.

Near Wendover, footbridges suspended by cable thirty feet above the water served as the main access to the Big House. After a heavy rainfall or melting snow, these swinging bridges were the only means of getting to the "yon side." Three of the five bridges eventually collapsed when the beams supporting them were water damaged from a swollen river that had risen almost to the level of the bridge. They were swept away along with trees, fences, and other debris in what the locals called tides. Special cases, those patients needing the care of a doctor or which required hospitalization, were often transported in foul weather. One nurse followed a father up Thousandsticks Mountain in a blinding snowstorm so severe that they had to dismount, throw the saddlebags on the grounds every few feet, and climb up after them while leading their horses.

At Wendover, a nurse was called out at four thirty A.M. the day after Christmas to assist with a delivery. The case was in Coon Creek, six miles away. The father warned her that flooding from the river had covered the roads and the horses might have to swim. Undaunted, she rode off into the cold misty dawn. She carried a lantern and medical supplies. Eight hours later her horse, Nellie Gray, returned to Wendover, riderless, dripping wet, with the saddlebag dangling. The nurse later showed up, unhurt but shaken. Breckinridge recalled the worry that set in among her and her staff but said they had to learn to take unforeseen events in stride. "If one's hair turned white every time something happened," she said, "we should all be crowned with snow."[7]

One winter the creek rose twenty-two feet and destroyed the trails to the point that no wagons could bring the mail for nearly a month. Yet somehow, the patients had to get out. There were five with special needs, including a pregnant woman who would require a Caesarean and Joe, an eleven-year-old boy with a heart condition. What they needed was to get to Lexington for care beyond the scope of the nurses. In her typical direct style, Breckinridge took action.

> A neighbor had planks and I had some pitch. In one day we built and caulked a flat-bottomed boat which we named *The Ambulance*. We turned the floods to our advantage and floated down the river from Wendover with our heart case and our expectant mother, picking up three other children whose homes were along the river banks. In the bow stood the builder of our boat, guiding us with the branch of a pawpaw tree. Next, on a plank sat Mallie, age three, and her sister, Hannah, eight. Joe and me were on the next plank; the expectant mother on the third along with a crippled, cross-eyed child of six. In the stern on the luggage, which included emergency supplies, sat Martha Prewitt, our secretary. She was alternately baling out our somewhat leaky vessel with a single tobacco can, and steering with a shingle.[8]

For sixteen miles they traversed the rapid currents downstream, finally coming to land at the mouth of Trace Branch. Their goal was to reach the railroad and get the patients safely onboard. All that stood between them was a mountain that seemed as wide as it was tall. It took three hours in a mule wagon to cross the ridge but at eight o'clock that night the entire party — patients, pilot, secretary, and Breckinridge herself — were waiting at the platform when the train thundered in. Since the children had never seen a locomotive they were both thrilled and terrified. Joe, the heart patient, gasped as the train wheezed to a stop. "Won't it git us?" he said. Once aboard, he turned to Breckinridge and asked if she would write to the friends who had helped care for him, for he was sure they would want to know how he was doing. His mother had died in childbirth and his father was no where to be found. Breckinridge, who said this was one young boy she would never forget, could not believe what happened next. "He pulled five cents out of his pocket, all that he had in the world, and said, 'If you bust this nickel, you kin git two cents to pay for a stamp for that thar letter.'"[9]

Several clinics were now underway that would boost the effectiveness of the nursing service. At first, only two or three patients showed up. Then a flu epidemic hit that led to pneumonia for some. "We nursed the sick," said Breckinridge, "and with the good nursing even the most desperately ill got well. After that, they began coming to the clinics seventy and eighty strong."[10] Beech Fork, built in 1926, was among the first of what would eventually become more than a dozen outpost centers. Funded by Mrs. Nathaniel Ayer of Boston, Beech Fork was a memorial to her Kentucky mother, Jessie Preston Draper.

A few small clinics, located in temporary quarters, had been opened in and around Hyden shortly after Breckinridge began the nursing service. The oldest, in Hyden, was a rented house with floors of unseasoned wood that warped and bent with human weight, and plank walls through which strong winds whistled and moaned. Over time, Hyden and other temporary centers either closed or moved to other locations. Sites were often selected based on donated land not convenient to much of anything. The Beech Fork site in Leslie County, for example, was thirty-two miles from a shipping center, located on the upper waters of the Middle Fork River. This was land that Daniel Boone had reportedly crossed, with colorful thickets of rhododendron that grew three times the height of a man. It took mule teams four to five days to get to the railroad, pick up supplies, and return. There were no professional builders anywhere nearby so Breckinridge ordered the facility ready-built from a manufacturer, had it shipped to Pineville, and hauled across to Beech Fork. Plumbing was included in the package. "The circular that came with it implied that a child could put it up with a little help from mummy and daddy," she joked. "So I sent a man to the site to drill the well. This was done so abominably that I fired him right there in the Middle Fork River while the water was rising around me and my horse. There wasn't time for argument. He went on his way on one side of the river while I went the other. A second man drilled a decent well later."[11]

There was still a foundation to be laid and a barn to be built. Breckin-ridge sent two of her nurse-midwives, one British, one American, to oversee that project. Neither knew anything about building. The first morning they arrived, twenty-five men were milling about among the beech trees, anxious to begin work while waiting for the women to instruct them on what to do. The English nurse, Gladys Peacock, was approached by the group's self-appointed foreman. "What about sills?" he asked her. "What about *what?*" she said. Surely he wasn't talking about window sills. They hadn't even dug the foundation. "Well, Mr. Hoskins," she said. "Mrs. Breckinridge may have said something to Miss Willeford about them. I'll go check." She rode down the hill to find her peer who was at the barn site. "What about sills?" she called to Mary Willeford, a well-educated nurse from Texas who within the next few years would become an assistant director of the FNS. "What about what?" Willeford repeated. "What the dickens are sills?" "Look here, old sport," Peacock replied. "Mr. Hoskins wants to know about sills. We can't let him think we don't know what they are. We've just got to bluff."[12]

The nurses returned to Hoskins who was waiting patiently for his instruc-tions. Willeford strode toward him. "You know these parts so much better than we do," she told him in her Texas twang. "What would *you* suggest?" He rubbed his chin and thought for a moment. "I reckon you can get all you want off Luther Moseley's land. He said you could have all the timber you needed."[13] It was the first and last time a ready-made building would be used by the FNS. Appealing to her practical side, the nurses convinced Breckinridge it was just as cost efficient to build a center from the ground up as it was to haul the con-tents of two freight cars in twenty-four mule-team wagons over thirty-two rough miles. And there was a lot less headache, they added, as every piece of manufactured board had to be mitered to make a decent fit.

To help raise funds for the outpost centers, Breckinridge decided to cap-italize on the Daniel Boone connection to the area. She made contact with an agency called the Film Mutual Benefit Bureau, which supplied companies with production locations for the benefit of nonprofits. The bureau staff was invited to the FNS to take moving pictures throughout the county and film the newly opened clinics. Two women arrived with the newest modes of portable cam-eras, accessories, and several thousand feet of film. With the aid of a pack horse and an able-bodied young assistant, they visited homes and clinics, crossing rivers and forks to produce their film. Several scenes were depicted of Daniel Boone (a local carrying a flintlock rifle and shooting at an Indian across the river). It was a raw, windy day and the unfortunate man playing the Indian had to fall into the freezing river three times in order to be properly shot. Breck-inridge used the finished film on a northern tour down the Maine coast, illus-trating the need for funds throughout her oral presentations.

The FNS fee structure, charging nominal amounts for medical service to ensure a measure of dignity, was set up similar to what Breckinridge had learned during her years in Europe. If people could pay even a little, she reasoned, it helped retain their sense of dignity. Investing in their own medical care also made them more willing to follow through with the nurses' instructions. Hyden residents were solicited for donations as well. Some gave a few dollars, others offered fence posts, stone, or free labor to help construct the outpost clinics.[14] Serving the entire FNS fringe area was Hyden Hospital, built on land donated by J.A. Alexander, who would become the hospital's first chairman. The native stone two-story structure, atop the steep Thousandsticks Mountain that overlooked Hyden, was dedicated on July 8, 1928.

Breckinridge had spotted the property on one of her horseback rides through Hyden. It was a chilly November afternoon warmed by sunlight dappling through the trees. Breckinridge stopped near the gate of a friend's home at the foot of Thousandsticks and was looking up at the future site when her friend came out to greet her. "Right there is where I want my hospital," Breckinridge announced. "You reckon I can have it?" "I'm sure you can because we own the land and my husband's nephew owns the adjoining land," the woman responded. She later told her daughter about the exchange. "You know how impulsive Mary can be," she said. "But she doesn't waste time. Once she makes up her mind, she can be very decisive. I think that's a great asset in her creative abilities."[15]

During and after construction, water had to be pumped from a two-hundred foot well at the foot of the mountain up to a cedar tank and a stone cistern. Upon completion, the new Hyden Hospital and Health Center facility covered a little more than thirty-five acres. Guest of honor for the official dedication was the distinguished Sir Leslie MacKenzie, a bespectacled white-haired gentleman and director of the Scottish Highlands and Islands Medical and Nursing Service. MacKenzie had helped establish a frontier nursing program in Scotland and had great empathy and admiration for Breckinridge and her efforts. Yet even he was taken back by the twenty miles of rough mountain road his entourage endured to get there. They arrived in a plush, private railway car from New York first which brought them as far as Hazard. Along with eight members of the Hazard marching band they were then subjected to a jolting ride into Hyden on buckboard wagons. The troupe also forded the heavy Middle Fork River still swollen with recent rains, another harrowing adventure.

Among the other influential guests, persuaded by Breckinridge to attend, were several local judges and Dr. William J. Hutchins. A handsome man with a thick mustache and side-swept, salt-and-pepper hair, Hutchins served as president of Berea College from 1920 to 1939 when his son, Francis, took over. He and Breckinridge corresponded regularly for many years and she considered him an excellent advisor and a dear friend. About a dozen mountain mothers either carrying or leading their small children were in the crowd as well, for the Frontier Nursing Service, they were told with great fanfare, was designed for them and their families. The *Courier-Journal*, of Louisville, Kentucky, devoted a two-page pictorial to cover the event. One photo showed a small band of visitors trudging up the rock-strewn mountainside to reach the site of the new building. Dressed in hats, coats, or flowing dresses, they appeared to be sweltering in the July heat. Another showed Breckinridge decked out in a beribboned straw hat, and sailor-style bodice (a popular style in the 1920s), all smiles as she posed beside MacKenzie. A caption describing the Hyden hospital read: "The institution is eighteen miles from the nearest railroad, with roads passable only on horseback or by mule teams."[16]

What the paper didn't report were the behind-the-scenes misadventures of a few high society guests attempting to reach the dedication. One of them was Martha Prewitt. Prewitt was the future sister-in-law of Breckinridge and one of her first part-time secretaries. Born into wealth like Breckinridge, ten miles from Lexington, she grew up on a farm built by slaves who constructed each brick by hand. Outspoken and blessed with a healthy sense of humor, Prewitt claimed (also like Breckinridge) that she never had a normal education. Along with her three incorrigible siblings, she spent most of her time thinking of ways to scare the governess into canceling classes. For instance, the woman hated snakes, so the children would hunt for reptiles and place them in conspicuous places to frighten their teacher into hiding. She knew Breckinridge through family connections but did not meet her until 1926 when she learned that Breckinridge was looking for administrative help in her new nursing organization. When Prewitt arrived in Hyden by horse, the Big House at Wendover was still a work in progress. Regardless, Breckinridge invited her to stay. "I was asleep upstairs about six o'clock one morning when I heard these loud noises coming from outside," said Prewitt. "I sat up in bed and suddenly this man stuck his head through the window. He was fixing the outside trim, hammering away while I was still half asleep. Then he climbed back down the ladder, laughing. Mary was already downstairs so I could hear them talking. "Your clerk sure does sleep late," he was saying. "Only he pronounced my title as c-l-a-r-k."

On a visit to the Beech Fork outpost, Prewitt was met by a woman also named Martha who looked her up and down and greeted her with: "I don't hold with women in pants or short hair. I was a-fixin' to milk the cows and chop wood. Which would you rather do?" "I knew damn well I couldn't milk a cow," said Prewitt, "so I told her I would take my chances with the axe. I was scared to death I was going to lose a toe or something. So I struggled with it a while and finally her husband stepped up and took over for me. Well, she was fit to be tied. He wouldn't chop it for her but he did it for me. That's *not* the way to get on well with the locals."[17]

On her next stop, she almost got railroaded into tying the knot with a young man in a bit of legal trouble. "I was in Pineville and met up with an older woman who asked me first thing how old I was. I knew she had a son who was considered the best-looking moonshiner in the county. "I'm twenty-six," Pre-

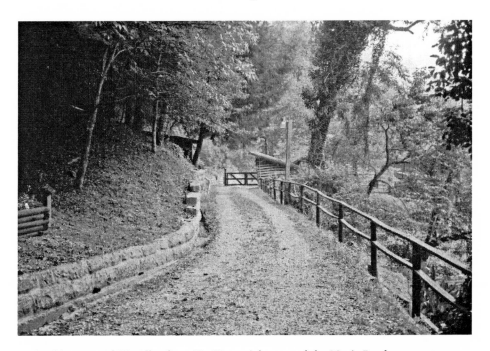

Looking toward Pig Alley from Big House (photograph by Marie Bartlett, courtesy Frontier Nursing Service, Inc.).

witt told the woman. "Ain't you never been married?" she asked. "No." "Well, can you milk a cow?" "Well, no, I haven't had much experience with that." The woman's brows furrowed. "Then can you chop wood?" Recalling her last stop, Prewitt answered that she could wield an axe if necessary. The woman shook her head. "Will is gonna have to marry somebody who knows how to do something. You ain't it."[18]

While out on speaking tours, Breckinridge would often leave Prewitt in charge at the Big House, where according to Prewitt, no one paid her much attention. She was, however, privy to the complex dynamics among Breckinridge family members. That was the summer Breckinridge's father, the Major, and his elderly sister came to stay at Wendover. Prewitt could hear them on the porch arguing vehemently about everything from which day in May their deceased mother had baked a cake, to whether or not it had rained the week before. "Then Mary would come downstairs for tea, walk over to her father, and put an arm around him. 'Isn't it lovely,' she would say, 'for these two dear old people in the sunset of their lives to share this harmonious time together.' And that would completely break me up because they just had another knock-down, drag-out fight over something totally inconsequential."[19]

One of Prewitt's most important assigned duties was to oversee a portion of the building at the still-to-be-completed Hyden Hospital. Not that she knew anything about construction, she said, or how to supervise a group of local builders. None of that seemed to matter to Breckinridge, who told Prewitt to do the best she could in her absence. She recounts what happened. "As Mary left to do her fundraising, she said the hospital roof *had* to be installed before the first snow, and to tell the men they could not quit work until that roof was on. The day I told them, I had been at Beech Fork Clinic all day taking supplies and was on my way back. It was a Saturday, a bitter November day; the wind was mean. My eyes ran from the cold and the wind."

She rode into Hyden and stopped at the hospital construction site, where one of the men approached to tell her the crew had quit. "It's too cold to work," he said. "They've already left to cash their checks." The roof was not yet on the hospital. Terrified of facing Breckinridge with the news, Prewitt rode into Hyden where the men were still at the bank. En route, she thought the best course of action might be just to leave town; disappear and not come back. "I got into town, walked in the bank, and I told those men, 'You have to finish this. You just *have* to.' And one of them said, 'Well, we ain't going to, Marthy. There ain't no sense in it. We've got enough to eat and to feed our families for the winter.' I was so tired, so exhausted, and so scared, that I burst into tears right there and then. I don't think they had ever seen a woman cry because one spoke up and said, 'Marthy, if you'll just stop making that noise, we'll do it!' And that's how the roof got on the Hyden Hospital."[20]

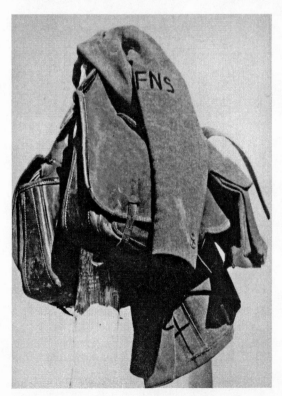

Standard winter uniform coat of the FNS nurse-midwife showing the easily identifiable insignia. The color of the uniform was a Confederate gray and the nurses said they could travel safely anywhere within the FNS territory once their uniform became recognized (courtesy Frontier Nursing Service, Inc.).

On the day of the hospital dedication, Prewitt had not planned to be there since she and Breckinridge's brother, James, were courting and preparing for a much-needed getaway to Florida. At the last minute, Prewitt agreed to help relay a small group of guests from Hazard to Hyden. They met for breakfast in Hazard and were told they would be transported in a buckboard wagon sitting atop bales of hay. "One of the women was from New Orleans," recalled Prewitt, "and she had never been in a jolt wagon. She kept telling us she was Mrs. So-and-so and of course no one had the faintest idea who that was. Everyone was dressed impeccably — I remember a festive purple gown and someone in expensive boots, and there was perfume all around." The refined group climbed aboard and set off for Hyden. Then it began to rain, a soft drizzle at first, followed by a typical mountain downpour.

Prewitt described what happened next: "The driver decided he didn't want all these people getting their nice clothes wet so he quickly looked around for shelter. The only place he could see up ahead was a pig sty on the side of the road. He drove the wagon straight into it, with Mrs. So-and-so waving her hands about and wafting her perfume over the stink of the pigs." Behind them was a banker dressed to the nines who was riding a borrowed mule. When the buckboard wagon went into the pig sty, the mule came to a sudden stop behind it, but the banker didn't. Instead, he dove headfirst into the mud. Unhurt, he got up, and to his credit, began to laugh about the whole thing. "But he sure smelled gamey," said Prewitt. "Most people like him would not have been amused."

Their mishaps were not yet over, she continued. Due to the sudden summer storm the river was now rising. Nearing Wendover, where the guests were scheduled to stop over and spend the night, they could not cross the water in their wagon. By now the rain had ceased and the hot July sun had turned their sopping duds into virtual sweat suits. So on to the dedication at Hyden they went, hair soaked, hats askew, as bedraggled a group as ever appeared from the backwoods. "After the ceremony, the problem was where to find a place for everyone to sleep," said Prewitt. "The river was still high and we couldn't get back to Wendover. Then it dawned on us. We're at a hospital with all these beds. There were about fifty of us, too many for the few beds available. One fourteen-year-old had no place to sleep, so Mr. Tillett-Cox of Louisville, a very important official, offered to let the boy share his cot." The young man, who grew up in eastern Kentucky, just looked at Cox. "Well," he finally stammered. "I think I'd rather sleep in the barn." "And then," said Prewitt, "I thought of all the people that would love to have slept with Mr. Tillett-Cox of Louisville and realized that was a rather wonderful reply."[21] But at least the building was now complete, a hospital at last that the little town of Hyden could call its own.

6

Building an Organization

By 1931, in addition to the hospital and Wendover, there were seven out-post nursing centers spread out over seven hundred square miles to serve nearly ten thousand people: Beech Fork, Possum Bend, Red Bird, Flat Creek, Brutus, Bowlington, and Beverly (a small evangelical mission on loan). A nurse was stationed at each, providing general nursing, midwifery, and public health services. The outposts were built nine to twelve miles apart so that one nursing station would overlap another and situated in such a way that a mountain gap could serve as the stopping point. Sites followed the two rivers—Middle Fork and Red Bird River—as the natural arteries of travel and trade. Red Bird Center, where Betty Lester worked, was considered the nicest. A roomy cabin with a peaked roof and warm brown logs, it sat on a hillside among the trees with a panoramic view of the valley below. Gingham curtains brought color to the large windows facing the banister porch. A stone fireplace with a hand hewn mantle beckoned visitors to come sit, while outside, round robins and fat blue jays flitted among the beech trees.

The FNS was particularly careful about two things when constructing a center. And it wasn't just about aesthetics. "First," said Breckinridge, "the building must reach solid rock so that the foundations will not sink. Second, every building down to the barns and chicken houses had to be well located above the highest floodwater mark."[1] There was great temptation, she added, to build on the relatively sparse and level bottom land. But that would never do. Wells had to be sunk and septic tanks installed. Sooner or later the bottom land would flood and a noxious mix of water and waste ensue. She also foresaw the day when the heavy forests would be depleted, with few trees left to hold back the melting snows and pounding rains. While fences might be ruined and pasture lands flooded, Breckinridge knew, in her visionary wisdom, that at least the FNS buildings would be safe.

For the clinics, land was usually offered free or at a discounted price, along with labor and supplies. One end of each center was devoted to a clinic and waiting room for patients, complete with appliances, a hospital-type bed, and

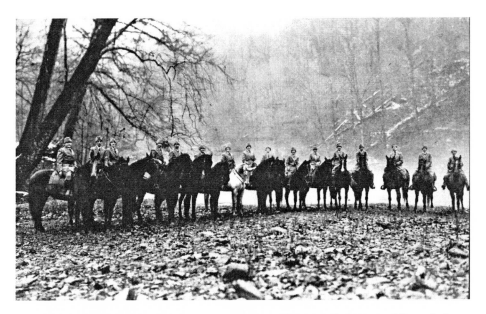

A brigade of the Frontier Nursing Service nurse-midwives in their FNS uniforms, led by Mary Breckinridge (extreme left). This photo was taken on Thanksgiving Day 1931 at the Mouth of Hurricane (courtesy Frontier Nursing Service, Inc.).

homemade furniture. The nurses had their quarters at the other end, softened by calico curtains, easy chairs, a desk, a homespun rug, a fireplace, and a dining table made from black walnut by one of the local craftsmen. Some had a bedroom for guests and a place for a live-in cook or maid to sleep. Without hired help, it was impossible for nurses, responsible for the care and grooming of their horses as well as patient care, to physically handle the dozens of other day-to-day responsibilities each center required. There were meals to prepare over a coal range, fires to tend, kerosene lamps to clean, candlesticks to refill, cows to feed and milk, and butter to churn. The housekeeper-maid tended the garden too and prepared foods for canning. Chicken coops were common at each location so that fresh eggs were always available.

Purchased supplies were supplemented by gifts and barter payments from grateful patients and their families. When a farmer killed a hog, meat was passed along to the nurses in that district. If someone had a good crop of beans or plenty of beets from their garden, it was shared. Sometimes a jar of homemade preserves was presented as payment. At Red Bird Center, the rugs and linens were woven on a hand loom at Big Creek and presented to the nurses. Split-bottom chairs, desks, and hand-planed tables were built by locals and offered as payment for services rendered. One man tried to pay his bill by handing over his .32 pistol. FNS nurse Betty Lester, thinking she would now have protection, accepted the gun. Then she remembered she wasn't much of a shot. In fact, target shooting at walnuts with a group of teenage boys led to them running for cover. The district supervisor learned of the barter exchange. "We don't have guns," she told Lester. "None of Mrs. Breckinridge's nurses carry a weapon. That's all there is to it."[2] She suggested Lester sell the thing. But currency was as rare as gun-toting FNS nurses. "We've had checks," said Breckinridge, "that went uncashed for nearly a year and then came back to us with scores of endorsements on the back. They had been circulated like cash."[3]

What the nurses missed most and wished someone would offer up was ice. While it was plentiful in January, butter melted and milk went sour in July. At the Big House in Wendover, Breckinridge had the same problem. She had a rock room built just behind the main house but the food still spoiled. It wasn't until 1937, when an anonymous benefactor donated a refrigerator fueled by kerosene that food could be kept on ice. "It was a wonder to me, who never studied physics, how the thing worked," marveled Breckinridge. "But it did, and there was no melted butter, soured milk, tainted meat, or warm drinks at Wendover from the time it arrived at our door."[4]

While midwifery was always paramount in importance to the FNS, baby and child hygiene were a close second. Between diet, nutrition, and teaching cleanliness, the nurses had their work cut out for them. This was true in most rural regions across America in the 1920s and '30s when unsafe water, infested foods, and lack of basic hygiene were not uncommon. But in the Appalachian Mountains, there were often other unforeseen illnesses and hazards: TB, typhoid, worms, cabin fires, and snakes. One mother under the care of FNS left her two-week-old infant on the floor of their small cabin while she worked in another room. Hearing her baby cry, she rushed in the room and discovered that a five-foot, nonpoisonous black snake was slithering across the infant. Running to the porch, she yelled to her husband outside. "Come kill this snake! It's crawling on the baby!" The next day, he built a wire-screened crib — something the FNS nurse had been asking him to do since the child was first delivered.[5]

Snakes made their appearance at the FNS headquarters too. At the Garden House near the Big House a large black snake crawled down the inside stairs from the second floor where the couriers slept—frightening the poor FNS secretary into a series of screams—which in turn frightened the remaining staff. At one point everyone in the building was screaming until a courier stepped up and finally killed the offending reptile. Breckinridge later told the staff to leave the black snakes alone as they were friendly, and kept the poisonous ones at bay.[6] There were three types of venomous snakes in the region, the copperhead, rattlesnake, and water moccasin. In the dense woods, rocky ravines, and watering holes, snakebites occurred frequently enough that the nurses eventually kept anti-venom serum at all the medical centers. As a result, most people survived. But snakes were so common, according to Betty Lester, that they even showed up as people were sitting down to dinner. One family told her they were ready to eat when one of a non-poisonous variety fell from the rafters of their cabin and landed in a sizzling pot of gravy on the stove.

It wasn't long before Lester was introduced to local snake handlers who used copperheads and rattlers in their religious services. One fundamentalist preacher grabbed a rattlesnake, wrapped it around his neck, and shoved it down his shirt, yelling, "See what ole Satan can do now!" It helped that he was drunk at the time.[7] After treating several snake handlers for venomous bites, Lester had her fill of reptiles. "We had one nurse who was always talking about how pretty they were and that she liked to watch them swim in the river as she was riding by," she recalled. "I told her that was fine for you but for me, no thanks. Someone is always offering me a set of rattles from a snake he killed but I never take them. I can remember a snake without a memento."[8]

Among the many people Lester worked with was Jean Tolk, a public health nurse for Leslie County. Tolk earned seventy-five dollars a month in 1919, knew the region well, and cooperated fully with the Kentucky Committee from the start. Breckinridge considered her a valuable resource, particularly during the early days when the organization had not yet gained the trust of locals. Tolk recalled a burn case she was asked to help treat after a homemade remedy was tried. "It just struck hard to my soul. It was a child who had stood too close to a wood stove. Before I arrived, someone had soaked the wet bark of an elm and applied it to the burns. They called it 'slippery elm,' and you can just imagine how that would stick. I had a dreadful time peeling off the bark."[9]

Cabin fires took their toll in other ways. One young mother of six was in her kitchen on a cold winter morning when she heard her hen squawk, ran up the hill to see if the hen had delivered an egg, and left the draft open on the hot wood stove. Wood was preferred to coal in many homes because it was cleaner. Suddenly, her three-year-old son ran toward her yelling, "Fire!" By the time she could get to the cabin, grab the baby, and herd the other children outside, the place was in flames. The baby, only two weeks old, suffered burns yet survived. With her home gone, the woman fell into a deep depression and hardly spoke a word from then on.

Besides the danger of fire, school-age children and some adults were afflicted with typhoid fever and tuberculosis. Tolk recalls sitting by the bed of a dying boy who was suffering from TB.

> He was beautiful, about eighteen, blond, with very clear skin. He lived with his grandmother, who was scared to death of him because he had TB. She would place a little plate of food beside him and quickly move away. I knew he would die because I'd done a year of TB work in Denver, Colorado, and my own brother died of TB.
>
> I was anxious that the young man be ready to meet the Lord. I got him a Bible but he wasn't interested. So I kept going back and one day he told me he now couldn't get enough of it. I stayed with him on the night that he died and we just read together and prayed.[10]

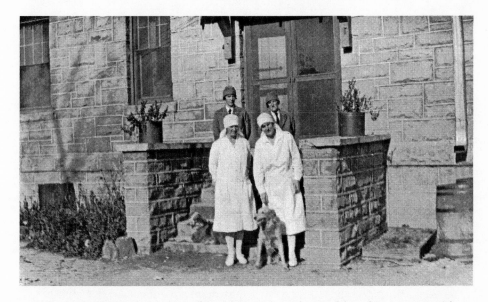

Two FNS nurse-midwives in uniform along with two hospital-based nurses pose with their dog in front of the nursing quarters at Hyden Hospital in the 1930s (courtesy Special Collections and Digital Programs, University of Kentucky Libraries and the Frontier Nursing Service, Inc.).

Breckinridge and her nurses were determined to rid the mountains of typhoid and other preventable diseases. Vaccinations were the only recourse, especially after a typhoid epidemic erupted at several local schools and twelve diphtheria deaths occurred. The superintendent of public schools wrote to Breckinridge asking for assistance. Once he received her affirmative response, he arranged for more than three hundred fifty children, many of whom traveled for miles by mule, to receive the shots. Nearly a dozen teachers volunteered to help. One took down the names of the children whose parents had agreed to have them vaccinated. Another collected the nickels of those who could afford to pay. A third sterilized needles while a fourth filled syringes. The physically largest teacher helped hold down the unwilling students, while another disinfected each child's arm with mercurochrome.

Jean Tolk, Betty Lester, and several other midwife nurses took on the role of public health nurse to complete the inoculation project. But not all school officials were as willing to cooperate as the superintendent had been. At one small school Tolk recalled that the students were scared to death and wanted to run home. "Someone told us if we vaccinated the children, the school would break up. It was really a problem." She also remembers a strapping six-foot adult keeling over in a faint because he so feared the needle.[11] Lester was appalled that any adult would attempt to frighten children about something so important to their health. Since 1900, vaccines had been developed or licensed against twenty-one diseases and were being used in most developed countries.[12] "A young teacher stood up before the group and said, 'Children, I am sure this is going to hurt very much. You don't want to have it, do you?' So of course all the children chorused a loud NO."[13]

Not to be outdone, the two nurses turned to the teacher and challenged her: "It's our personality against yours." For the next half-hour they stood before the group and talked in glowing terms of how to set an example for bravery. Then they led the youngsters outside and lined them up. A few parents had shown up as well, curious about this new procedure, though understandably anxious for their offspring. Finally, a boy of nine stepped forward. "I'll be second if someone else will be first," he said. His father, a tall, lean man standing near the schoolhouse doorway, moved toward the nurses, rolling up his sleeve. "Take me first," he said. By the end of the afternoon, the nurses had vaccinated more than one hundred children and adults. And the young boy who volunteered to be second grew up to become a respected family doctor according to Betty Lester.[14]

Eventually, more than fifty thousand inoculations and vaccines for typhoid, diphtheria, smallpox, flu, whooping cough, and pellagra were administered. The Kentucky Board of Health and other agencies deserved at least half the credit for their cooperative and educational efforts. But the real heroes and heroines were the eastern Kentucky parents themselves—many of whom had never seen a shot other than one that came from a gun. By swallowing both pride and fear, they allowed their children to receive the benefits of modern day medical cures, and possibly saved their lives in the process. It was one of several victories the fall and winter of 1929 on the part of the Kentucky Committee team, the generous people who supported them, and the local communities. Yet there were still too many unfortunate, preventable cases.

A ten-month-old baby from Coon Creek, "covered with carbuncles head to toe, his torture patiently borne with old, sad eyes," was transported on horseback atop a pillow on the nurse's saddle. He wasn't expected to survive. But after transfer to the Children's Hospital in Louisville and then to a patron's spacious country home for six weeks, he made a complete recovery and is now, said one of the nurses, "a radiant toddling baby."[15] Diabetic patients were a special challenge. Many remained unaware of symptoms and the insidious effects of the chronic disease. One woman had gone untreated until both her legs ulcerated. The nurses got her to the hospital where she stayed for two weeks, the twenty dollar fee charged by the hospital ultimately covered by her poor but grateful family. Before her discharge, she was taught how to control her diet and give herself insulin. A four-year-old, badly burned in a cabin fire the year before, had so much tissue damage on his arm that it grafted onto his side as though he had grown a wing. The nurses carried him on horseback twenty-five miles from his home to the train station where he rode with a nurse to St. Joseph's Hospital in Lexington. There he received a free room and surgery that released the imprisoned limb. He went home with a new blue coat, complete with shiny brass buttons, and an armload of toys— all donated by patrons of the Kentucky Committee for Mothers and Babies. And finally, as the year ended, a boy of sixteen came to the midwives with a crushed right hand. His job was felling timber and preparing rafts to float down the river during "high tide" events. Now the hand lay useless, in danger of amputation. A doctor in Lexington who treated him performed a technique involving curetting and deep drainage. Not only was the hand saved, the young man returned to work within a matter of weeks.[16]

Among her initial accomplishments in 1929 was a film detailing the inception of the Frontier Nursing Service. *The Forgotten Frontier* was the brainchild of Breckinridge, who was always looking for new ways to raise funds for the FNS. She wrote to her cousin, Mary Marvin Breckinridge, a film student in New York, and asked if she would be interested in producing the project. The end result was a powerful tool the FNS used in its fund-raising efforts. "I came down first in December of that year to capture snow scenes and to practice on my camera, a hand-cranked thirty-five millimeter," cousin Breckinridge said. "I would wind it up like a clock and it would run for so many minutes." All the participants volunteered to recreate scenes as she captured midwife deliveries, floods, elderly patients, childhood vaccinations, and the cinematic climax — a shooting between two men that required the services of Betty Lester, who would have a starring role in the film.

Lester, however, refused to call it a feud. "But if a man shot someone's relative, there was going to be a retaliation," she said. From her recollection, the two men — one she referred to as "just a boy"— met on a ridge at Thousandsticks Mountain and began to talk. One accused the other of shooting his brother. The younger man denied it, whereupon the other drew a gun and shot him in the stomach. The bullet exited after passing through a lung. The boy toppled off his mule onto the trail. Someone riding the ridge spotted the victim, and took off to get Lester at the Bull Creek Clinic. She followed him on horseback to the site. "By the time I arrived

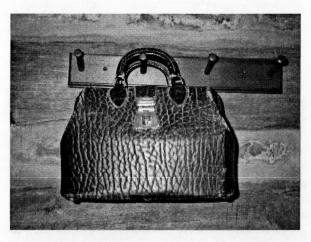

Medical bags like this were kept ready for home visits, including deliveries of babies (photograph by Marie Bartlett, courtesy of Frontier Nursing Service, Inc.).

and got the boy fixed up, a whole crowd of men had gathered," she said. "I told them they'd have to make a stretcher. So they cut down two small trees, put them side by side, took off their coats and buttoned them over the poles to make a sort of stretcher. We then carried him to Hyden Hospital. And he did recover."[17] Ironically, the boy would be shot again two years later in another dispute, this time fatally.

Mary Marvin Breckinridge wanted to recreate the entire scene for the film including the emergency ride to find Lester, the first aid administered, and the dramatic rescue down the mountain and across the river to Hyden Hospital. All the parties involved — with the exception of the two gunmen — agreed they would do what they could and try their best to appear natural. But things didn't go exactly as planned. "Mary Marvin was trying to show how we had to cross the river in a boat with a man on a stretcher," Lester recalled. "So we're all going across the river which wasn't very high, on this very nice day. We got just about to the middle of the river and Mary Marvin yells 'STOP! Stay where you are. Don't move.'" The camera had jammed. Fifteen minutes later, the little band of actors was still sitting in the middle of the river, waiting on Mary Marvin to restart the shoot. "And she was such a perfectionist," said Lester, "that we'd start and stop, start and stop. By the time we got to the river bank and back on the trail, we were exhausted, stumbling up and down the hillside trying to hold onto this stretcher."[18]

Since there was no electricity yet at Wendover, and thus no lights, the indoor scenes were filmed at Hyden Hospital. It took more than a year to produce. Throughout the experience, Mary Marvin was exposed to many of the conditions the FNS nurses encountered daily, including a night so cold that when she took off her rain-slicked coat, it stood in a corner by itself. She also worked as a temporary courier helping groom the horses, greeting visitors, and conducting errands, for Breckinridge was nothing if not a practical woman. Why not put Mary Marvin to work while she was here to film? There was only one argument between the two women and that was when her cousin tried to convince Breckinridge to appear in the movie. "She said no, she couldn't be in it and still show the film," Mary Marvin recalled. "And she didn't want to be pictured as a heroine. That would be embarrassing. So we went back and forth on that." To compromise, Breckinridge agreed to a cameo appearance.

However, one of the things the filmmaker believed she did capture was the spirit and independence of the women enrolled in the Frontier Nursing Service. "They were not self-conscious about being women in this difficult outdoor role, but neither were they antagonistic toward men," she observed. "They just went out and did their jobs and got along well with about everyone. It was a real demonstration of what women could do during that time."[19] She also noted while most were excellent nurses, they were not all excellent horsewomen. One nurse had only undergone six riding lessons in preparation for the FNS and was still terrified of horses.

After completion, the silent film was shown in New York in 1931 at Mecca Temple, eventually the home of the New York City Ballet. The house was packed that night, thanks in part to promotion on the part of the New York FNS Committee, which strongly supported the organization due to early speeches and visits made by the charismatic Breckinridge. In addition, coal mining was just beginning to gain momentum in the eastern Kentucky mountains and a union strike in Harlan County had made national news (Harlan County was considered the center of the earliest union struggles), finally putting the obscure region on the map. At least now, people knew that eastern Kentucky existed.

The film was well received. Mary Marvin Breckinridge went on to become not only a trustee of the FNS, but also a successful photojournalist and then a broadcaster whose boss, during World War II and the London Blitz, was Edward R. Murrow. Nationwide, more than 37 percent of births now occurred in hospitals, a number that would rise to 75 percent by 1939.[20] In Hyden, all children under the age of sixteen were provided with free hospitalization, though Hyden Hospital did not yet have an X-ray machine. A cook stove in the nurses quarters served as a sterilizer, much to the annoyance of the staff who had to run back and forth to sterilize instruments, in addition to keeping it filled with coal. When the nurse-midwives went into town to run errands or pick up supplies, hogs rooted on the dirt streets and had to be shooed away before a place was found to hitch a horse or park the occasional Model T.

Despite these difficulties, hospital superintendent Ann "Mac" Mackinnon had a reputation for being an excellent administrator and a fine FNS nurse. It was not uncommon that following a difficult case, she would prepare tea for her colleagues, or insist they take a break to stop and eat something. One of the more challenging cases these nurses faced was caring for a set of undernourished twins whose mother had died in childbirth. The woman's niece, Sadie Stidham, said the babies' teenage sister had taken over their care but the young girl needed help. "My dad went over to check on them and came back telling us something had to be done about those babies. He had heard there was some kind of hospital at Hyden and he asked the children's daddy if he could take them. If not, they would surely die." The infants, a boy and a girl, were transported on horseback and handed over to two of the FNS nurse-midwives at the hospital, along with a cow for payment. Within two months, they were healthy and thriving. One grew up and went to work in nearby Harlan. The other married and moved to Indiana. And both, said Stidham, owed their very lives to the Frontier Nursing Service.[21]

Shortly after, another set of twins was born, this time at Dry Branch, and delivered by Betty Lester. She had everything in place for the coming birth; cotton, rubber gloves, a spirit lamp, cord clamp and ties, scissors, hypodermic syringe, and five kidney-shaped basins. The cabin leaned at a weary slant against the granite mountain, as worn out as the young mother inside. This was her fourth baby. Lester made a quick abdominal exam and confirmed her suspicions. There were two babies, both full sized, which would put her nurse-midwife skills to the test. "Time for you to push, Hattie," she said. "With the next pain, hold your breath and push hard." The woman's husband stood nearby, ready to help. Lester found his presence unusual. Most fathers did not choose to be on the property, much less in the same room. A baby girl slipped out first. Lester tied off the cord and began to clean the infant while waiting for the next one. Second babies usually arrived within five to six minutes. Now might be the time to inform the waiting father. "There's another baby coming, Jude." "What?" he said. "Aw now, not really! There's never been a set of twins in our family." "Well, there will be tonight," Lester said, as the baby's head appeared. A moment later she announced, "It's a boy." "Ain't that grand," said Hattie, "a girl *and* a boy. But I don't even have any names." "No trouble at all," Jude told his wife. "We'll call one Betty, and the other we'll call Lester."[22] It was not the last time a newborn child in Leslie County carried the name of a British Frontier Service nurse.

Lester went from one birthing to another that same week. Just as she completed her last delivery one Friday night, a four-year-old boy peeked inside the cabin door. "Has the new baby come yet?" he whispered. "Yes it has," Lester answered. "Would you like to see your new brother?" The youngster stepped inside the room and gingerly approached the bed. "Nurse," he said, "I'd rather have a sister. Do you suppose if you washed your saddle bags out real well, you could bring me a sister next time?" Babies in saddlebags—the Kentucky version of the stork. "We'll see what we can do," Lester said, laughing. "Just take good care of this one while you're waiting."[23]

Its first few years in operation, the FNS had obviously proven its worth. Some now called it a beacon of light in a geographically, poverty-stricken place. At a Lexington Country Club annual meeting for FNS directors and trustees Breckinridge delivered a progress report to an enraptured audience who referred to her as "this charming woman." "It is significant," she began, "that of the three hundred seventy maternity cases we had last year, there was not a single maternal death. And of the 1,950 deliveries in the past nine years, we've had only two deaths of mothers. Those were heart cases."[24] She went on to report that five thousand children were cared for in the prior year and more than seven thousand vaccines administered. Babies were now brought to the centers at six months of age for inoculation against diphtheria—a major accomplishment as the 1930s began. And now, said Breckinridge, for the first time in the history of the FNS, more calls were received at the nursing stations than were made by the nurses.

She gave due credit to the couriers—"a most valuable feature of our work"—especially when the few telephone lines were down, as they were often were. "These girls," she said, "ride horseback relaying important messages or emergency calls quickly, saving us time and even lives."[25] At the Hyden Hospital, the wards remained full, some patients sitting on chairs with no available bed — another justification for much-needed home visits and public health care by the FNS nurses. The organization now had the resolve, good intent, and clear direction that Breckinridge envisioned. Yet due to worldwide events that Breckinridge could not control, all of that was about to be sorely tested.

7

Hard Times

The stock market crash in 1929 wrought havoc to the country by 1931 when rising interest rates and reduced money sources ushered in the Great Depression. Rural areas like eastern Kentucky with subsistence economies felt an extra-hard punch. The worst hit sectors were industry, agriculture, mining, and logging. Roe Davidson, a Leslie County farmer and coal miner, recalls a period in Hyden during the early 1930s when dry goods were carefully rationed and food was so scarce, "you couldn't maintain a bread line." "At the store, where there was no credit, they wouldn't let you have a whole bag of meal, a whole can of lard, or a bag of sugar. It was divided up among everyone. That made it really hard on the moonshiners, having only so much sugar to come by."[1] Producing whiskey, especially in a dry county like Leslie, was one form of revenue for the locals, but the subject was seldom discussed. In fact, Breckinridge issued a standing order that her nurses were forbidden from raising three subjects—politics, moonshine, and religion.[2] Their focus was medical attention, not offering opinions that might incite a riot, or interfere with federal law.

There was little work to come by in Hyden, before, during, or after the Depression. Hyden residents had yet to own cars, so there were no autos needing gas or maintenance. The first time a small plane flew over, someone said it must be the end of the world. Women still washed their families' laundry in tubs made from logs and used a paddling board called a battling stick for lifting and scrubbing. Homemade soap was made from lye and ash. Farmers marked their hogs by cutting off an ear and fattening the pig with corn before slaughter. For entertainment, people went to church, to court, sat on the porch and swapped gossip, attended square dances or gathered for a molasses-pulling event. In other words, the only real progress that had come to Leslie County since 1925 was the Frontier Nursing Service.

Breckinridge and her administrative staff were struggling to keep the organization's finances afloat, often waiving medical fees and suspending their own pay to cover immediate expenses. By May 1931, the nurses had made more than

97,000 home visits and received nearly 57,000 visits by patients during their six years in operation, at a cost to each patient of only $10.92 a year[3] The FNS staff included two assistant directors, three supervisors, relief nurses, secretaries for the various locations, volunteer couriers, and twenty-one field nurses. There were also three nurses and a physician on staff at the Hyden Hospital. In an effort to balance the budget during the Depression, Breckinridge reduced personnel and strengthened her fund-raising efforts by agreeing to travel more and better utilize her large network of friends and wealthy acquaintances. Plans to increase the FNS region to a one-thousand square mile radius by the end of the organization's first decade were put on indefinite hold.

In budget matters, the FNS was operating on receipts totaling just a little over sixteen thousand dollars, with indebtedness owed primarily to the nurses and secretaries who agreed to work on reduced salaries, some for as little as twenty-five dollars a month. It was because of their sacrifices, Breckinridge emphasized, that none of the outpost nursing centers had to be closed during the Depression. Locals were kept on the payroll as long as possible, especially one man, a carpenter, whose neighbors told Breckinridge they heard his children crying for food. She found his pregnant wife and five children with only a few potatoes between them and nothing but polluted river water to drink. She did what she could to keep him busy even when it meant making work. Another local was unskilled as a laborer but proved hard-working and reliable. The Wendover staff gave him two weeks work white-washing the barn and performing general cleanup. So many men were asking for work that Breckinridge could hire them only in two-week shifts in order to give as many as possible a payday.[4]

The volunteer couriers—mostly college students from wealthy families who chose to spend their spring and summer breaks at the FNS—were critical to the program's success. Their duties entailed caring for the horses, transporting patients, relaying messages, and even assisting with cases. A sixteen-year-old boy, one of the few male couriers, was considered an expert in transporting expectant mothers over the harsh mountain trails by mule. He brought one woman expecting twins. It was an eleven-mile trip by mule to Hyden Hospital. The hardest part, he said, was convincing her to leave her other children at home. She insisted on bringing "the least one" with her and continuously fretted over the others. "So there were practically four of them," he said, counting her unborn twins. "Some job for me and the mule!"[5]

When they arrived at the hospital, he thought his role with this patient was over and returned to Wendover. A couple of mornings later he was grooming horses at the barn and looked out to see the woman, still pregnant, her baby in her arms. She was walking toward her home. He called for help but there was no one at the Big House except a cook. "Here comes that woman with twins!" he told the cook. "And they haven't got a chance of a snowbird if she makes that hike today. You make some tea and I'll 'snake' her in." He hurried toward the mother on the dirt trail below the Big House. "Good morning," he called. "Why don't you come in with me and have a good hot cup of tea?" Once she was in the house with her baby in tow, he locked the door and kept her hostage until a FNS nurse arrived. Together, they took her back to the hospital where the twins were born later that same week.[6]

Making matters worse was a drought that hit the region, creating dire conditions for the farmers, loggers, and tradesmen. It also affected the Frontier Nursing Service. Neither rain nor snow fell during the early spring and summer of 1930. By August, pastures had turned brown and wells and springs had dried up. The Middle Fork River morphed into a shallow pool. By fall, the only drinking water available was tinged with green slime. Dysentery and typhoid spread, then smallpox and diphtheria, followed by flu and pneumonia when the weather turned cold.

When the Depression got so bad the FNS could not meet its nursing payroll, Breckinridge called the women together and told them she would have to cut their salaries by one-third and eliminate paid vacations. The family money she used to start the FNS organization was running out and she had placed herself on a flat salary of a hundred twenty-five dollars a month.[7] She offered anyone the chance to leave if they felt it necessary. Three of the nurses took her up on the offer. When payday came, Agnes Lewis simply divided up what was left and gave each FNS nurse a proportionate amount. An emergency letter went out to donors stating there was "a desperate need of funds to continue our work." Citing the drought as one of "the worst disasters in the history of the American people, with Kentucky among the hardest hit states," the FNS appeal included descriptions of hungry children and perils of childbirth made worse by the Depression and the drought: "Some of the cherished funds for the maintenance of the Nursing Service have gone for food to starving families. Will you give to save human life?"[8]

Despite their reduced pay (only twenty-five dollars a month on average) the FNS nurses ministered to their patients day and night, treating them as best they could, some with no access to clean water. Safe water was often more than a mile away from a patient burning up with fever. But old habits die hard, and it was a slow, uphill battle to get the mountaineers to understand the importance of good sanitation and clean drinking water. Screening cribs and windows, opening cabins to fresh air and sunlight, moving outhouses away from the main living quarters—eventually became the norm but that was not the case in the 1930s. One nurse complained that her biggest problem during deliveries was dealing with chickens. "I would sterilize my supplies and lay them out on a table or a board between two chairs. But right at the critical moment, I'd turn to pick up something and find a couple of chickens parading their dirty feet over the lot, which meant of course I had to stop and sterilize all over again."[9] This same nurse said it once grew so cold in a drafty cabin that she reached for a tie to secure the baby's umbilical cord and found the cloth frozen solid in the sterilizing pan. Despite the primitive conditions, or perhaps because of them, the FNS nurses gained a genuine admiration for the stoic nature of the men, women, and children who battled harsh elements daily and suffered their various ailments and conditions without complaint. When a young boy of ten accidentally speared his foot while fishing, the nurse was not able to reach him for two full hours. He lay on the ground with the barb caught inside the tendon. "I had to probe deep," she said "and it took me some time to get it out. I even had to move some of the tendons where it was caught. But though he nearly fainted from the pain and was white as a sheet, the little chap made not a sound at all."[10] Other British born nurse-midwives concluded that the locals bore pain as unflinchingly as the sturdy souls who lived in the Scottish Highlands.

Living in cabins with pests buried in the soil both inside and out, more than a third of the local children suffered from hookworms and roundworms. Symptoms of worm infestation were paleness and fatigue. Or as a parent might describe their children, "They would puny around." A six-year-old reportedly had more than two hundred fifty roundworms, while a sixteen-year-old had more than two thousand hookworms squirming inside him. Breckinridge enlisted the help of outside federal and state agencies including the Rockefeller Foundation and Vanderbilt Universities, along with regional researchers who began an active campaign to eliminate worms in children within the FNS district. At a field laboratory, eight hundred and twenty worm cases were treated with a new drug (possibly tetracholrethylene which, unfortunately, turned out to be a carcinogen) that led to "miraculous results."[11]

Mother Nature had other things in store that year. Due to the drought, no corn grew and famine soon hit. With little fodder, the cows delivered only a small amount of milk for the children. Mules and other farm animals grew slack from poor diets. The Middle Fork River dried up. Families suffered in silence, too proud to ask for help. Even then, there wasn't much anyone could do from the outside, for the Depression had robbed miners, railroad workers, and loggers of their jobs. No streams were flowing to float the logs down the river anyway. In desperation for the mountaineers for whom the FNS felt responsible, Breckinridge reached out for help to the American Red Cross. Prior to asking for assistance, she sent a few of her staff around on mules to conduct a survey on how much food each family had in stock. With results in hand, she went to Washington, D.C., and requested the Red Cross send a field representative to Leslie County. The agency responded and before long two-thirds of the patients in the care of the FNS received an allowance ranging from $1.50 to $2.50 each per month. A family of ten or twelve might be given up to fifteen dollars a month to purchase lard and cornmeal, two of their staples.

It wasn't enough to cover all their essential needs, so Breckinridge borrowed (and begged through fund-raising) thirty-five thousand dollars for buildings and supplies that not only provided work for local laborers, but canned milk, cod liver oil, shoes, and clothing for more than two thousand needy expectant mothers and children. Breckinridge hated being in debt and knew many of the locals did not like it when she went outside the region to ask for help, but she felt she had no choice that year. The Brown Shoe Company in St. Louis donated over two hundred pairs of shoes to needy children when they learned that 6.5 percent of youngsters in Leslie County had no footwear at all.[12]

Among the few other bright spots was a new records secretary Breckinridge hired in 1930 who would become one of her most loyal and trustworthy employees. Her name was Agnes Lewis, from Montgomery, Alabama, and she was thirty years old. Lewis had heard of the FNS through one of its committee members. Enthralled by romantic visions, she plastered her walls with maps of Kentucky, circling a blank space called Leslie County, where no towns and no roads were yet marked. When her employer learned that she was leaving for the Appalachian Mountains, he came to her and told her she probably wouldn't like it there, so he would hold her job for at least a month.

Once Lewis arrived in August, the reality of the place rattled her to the point that she almost became physically ill. She recalls her first impressions.

> I felt sicker and sicker as I neared Hyden, for the road from Hazard was just dirt and still under construction. We had to go through a river, which was dry but rough. The hospital superintendent rode a mule to meet us and took one of my suitcases. I had to carry the other one up Hospital Hill, which was nothing but a rocky wagon road. I didn't have sense enough to bring my walking shoes so I was still wearing heels. That didn't make it any easier.[13]

Complicating matters further, she had received instructions at the last minute to pick up two children at the big city hospital in Lexington. The youngsters, Lewis learned, were more than ready to come home, but she wasn't sure exactly where home was. She was told simply to bring them back to the mountains on the train, transport them in the motor car pick-up, and make sure they both arrived in the right place. One was an eight-year-old girl who, along with Lewis, did not sleep a wink on the eight-hour train ride, nor on the twenty-five mile stretch over the steep, bumpy road in an antiquated, overloaded car. The other child was a four-year-old that she was almost forced to leave at a train stop prior to arriving in Hyden.

> It was five in the morning, and the nurse wasn't there to meet us. I told the conductor I could not put this child off in the woods. He told me he could only hold the train so long. We waited about five minutes and then he said, "Lady, I've got to get to Hazard. I can't stay any longer." About that time a young mountain boy who lived nearby was watching the train and offered to take the child to the nurses. He said they had been detained. So I turned the child over to the boy, and he cried and cried. Of course, that was my undoing.[14]

The eight-year-old was scheduled to be readmitted to Hyden Hospital, so along with her luggage and lack of comfortable shoes, Lewis had the child in tow as she trudged up Hospital Hill. By the time she arrived, she was stressed and exhausted. From Hyden Hospital, she set off for Wendover accompanied by the FNS donor secretary. Lewis, always skittish around animals, was handed the reins to a horse named Silver and told to be careful as they passed the general store in town. "Why?" she asked. "Well, the nurse who usually rides her spoils her by stopping for an ice cream cone. She might rear up if you don't stop." The horseback ride to the Big House, however, was uneventful.

At Wendover, Breckinridge came outside to greet the new employee. "She was warm and gracious and told me to come in, sit down and have my supper," Lewis recalled. "But I didn't want it. It seemed there were a lot of people there but really there were only six or seven. I was very homesick and just wanted to go to my room."[15] The next morning one of the nurses asked Lewis if she had been inoculated against typhoid. She answered yes, having traveled to Europe two years before. But she had brought no records with her. "Then we'll have to do it again," the nurse said. Lewis groaned. Could her introduction to the Frontier Nursing Service possibly get any worse? "I didn't know it then," she said, "but I'm allergic to horse serum. So as soon as they stuck the needle in, I blacked out. The assistant director thought I was just being a sissy and fainted too easily, which I guess I did. When Mrs. Breckinridge found out, I was ordered to bed for a week and placed in one of the guest rooms."[16]

Embarrassed by all the fuss, Lewis insisted on getting up the next day and told Breckinridge when she came by her room that she was ready to get on with her duties. "In fact," she added, "I felt as well as I ever had and resented being put to bed." Her first impression of Breckinridge, besides her welcoming manner, was her physical appearance. "She had short gray hair and not a wrinkle in her face. It seemed to me those big blue eyes could cry or laugh at will. I found her delightful — when she wasn't upset about something. She really did have two sides to her personality."[17]

Through the many years that Lewis worked in her various roles as administrative assistant and finance director to Breckinridge, she remembered times she was on the receiving end of her boss' wrath. Once, when she gathered data at Breckinridge's request and sent the information to Washington, D.C., where Breckinridge was fund-raising, Lewis added a personal note at the end of the letter. She thought her report, and possibly her two cents worth, would put Breckinridge at ease. In reply, she received a four-page letter that began, "Dear Agnes, I do not want your opinions with facts. I will form my own opinions."[18]

Many who knew Breckinridge well and worked closely with her said people were, by and large, intimidated by her presence and demeanor. For one thing, the word "can't" was not in her vocabulary. And for another, she expected things to be done *yesterday*. She was also a woman of such vision that some said she was a hundred years ahead of her time, and seemed to know something about most every subject, large or small. Martha Prewitt, future sister-in-law to Breckinridge, says her personality was "very autocratic."

She could really put you down fast and hard. And she had that almost regal way about her — like she was Queen Victoria or something. If you recall the very proper character "Winchester" on the TV series *MASH,* she had a touch of that. Every now and then, I'd want to slug her.

And yet, she could also be very loving and compassionate. I remember a woman who had several children and was getting ready to have another. Her husband threw her out because he said it wasn't his. She was about eight and three-quarters months pregnant when Mary took her in.[19]

Prewitt claimed she nearly ended up delivering the woman's baby. "She was helping me fold letters one day when she looked up at me and said 'I think it's time.' I didn't know where the nurse was, so I put her on a cot and started trying to do things while terrified. The baby's head was showing. And of course the woman had four or five children. She probably could have delivered it herself. Finally the nurse got there, just in time to wash her hands and catch the baby."[20] Prewitt said Breckinridge could also be great fun, especially at other people's expense. "She liked shocking people. I remember we had two men visitors at Wendover and Mary decided to start lecturing them on breastfeeding. All they wanted to do was look anywhere but at her. She loved it!" Another time Breckinridge, according to Prewitt, while wearing a dress was describing a battle scene in France in which a wounded solider hiked his leg in the air to attract medical attention. "Everybody's eyes popped out of their head when she threw her leg up with that dress on," Prewitt said. "But she enjoyed being just a little out of line."[21]

Agnes Lewis — a tiny woman timid and shy in contrast to Breckinridge's dominating chutzpah — alternated between pride in her work and an overwhelming sense that she had overstepped her limits. She said she seldom felt that she was good enough to work for Breckinridge. "I routinely felt that I was asked to do things I was not qualified to do. I was really not fitted for the life, had no real training for it."[22] She also realized before long — through Breckinridge — that the mountain people to whom the Frontier Nursing Service was dedicated were intelligent, highly resourceful, and kind-hearted people who simply lacked the opportunities afforded to those who lived outside the region.

Lewis recalled she felt totally out of place at first and spent the first few months on the job near tears. Along with her fear of horses and the harsh conditions in which she found herself, she often wondered if she had made a huge mistake in coming to eastern Kentucky. One day while making an errand run to Hyden, a downpour began that resulted in the Middle Fork River rising. Kermit Morgan, in charge of the FNS horses, took time to ask one of the Wendover secretaries to contact Lewis in town and tell her to come home. The message was relayed by phone. "When I heard that I would probably have to swim my horse, my heart sank," said Lewis. "But I didn't lose any time in getting on Glory and heading for Wendover. I rode down Muncy Creek and it was already roaring. It was rocky and I was trembling all over. When I got to the edge of the river, it was now raging and I knew I'd have to swim. I looked across to the other bank and there was Kermit sitting on his horse. He met me in the middle of the river."

As her horse plunged into the water Lewis burst into tears. "What are you doing here, Kermit?" she wailed. "I knowed you would be scared," he replied. "You don't forget something like that," said Lewis. "These mountain men, gentlemen under every circumstance, would do anything for you."[23] Lewis believes that because the mountain people were inherently kind to those they came to trust, Breckinridge exhibited a genuine gratitude toward them, while she could be curt, demanding, even condescending with her contemporaries. "If you had a degree after your name you were expected to be able to do almost anything," Lewis said.[24]

The few locals to whom Breckinridge addressed any wrath were handled with utmost diplomacy. After all, it behooved her and the FNS organization to stay in their "good graces," said Lewis:

> In the early days, Mrs. Breckinridge had great opposition from one of the rural doctors. He had come into the county before the FNS and he resented their presence. It was just something she put up with, but her goal was to always put the patient first. I remember him writing her a nasty letter. When I walked into her room, she handed it to me. I rose to her defense, indignant that he would write that kind of letter.
>
> "Never mind, child," she said. "It'll take me about three days to get in the spirit to answer it, but I'll show it to you when I do."
>
> And she did. It was the most courteous, kind, sincere letter that one could have written. That's the way she replied to such things.[25]

When a young man was rejected from the military due to his low intelligence, Breckinridge took him in, hiring him to help her feed the chickens. "He was more trouble than I wanted to put up with," said Lewis. "I had little patience with him as it took him so long to understand things. You'd say something to him and forty-eight hours later, he'd get mad at you. But Mrs. Breckinridge liked talking to him, and to all the locals who worked for her. She always came out and spoke to each one."[26] Lewis concluded that Breckinridge had a special talent for bringing out the best in people while demanding the most from them. In return, she earned their loyalty, respect, and lifelong devotion.

Lewis ended up staying with Breckinridge for thirty-seven years. Throughout her tenure, she was perhaps one of the few people who really got to know Mary Breckinridge — knowledge the other nurses would periodically attempt to coerce out of Lewis — for few had the nerve or opportunity to explore this imposing woman's nature. In time, Lewis would become one of her closest confidants, even offering to destroy personal correspondence for Breckinridge. Among the letters and personal artifacts shared were the small worn shoes of four-year-old Breckie, one of her first husband's shirts, and a journal that Breckinridge had kept from the time she was a girl. "She could be highly emotional and sentimental," said Lewis. "And there were things she wrote in her day book at the tender age of thirteen. I never read it. But she read parts of it to me, as I was a romantic too. So I appreciated it. It was about her young inner life and I understood why she would not want it published or open to anyone. I was delighted to burn it on her behalf."[27]

Another part of Breckinridge's psyche known only to Lewis and a handful of others was the fact that she had a spiritual advisor — not uncommon in the early twentieth century when magic, séances, and other faith-based activities gained popularity. The woman's name was Sister Adeline. Breckinridge met her in England, recalling the day the sister descended from a flight of stairs appearing almost other-worldly. Lewis said Breckinridge told her that Sister Adeline was "the most radiant woman she'd ever seen."[28] The two women corresponded for years and through her, Breckinridge felt sure she could communicate with her two dead children. The sister convinced her that each night before she went to sleep, she was with her beloved Breckie and that he was well cared for "on the other side." She also helped Breckinridge through various personal and medical crises, serving as a counselor, a mentor, and a close friend.

On the surface, Breckinridge minimized her relationship with Sister Adeline, fearing that disclosure would somehow hurt the reputation of the FNS. Nor did she believe most people would understand the need to consult an advisor of the spirit. Pragmatic by nature, Breckinridge often said she didn't have a lot of time for spiritual matters — though she was a devout Episcopalian and held chapel services at Wendover when the nurses couldn't get to church. Sister Adeline suggested Breckinridge do "short meditations rather than long prayers," and remained an important part of her private life until the day Breckinridge died.[29] Sometimes cases came to the Frontier Nurses. Anna May January, a supervisor at the Hyden Hospital Clinic, said children always made a lasting impression. "As I entered the clinic one day," January recalled, "two of our nurses from an outpost handed me a tiny bundle and said, 'We brought you a dying baby.' One look told me this tiny mite really was dying. The only sign of life was a faint gasp now and then. And I thought, as long as there is a spark of life, there is hope." The nurses set to work applying external heat, oxygen, and mouth-to-mouth respirations. A hospital physician was consulted who determined the baby needed fluids to counter severe dehydration. "With shaking knees and prayer," said January, "I passed the gavage tube into the child, aspirating about an ounce of what looked like coffee. As hour after hour went by, we somehow managed to keep the spark of life intact. Little Beth was placed in an incubator upstairs and soon became known as our 'miracle baby.'"[30]

A few weeks later a local grandmother rushed to the clinic with a blonde, curly-haired two-year-old in her arms. "My baby done swallowed rat poison!" she cried. The child was in convulsions from strychnine she had ingested. The staff worked furiously over the toddler until the convulsions ceased. She was admitted and made a full recovery. Less serious was the case involving little

John, who had inexplicably shoved rice into his right ear. As his ear canal was deluged with water, an entire basin full came tumbling out. "Now John," the FNS nurse admonished, "next time you decide to plant a rice patch suppose you find a bit more acreage?" "I reckon I will," the child said with a sheepish grin.[31] At last, in April, the rains came and ended the year-long drought. Wells and springs were renewed and people cheered as great rafts of poplar, oak, and walnut that were scorched dry in the hills floated once more down the river. Families were soon back at work, planting gardens, mending fences. "But it will take years," maintained Breckinridge, "to overcome the effects of this colossal calamity. And the brunt of it, in our district, will fall on the Frontier Nursing Service."[32]

In fact, bad luck continued to dog the Frontier Nursing Service. In 1931, the first of several FNS nurses died in the line of duty. A red-headed Irish woman named Hannah O'Driscoll, known to the nurses as "Nancy," had come to the FNS in the previous fall after training with the Queen's Nurses in Manchester, England. Shy at first, she had a good sense of humor and soon made friends among the staff. Breckinridge and the other nurses considered her a hard worker and a quick study. They also liked that she wanted to ride the wilder horses as opposed to some of the nurses who were still somewhat hesitant horsewomen. In fact, it didn't bother O'Driscoll when her horse, Dixie, threw her off, as she often did. She would simply get up, dust herself off, and climb back on. She broke her nose during one fall but dismissed it as "just a nosebleed," according to her colleagues.

On a midwife case in the middle of the night with another FNS nurse, O'Driscoll's horse took a wrong turn and was soon wandering the woods with O'Driscoll astride. Working her way toward the right path, O'Driscoll lost her FNS hat and cut her face on the heavy branches that slapped her in the darkness. When she finally caught up with the other nurse, she noticed that her face too was bleeding from scratches. She burst out laughing, saying what a sore sight they would be for their patient. Her favorite horse was Raven, a spirited black steed that she loved taking on rugged trails and into deep ravines. One early spring morning in heavy rain, O'Driscoll and her friend, Scottish FNS nurse Ann P. MacKinnon ("Mac") were attempting to get to the river. The women found themselves on a trail so steep that the horses slipped and slid, rearing back on their haunches, all the way down. O'Driscoll found the entire trip amusing. "I could hear her ringing laugh through the heavy rain," recalled Mac. "Here she came, her service cap dangling over one ear and the layette, tucked in heavy brown paper, under one arm. When we came to the roaring river below three men were waiting with a small flat boat. In we got, with our saddle bags weighing nearly fifty pounds each and the layette held over our heads to keep it from the waves that splashed into our boat. Nancy, of course, considered it all grand sport."[33]

Known for her meticulous record-keeping and high energy, she also liked

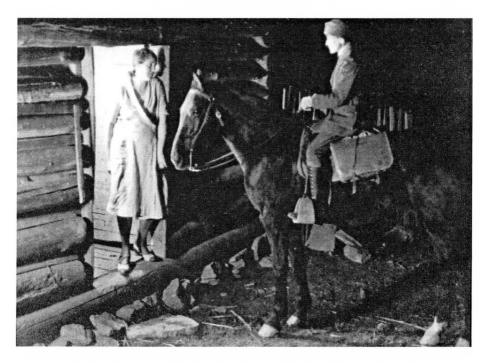

A Frontier Service nurse-midwife arrives for a midnight delivery of a newborn in Leslie County, 1930s era, and is greeted at the door by a neighbor who tells her the woman is "punishin' bad" (courtesy Frontier Nursing Service, Inc.).

to have a good time. Whenever an Irish tune was played on the Victrola at the Big House she would dance about the room, tossing her flaming red hair. A collector of wildflowers on her many trips through the woods, she dried and pressed them into a book for safe-keeping. On clear nights, she liked nothing better than star-gazing from the crest of a hill, alone atop the dark ridge. So seldom did she wear her FNS cap that the other nurses teased her, asking why she bothered to carry it at all. "Oh, I think the world of my fine cap. I just don't want it on my head," she responded. They also gave her grief about her poor eyesight. The girl was so near-sighted she could hardly spot what was on the ground beneath her. "Look out!" Mac called to her one day. "There's a copperhead below you!" "I don't see any snake," O'Driscoll replied. "Well he's right down there in front of your horse." "I'll just have a look then," she said. And before Mac could stop her, she climbed off the horse and leaned toward the ground. The snake hissed and struck as O'Driscoll jumped aside. "Oh, so *that's* a copperhead," she said, nonplussed.[34]

The day she fell ill she was en route on horseback to attend an expectant mother. She hadn't felt well lately and the intermittent pain had been present for a while. "There's this intestinal infection going around," O'Driscoll told a courier just prior to her trip. "I may just have indigestion." True to form, she made light of it, going on about her business. This particular patient, several months pregnant, was not progressing and she wanted to keep an eye on her. She dismounted at the woman's home, opened the gate, and felt another stab of pain. Then it subsided. She also had a splitting headache. Dismissing her discomfort, she performed her nursing duties and returned to the FNS headquarters at Wendover around dusk. Along the way, she was so exhausted, she had to get off her horse and sprawl on the grass to rest. The local FNS committee members were coming to dinner that night but O'Driscoll excused herself, explaining to Breckinridge she wasn't hungry, that she would just have some tea and go to bed. The next day, as her condition grew worse, a doctor was consulted. He diagnosed appendicitis and transferred her to Hyden Hospital. A surgeon from Hazard performed the operation and found a ruptured appendix. Without the advent of antibiotics, there was nothing they could do. She was thirty-nine years old.[35]

As she lay near death, O'Driscoll asked Mac to check on her patients, especially the prenatal cases she worried about. Then she inquired about Raven, her horse. In her delirium, she rode him up and down the trails, and through the swollen river. The next day, Nancy O'Driscoll died. She was taken to Lexington for burial. But not before her body was placed on a stretcher and carried down the winding path from the hospital, through the town of Hyden past three hundred mountaineers standing in a solemn line to bid her farewell. Her horse, Raven, followed behind the stretcher, stirrups crossed over the empty saddle. "I don't feel like I ever want to come to Hyden any more," said one mourner. "She saved my woman."[36] The loss was a devastating blow to Breckinridge and her staff. O'Driscoll's colleague and friend, Mac, was grief-stricken. But the women could not be deterred long from their mission — for there was always another patient, another family in need.

By May 1931, they had attended more than seventy-five hundred men, women, and children, including two-thousand babies and toddlers. Bedside nursing was provided to nearly five hundred serious cases, mostly at Hyden Hospital. One was a young husband whose wife walked miles to the hospital barefoot on a cold autumn day, two small children at her side. She lived outside the FNS region and could not afford to call in a doctor when her spouse became ill. He had, she reported to the nurses, swelled up with "a terrible pain in his side." All she could do was leave him in their cabin while she went to gather corn each day. On the third day of his illness, she came in after working all day and found him dead. With winter coming, she had no idea what to do except gather her children and walk to Hyden Hospital. She had heard of the Frontier Nursing Service and hoped maybe they could help. The nurses on duty went into action, locating a temporary home for the young widow and her family, and giving them free medical care.

Tuberculosis was running rampant, especially among the children living in crowded, drafty homes. Some called it the "Great White Plague." For once, Breckinridge felt overwhelmed, almost helpless in the face of such an opponent. She recalled a child of ten who came to Wendover for treatment. Two of his brothers had already died of T.B. "Well, now I'm going home to die," he announced. "Everyone in our house dies."[37] The nurses were able to assist most by getting the children out of infected homes and into the few T.B. facilities where adequate care was provided. "But for every life we save, ten are lost — needlessly lost," Breckinridge said, "all because we haven't the funds to tackle this problem in a big way. The state is poor and gets almost nothing in taxes here. I am hoping to at least make a start in an anti-tuberculosis campaign."[38]

Her ambitious plan was to build a summer camp on a high plateau in the sun, away from the dark, dank cabins she believed were harboring the disease. She hoped to take three to four hundred children in the early stages of T.B. and house them in open cabins around one central large building from late spring until late fall. The idea came to her while riding her favorite horse, Teddy Bear, accompanied by a friend and writer from New York City, also on horseback. Breckinridge loved these occasional jaunts through the mountains with visitors, saying that it was one of the few times she could get escape her work-related problems. They had come to a spot on a ridge that Breckinridge considered a perfect place for a camp. "Of course later on, we shall need other camps and a special hospital too," she mused. "But we'll have to wait some time, I'm afraid, for money is so hard to find these days."[39]

There is no record to indicate the camp was ever built. It could have easily been because of the perpetual lack of funds. Or perhaps that Breckinridge had too many other pressing matters. By November, 1931 was turning out to be a very bad year for the Frontier Nursing Service. Not only were there past and pending money problems, the nationwide Depression still looming, effects from a year-long drought, famine, infectious diseases running wild, and the loss of a popular, capable nurse, there was one more disaster waiting in the wings. And it was poised to strike Mary Breckinridge herself.

8

Setback

The trouble began on a rainy November day at Wendover when Breckinridge mounted a young Bluegrass horse, one she simply wanted to try out. Her favorite horse, Teddy Bear, had taken a bad fall earlier that year and had to be destroyed. To comfort Breckinridge, and to help a local neighbor needing to sell a horse, the Wendover staff, led by Agnes Lewis, agreed to buy the animal. With money so tight, it was a true luxury. Lewis, who didn't care much for animals, rode him twice herself and announced he had a beautiful gait and "a good personality." The final price was one hundred fifty dollars, money definitely not in the budget. So Lewis gathered the staff and asked if they all wanted to contribute. They agreed and decided to present the new purchase to Breckinridge at a Thanksgiving dinner scheduled at Hyden Hospital. "She was very pleased," recalled Lewis, "and said he was more like Teddy Bear than any horse we since had in the stable. She thought Traveler would be a good name for him and that she should take him on her upcoming fall tour."[1]

The next Sunday afternoon, Breckinridge prepared to leave from the Big House at Wendover. She was en route to meet a car that would take her to the train, then on to Lexington, Cleveland, Chicago, and Detroit for her annual fundraising tour. Lewis explained what happened. "It was just beginning to drizzle," she said. "We went to the barn to watch her mount. The courier was there along with Wilma, a secretary, and a girl who was taking the pack mule out. Mrs. Breckinridge wore a coat and a rain cape with arms slits, fashioned after Canadian police apparel. But she wouldn't button it; just let it flop about." As the small group watched Breckinridge ride off, Lewis turned to her co-worker. "Wilma," she remarked, "isn't it a comfort to see Mrs. Breckinridge get on a safe horse?"[2]

Riding toward the trail on which the car was scheduled to pick her up, she looked forward to meeting potential new donors. And no doubt, she would impress them with her speaking style. People who witnessed her engagements described her as "magnetic," and a "truly gifted speaker." There was only one instance in which she was not at her best and that was on a New York public-speaking tour. Tired and frazzled from her trip, she was sitting on stage waiting to be introduced. The hostess, however, went on so long that when she turned to say, "And now I give you Mrs. Breckinridge," they found the guest of honor was fast asleep in her chair.[3]

Yet Breckinridge had a knack for drawing people in. To emphasize a point or get someone's attention, she was not above using affectations — tousling her short, cropped hair until it stood on end — or singling out someone from the crowd. One witness at a Lexington Country Club fundraising event recalled Breckinridge getting up to give a report and motioning to a woman in the audience who was dressed in a white lace smock and a large red hat. "That handsome woman there," said Breckinridge, pointing her out. "I wish for her to stand up so that everyone can see her, for she has done so many things as a volunteer. And we are so grateful." The lady received a healthy round of applause and the group, now eager to listen, gave Breckinridge their full attention.[4]

The trail on which Breckinridge rode that fateful Sunday afternoon took several twists and turns, wending along Hurricane Creek, where huge, irregular rocks and smooth granite boulders lined the riverbank. She had donned her heavy rubber cape to protect her from the downpour. Suddenly a gust of wind blew the cape forward, spooking her frightened animal. It bolted with Breckinridge astride. Driven by fear, the horse pushed forward up a rocky trail. At first, Breckinridge hung on for dear life. Then she realized he was literally running out of control. An experienced rider, she knew her only chance was to throw herself off. She glanced down, looking for the least rocky place to land. She dove from the saddle and landed on her back, crushing two vertebrae in the fall. Still conscious, she managed to crawl through the brush in the rain toward the nearest cabin. The two men inside rushed out as this rain-slicked apparition snaked toward them, shocked when they realized who she was.

Breckinridge calmly instructed them how to properly lift her. They carried her to the car still waiting at the head of Hurricane Creek where she was transported to Hyden Hospital. The next day, doctors decided she needed more specialized care and called for an ambulance to send her to Hazard. But the only one available couldn't get up the steep winding hill at Hyden. So the Hazard medical team sent a hearse in its place. Breckinridge balked, flatly telling the physicians she wasn't about to go to yet *another* hospital. She had work to do and would instead find a room at the Lafayette Hotel in Hazard. Finally, knowing she needed X-rays, she agreed to be seen. At the hospital in Hazard the surgeon told her she had a few broken ribs and a wrenched back. When the pain failed to ease, she sought a second opinion with an orthopedist in Lexington who diagnosed her with a fractured vertebra and ruptured ligaments. He cautioned that if she did not remain in the hospital for up to eight weeks encased in a rigid frame, followed by a back brace, she could be looking at a crippled condition for the rest of her life.[5]

She summoned Ann MacKinnon, superintendent of the Hyden Hospital, and her secretary Wilma to accompany her to a local hotel while she recuperated. Her doctor, reluctant about releasing her, agreed to place Breckinridge in a Bradford frame, designed from a rectangular frame of pipe attached to a heavy sheet of canvas. Set up in the hotel room, the device kept Breckinridge immobile. It was there she stayed for the next several weeks, along with her companions. "We'd get letters written at two, three o'clock in the morning," said Agnes Lewis, who had stayed behind to manage the FNS headquarters at Wendover. "Whatever time she woke up and felt like corresponding, poor Wilma had to get up and take diction for Mrs. Breckinridge while Mac nursed her." Lewis said Breckinridge was determined not to come home until she could ride a horse again. "When she was ready, we sent Carminette, just a pony really, and Kermit Morgan to lead her," said Lewis. "We had a rubber cushion for her to sit on and Kermit was to lead the pony as slowly as possible. It was a terrible experience for all."[6]

While Breckinridge worked to regain her strength at Wendover, a new nursing center was underway in Brutus several miles away. Because of the Depression, fees were reduced to two dollars a year rather than the standard five. Grateful for the almost-free medical care provided by the FNS, community members stepped up to help the nurses any way they could. Among them was Alden Gay, who offered to work with the horses for free. "The land for the center was donated by a local man named Frank Martin. It took about six months to complete the building. My job was to water the horses but the nurses saddled their own. I wasn't too concerned with pay. I was proud to get a chance to take care of the animals. We were enthused that we were having a center built because the community realized it would benefit us all."[7] When Gay cut his leg in a work accident, he recalls one of the FNS nurses attending him. "It impressed me how devoted she was to taking care of my wound. And the caution that she gave me about keeping it clean. *Everyone* was impressed by the nurses' duty and devotion, not only to the mothers and babies, but to the elderly. They were constantly cautioning people about better foods, better health care, and all kinds of preventive medicine."[8]

One weekend in early fall, a major flood banked the rivers of the Middle Fork on both sides. At nine o'clock that Friday night, a father arrived from Wolf Creek after literally swimming his way to the center. Finding the FNS nurse on duty, he told her his wife was ready to deliver and he would accompany the nurse to his home. But she had better be prepared to get wet. "We had to swim the creek, sometimes wading up to our neck," she wrote in her follow-up report. "We reached his cabin about midnight and I delivered the baby early next morning. I got back to the center that afternoon and was just dozing off when another call came. This time, we had to take a boat. The river was now so swift the boat skimmed right past the landing like a piece of driftwood. We landed safely below the ford in a bottom field and reached the cabin that night. At two

A.M. I caught an eleven pound boy."[9] Another nurse reported a "fruitful time, five babies in three days, one false call, and a sixth baby two days later. In three days I've had only four hours sleep, two fried eggs, and a spoonful of rice to keep me going."[10] One of her delivery cases lasted more than thirty hours while a bitter wind blew down the chimney, filling the windowless cabin with smoke. Once the mother was safely delivered, the FNS nurse and the woman's family sat around the fire rubbing their burning eyes.

Christmas Eve, that same year, amid slick boulders and sheets of ice in a gulch called Hell for Certain, FNS nurses set out to administer to a woman in labor. The gulch was named for its treacherous grade and mammoth rocks. (Eventually, the U.S. Postal Service changed the name to something they considered more respectable). When the nurses arrived, they carried their saddle bags and layettes into the cabin. The single room was lighted by a coal oil lamp and a log fire. For insulation, the walls were papered with pictures from magazines and headlines from newspapers.

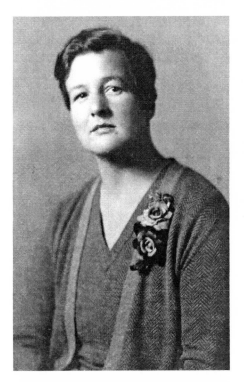

Two neighbor women had already arrived and placed an iron kettle on the stove to boil water. A corner bed had clean sheets in preparation for the newborn. A patchwork of quilts, stitched together with bits of odd fabric, lay across each bed. The mother, married at sixteen, was known in the community as the "sewinest an' workinest woman on the creek." She was now twenty-six and had been in labor for three hours. A little after midnight, an eight-pound girl was born, referred to by her mother as "a right pert young 'un." The proud father then climbed a handmade ladder into the small loft above the one room. And there, he told the news to the four little boys all sleeping in the same bed. One of the nurses asked them what they'd like to call their new sister. They couldn't think of a name. "Since it is Christmas, what about Noel Mary?" she suggested. And that's how the child became known.[11]

Edith "Johnny" Matthams was born in Malden, Essex, England, in 1898. She immigrated to New York in 1931 and it is believed she joined the FNS at that time in Kentucky. It is unclear how long she was with them (courtesy Gary Matthams).

At Wendover, Breckinridge spent Christmas Day in bed, encased in a steel brace as a result of her back injury, but still in command. Her assistant Agnes Lewis had been up late the night before, catching up on correspondence or going over the latest FNS budget. Lewis said half the time she could barely make it to breakfast at seven-thirty and into her boss' room by eight. "I wasn't always at my best that early in the morning and she would start with me, firing questions. Of course, she'd want the answers just *like that*. If I was slow in responding, someone else would answer. That was always a great help."[12]

A rapid eater, Breckinridge spent little time at the dining table. With her back pain, it was hard to sit in a straight-back chair for long. Afterwards, she would go to her easy chair in the living room, smoke a cigarette, and read the mail. If she wanted something, had a comment to share, or simply needed someone in the room, she would call for Lewis, Betty Lester, or anyone else who might still be at the table attempting to finish their meal. Few of them got through a meal without interruptions. It had been a tough year, donations down, the FNS director disabled, and another year ahead with no assured financial support. There would be no Christmas party this year either, nor would Breckinridge be making any personal appearances for a while. But the FNS work had to continue.

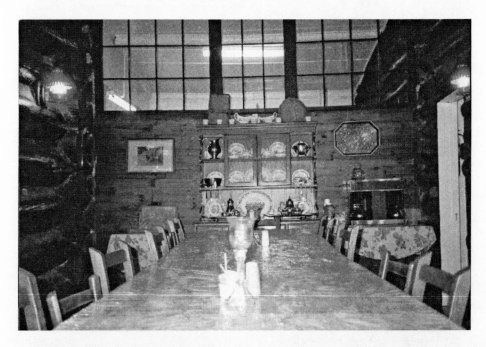

The dining room in the Big House where FNS staff and Breckinridge had their meals and discussed cases; often referred to as "the dogtrot," it was an add-on to the original structure (photograph by Marie Bartlett, courtesy Frontier Nursing Service, Inc.).

In a letter dated December 8, 1931, written by three FNS trustees who said Breckinridge had no knowledge they were sending the appeal, a fund-raising plea went out asking for donations. They needed $150,000 to cover next year's budget. Three Kentucky friends of the FNS had offered $5000 each. But that was a drop in the bucket compared to their shortage. They reminded the letter's recipients that Breckinridge was on a fundraising campaign that would have alleviated the current budget crunch when she broke her back. "How to meet this budget will be the burden of her thought until she is assured that it has been met," they wrote. "Notwithstanding the unemployment situation, notwithstanding the business and financial depression, and the many increased demands upon the generosity of the public on all sides, her faith has never faltered that the people of America will not fail to support a work of such primary and vital importance as the Frontier Nursing Service."[13] Despite the hardships, the organization was growing in size and credibility. Nine nursing centers served by twenty-eight trained nurse-midwives had ministered to more than seventy-eight hundred patients during the past year, and recognition was finally forthcoming from renowned public health and sanitation officials.

Elsewhere across the nation, making do and trying to forget the Depression was the order of the day. In Chicago, unemployment had hit 50 percent and men were fighting over bags of trash. In the Dust Bowl, farmers threatened anyone who tried to foreclose on their land. The words "soup kitchen," "relief office," "government cheese," and songs like "Brother, Can You Spare a Dime?" became part of the American lexicon. Women and children wore cardboard in their shoes. Men took overcoats from the dead. Immigrants got on the boat and headed back where they came from for this was not the America they envisioned.[14] Things could only get better for everyone. Among the few bright spots: Jesse Owens won gold medals for the U.S. at the Berlin Olympics, and in Hollywood there was always Shirley Temple. Prohibition was also about to end.

By February of 1932, X-rays showed some major improvement but Breckinridge still suffered frequent pain, particularly when she was tired. Her specialist in Lexington urged her to take a long-delayed holiday in order to prevent her back injury from becoming a chronic condition.

"So," she wrote in an open letter to her constituents, "I am leaving work on June first and not returning until September. My present plan is to sail on a freighter for some point in the Mediterranean, get a long sea voyage, and then to England where I will spend the summer visiting country places and motoring with friends, including some of the 'old girls' with whom I went to school in Switzerland in the 1890s." Sailing on a liner or freight ship was not a luxury, but just another form of transportation in the 1930s, albeit one that allowed for more leisurely travels. Breckinridge looked forward to the voyage so she could catch up on correspondence and perhaps do some reading. In her absence, she put one of her assistants in charge of the field nurses, the administrative staff in charge of Wendover, and the "old guard," including the medical director and supervisory nurses, to carry on their normal duties. It was her longest stretch of time away from the FNS since its inception. "But as a nurse," she wrote, "I cannot disregard the orders of my medical advisors. I request all the friends of the Frontier Nursing Service to stand by during my long absence, to renew if possible their support, and to keep the thoughts of the work constantly alive in their loyal hearts."[15]

9

Life in the Mountains

Divorce mountain style: A one-room cabin sits atop a ridge. Another smaller structure more similar to a hut than a house sits ten feet away. Inside the two cabins are two adults, one in each cabin, and a new baby boy. The husband is not sure he's the father. In time, he is convinced that he is not. He decides he cannot shoot his rival — primarily because the man has run for his life and is nowhere to be found. But he wants a divorce from his unfaithful wife, one he legally obtains from the local county court. Trouble is he needs a cook and someone to fend for the child. So he divorces his wife but builds her a cabin close by. And there they continue to live, happily or unhappily ever after. Problem solved.

* * *

Despite the stereotype of a violent and backward people, the truth is, eastern Kentucky mountaineers in the 1930s were by and large a quiet, respectable group who led the same kind of lives found in most of rural America. They sat on the front porch and smoked; swapped gossip and current events. Going to town, or sitting in the courthouse watching the more educated folks do their fancy talk was a rare form of entertainment. Generally, they retired by dark and were up at three or four in the morning ready for chores. If food was scarce, they ate whatever they had —cornbread and pork for breakfast, potatoes for lunch; often the same at dinner. If literate, reading the Bible might be the only form of book they had. Seldom did they become rattled about little things or allow themselves to get in a big rush. They were resourceful, tough, brave, and despite their spiritual side, fatalistic. Death could easily come in the form of a hunting accident — one man fell on a sharpened pole he was using to "stir up possum," rupturing his internal organs. A mule might kick a boy in the head, killing him before he turned fifteen. There were relatively few shootings— though locals did carry guns and were not afraid to use them. But when one man aimed his rifle at another he usually meant it. A family feud could end in gunshots without injury only to be revisited months or years later, this time with fatal results.

When a death did occur neighboring families would sometimes wait until there were several deceased members before they held a funeral. It could be two or three years. A preacher was then summoned and hundreds rode in from miles around. From morning to night, "funeral orators" assisted with sermons, many of them lasting for hours. It was strictly ceremonial, communal, and designed for the living. Helping neighbors came just after family. And making do was just a way of life. But when company arrived — whether it was someone dropping in from a nearby ridge or one of the Frontier Nurses, nothing was too good for their guests. "If you consented to stay for a meal," said one nurse, "they would cook for you fried chicken even if they had only a little. With the corn and the potatoes were turnip mustard greens, biscuits, stewed fruit, and jam. They were the most hospitable people I ever knew."[1]

Older children pitched in to care for younger children, and sons cut wood and hauled timber with their fathers. The nearest school might be miles away, open only from July to January due to bad weather and poor weather conditions. Wood stoves provided the only source of heat. Nearly everyone had an outhouse. With no electricity, lanterns cast both light and shadows as darkness fell. There were no radios except for the one at the post office; no TVs, movies, video games, or other forms of artificial entertainment. There *was* a hand-cranked phone at the Hyden Hospital but it worked only part-time. Set up on a party line, current was weak as it attempted to travel from Hyden to several of the FNS outpost centers. What made the connection weaker was that whenever the bell rang, everyone on the line picked up and listened in, especially when it was an emergency or there was news of a forthcoming baby. So to entertain themselves, stories abounded throughout the hills, passed from one generation to another, especially those involving ghosts. Most were homespun tales that revolved around rides which took place at night in answer to emergency calls. The spirits were called "buggers" and "hants."

When the dog barked at Wendover one cold windy night and a horse neighed to indicate someone was approaching, the FNS nurse on duty knew that it was her signal to grab her bag and saddle up. "This man had come to fetch me for his wife," she recalled. "The first thing he said was that he'd had a 'turrible time' for a 'bugger' had jumped on him from behind, attempting to join him for the ride. He had tried valiantly to shake him off but the ghost then grabbed the horse's tail and rode a good long distance."[2] Granny midwives contended this never happened unless the husband was riding with a guilty conscience. Others said it wasn't his conscience — it was corn liquor.

Betty Lester was a natural storyteller who loved sharing her high adventures on the trail, especially on rides after dark. One night she reported coming across Thousandsticks Mountain when her horse suddenly halted. Raven snorted, ears pointing forward, body rigid. Lester reached out and patted her, though she was beginning to feel nervous herself. There was something not quite right about this place. "Come on girl," she soothed. "It's okay." Through the darkness she could see the faint outline of an abandoned cabin up ahead. She spoke to her horse once more. "No one lives there. Let's go now." Reluctantly, the horse moved forward, the trail widened, and Lester's trepidation began to lessen. She knew there were bears and other wild animals in these parts, possibly even some bad men, though she hadn't met any. If only she had brought a lantern or a flashlight. All she had were the midwife supplies in her bag.

Up ahead at the cabin where she was scheduled to deliver a baby, Lester arrived to find a neighbor, Sue, waiting on the porch to assist her. She was staring at the nurse's approaching form. "You come by that holler alone?" the woman asked, incredulous. Lester tied her horse to the post and stepped up on the porch. "Why, of course," she said, "Why not?" "Don't you know it's hanted?" Sue said. "A man was killed there years ago and if you pass close by you can

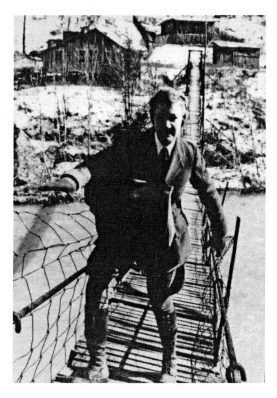

FNS nurse-midwife Sally Ann Tyler Dyrez on the swinging bridge that spanned the Middle Fork River and connected the Hyden community to Wendover where the FNS headquarters were located. Undated photo taken in the 1940s (courtesy Frontier Nursing Service, Inc.).

still hear him moaning. I wouldn't go by there day or night!" Lester gave a nervous laugh, ready to forget the whole thing. Then she decided against it. "I didn't see anything but my horse did get spooked." "And you didn't see or hear nothin'?" Sue repeated. "No, Sue, not a thing. Raven just ... *stopped*." "Well, hit was thar!" Sue insisted. "Your horse seen it."[3] Though most of the FNS nurses scoffed at such tales, Lester did refuse to ride through the area again at night alone. Nor, when she later became a midwife supervisor, did she want her nurses going solo.[4]

Part of her problem, as it turned out, was that she had no sense of direction. In strange territory with no maps, and up against unfamiliar hazards, it seemed only practical to have someone with you who might know the way. The other reason was pure common sense. Traveling alone on an isolated trail, especially at night, was a recipe for disaster. If a nurse fell off her horse and was injured, she could lie there for hours unattended. Some nurses were more accident-prone than others. One was Mary Harry, who hailed from England. Prone to getting lost like Lester, she usually managed to return to her district, but with scrapes, scratches, bruises, or other forms of minor injury. She still harbored an abdominal wound — and had the shrapnel to prove it — from World War I when she was in the wrong place at the wrong time.

One evening she was at the barn discussing the condition of a cow with its owner, blithely ignoring the fact she was expected at the nursing center. Lester joined in the search to look for her, inwardly seething at Harry's cavalier attitude toward time. When an FNS nurse didn't return on time, everyone had cause to worry. Meanwhile, Harry was leaned against the barn wall chatting. Just above her head lay a copperhead coiled around a rafter. Suddenly she cried out. "Ow! I think I've been bitten!" Her companion grabbed a hoe and quickly killed the snake. Lester arrived soon after and examined the bite just above Harry's arm and high up on her shoulder. "Lie down," Lester instructed. "It's a good thing we got here. A bite that close to the head could have been fatal. I'm going back to get the anti-venom. Don't move."[5] Harry survived the snakebite with only a few days of feeling poorly. But there was deep tissue damage and it was months before she was able to return to work.

Though the nurses generally felt safe within the confines of the hills and had the protective local men to assist them whenever there was trouble, one nurse was the victim of an attempted shooting, prompting Breckinridge to call in law enforcement. The woman was stationed at Flat Creek and heard a noise one night. She stepped outside and looked around but saw no one. She scanned her lantern over the bushes near the porch and spotted a crouched man, a revolver in his hand. So she ran inside the clinic and slammed the door. A shot blasted through the wall, followed by another; there were six shots in all. Then there was total silence. Unsure if he had left, or was reloading, the nurse hid under a bed and remained there wide awake the rest of the night. The next morning, as she gingerly stepped outside, there was no sign of the shooter.

With no phone, she had to ride the several miles to Wendover to report what had happened. Breckinridge summoned the district committee for an emergency meeting and all eighteen members showed up, expressing genuine shock and concern. They also offered their help in catching the offender. Several men were arrested on suspicion but none were charged. One told the investigating sheriff, "You know I wouldn't harm them nurses. They helped me raise my children."[6] And that was true. Throughout the long history of the Frontier Nursing Service, when nurses were often put in what today would be considered perilous situations, not once did they report being accosted, threatened, or physically harmed in any way by the fathers, husbands, or sons of the many families who depended upon them for help. In fact, most men went out of their way to ensure the nurses' safety, even providing a shortcut through the woods for Betty Lester after they learned of her ride past the "haunted" cabin.

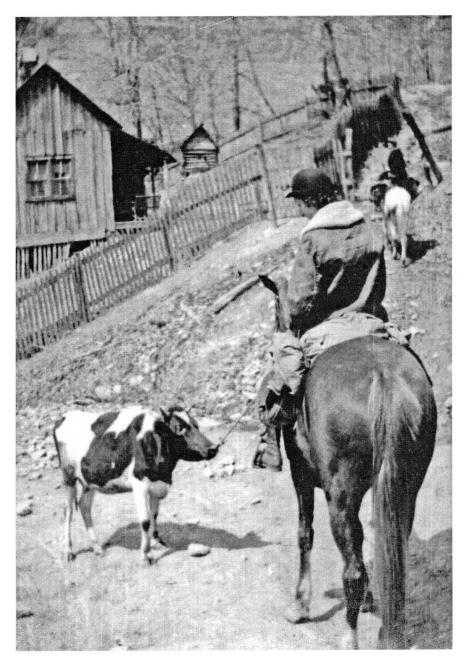

An unidentified FNS nurse-midwife making rounds sometime in the 1930s. The nurses often served as the only healthcare provider to families throughout the seven hundred square mile region of the FNS (courtesy Frontier Nursing Service, Inc.).

One full day was set aside for "workings," in which entire families showed up to saw wood, haul trees, and clear brush. They brought covered dishes brimming with dumplings, beans, salad, plates of fried chicken, and cast iron pans of hot cornbread. At midday they had a picnic, inviting the nurses to join them. When this particular shortcut across the ridge was completed they dubbed it "Betty's Trail." Coincidentally, it led to "Betty's Branch," named for a long-ago resident in the mountains. But what Lester needed most was a clinic. Up until now, she had been working out of borrowed space, a room in a teacher's home for clinic once a week in the winter; and the one-room schoolhouse in the summer. Riding through the Bull Creek District on rounds, she pondered the idea of how to get her own building. She knew the Frontier Service was hard pressed for cash, so asking for funds from Mrs. Breckinridge was out.

Lester stopped by the school to see Charlie, the teacher whose wife, Edith, had graciously provided a room in their home. Having taught in the area for years, he knew the locals well. And Edith, despite a lack of medical training, had accompanied Lester on several deliveries. Her role was to build a fire, fetch supplies, or comfort the mothers. "Hey Charlie," Lester called. "Do you think people around here would build me a clinic?" "I sure do, Miss Lester," he said. "Not that we mind having you use our house!"

They decided to call a meeting that evening to get a consensus. A group of parents filled the small school. Lester stood at the back of the room while Charlie got up to speak. "You all know that Miss Lester has been coming over that mountain every week to hold a clinic for us. We're mighty glad we have our own nurse because most of you remember what it was like before the nurses came." Heads nodded. The majority of the younger children present were delivered by Frontier midwives. Lester smiled. "Now she needs our help," Charlie continued. "She needs a place where she can leave her equipment and visit with the mamas and the babies every week. I think we could build her a clinic, don't you?"[7] There was complete silence and Lester's smile dropped. This was not what she expected.

Finally, one man spoke up and Lester realized these were people who made up their minds only after careful deliberation. "Sure," he said. "We can help Miss Lester. Where does she want this clinic?" Charlie pointed out a spot near the schoolhouse and several people raised their hand to volunteer materials. He made a list: white oak, four hundred feet of black walnut, two windows, and lots of nails. They would figure out later how to get the remaining supplies. "Well, Miss Lester," he said, "it looks like you'll have your clinic."[8] Lester was ecstatic and couldn't wait to tell Mrs. Breckinridge and the other nurses. But as weeks went by and nothing happened, she began to wonder if she had imagined the whole thing. "I wasn't very patient in those days," she said later. "Nobody was bringing any lumber and I thought this clinic is never going to get built. I yapped and yapped and talked about nothing ever getting done."[9]

Finally, one day Lester was on the trail doing rounds again and met up with a young boy. He was on a mule with a chain attached to a log. "Where are you going with that?" Lester asked. "Down to the mill," the boy responded. She eyed the log closely. "Is that by chance for my clinic?" "Yes." She rode off, hopes flying high, telling everyone she encountered that the first log for the clinic was going to the mill and that they should start moving, for they were all behind schedule. "That kind of woke everybody up," she said, "and before long, we got all the lumber there, ready to saw."[10] But her hopes were short-lived.

Days passed and she decided to visit the sawmill where logs had been delivered and work was finally taking place. Along the Thousandsticks trail, riding her horse Raven, she crossed the ridge top only to meet up with someone galloping toward her. "You've gotta come quick, Miss Lester!" he yelled. "The mill blew up and Hiram is killed. They want you down there right away!" Lester remained calm. "Get on down to the hospital for the doctor," she told him. "Bring him back as soon as you can." Then she rode off toward the mill, her thoughts turning to Hiram Young. She hoped it wasn't as bad as it sounded, for sometimes mountain people used the expression "killed" when they meant a person was badly injured. If the accident was fatal it was more likely "killed dead."[11]

When Lester arrived at the mill and examined Young she found he was badly burned, had a broken arm, and several lacerations, but was still very much alive. She wanted to get him to the hospital right away but he refused. Even when the doctor came and saw there was little more to add to the medical aid Betty had provided, the patient still said no. "Hospitals are places you go to die," he insisted. Lester promised to return the next morning. She brought FNS nurse and friend "Al" Logan with her. Both nurses tried persuading Young that he would be better off at Hyden Hospital. With encouragement from his wife, he finally relented. Now the challenge was how to get him there.

Neighbors gathered and discussed a method for transporting Young. They decided to concoct a "mountain stretcher" from two cut poles and a heavy fabric coat. Each set of men would take turns bearing the patient. The trip would take six hours over the mountain and up the hill to Hyden Hospital. Lester administered sedation to Young and the group set off, the nurse following along on her horse. When they arrived, Logan had food ready for them and the patient was transferred to a hospital bed. The nurses alternated their care of Young during the night, including a few who volunteered to come in from other districts. As Lester stood at Young's bedside, he opened his eyes and looked up at her. "Are you the nurse that's building that clinic?" he asked. "Yes, Hiram, that's me." "Well," he said, "when I get better I'll help you."[12] A little after midnight, Young died. Lester took his widow into an adjoining room and sat with her for hours in front of the fire. "She wasn't really that old," Lester recalled. "But she looked old. We put her in a rocking chair and she sat there smoking her pipe, telling us stories about her life with Hiram."[13]

Eventually, the Bull Creek Clinic was completed — the first FNS clinic built entirely by the community itself. Lester called it "the people's clinic" and swore that it would stand not only as a fine example of how the people of Bull Creek came together, but as a monument to Hiram Young as well.

10

Animal Farm

No one knew exactly how it happened but they blamed it on Ann "Mac" MacKinnon, the Scottish nurse-midwife who served as the Hyden Hospital superintendent. The group had gathered in the hospital dining room for a serious committee meeting. They came from Louisville and Lexington, important, upstanding people within their communities, enduring the strenuous trip to brainstorm ideas. Their goal: find new ways to raise more funds for the Frontier Nursing Service. Breckinridge was there as well, leading the discussion on first one financial topic, then another. Down the hallway, in the nurses' quarters, Mac had the door shut for privacy. That is, until someone noticed there was a foul-smelling liquid seeping from beneath her door. It began as a trickle, then a stream, followed by a foamy concoction that bubbled and raced down the hall. "And all of a sudden," said Anne Winslow, committee member who conducted public relations for the FNS, "here comes this huge cascade of beer into the room. Everyone kind of jumped up and hopped around. She must have been making the stuff in her room because it was just a river of beer. It was the funniest thing."[1]

Whenever a party ended, or at the beginning of a good meal, Mac's favorite Scottish toast was: "Here's to us; Who's like us? Damn few. And they're all dead." Even Breckinridge would leave amused whenever she dropped by Hyden Hospital and found the incorrigible Mac piled up on a cot outside the ward after her shift had ended. To the superintendent's way of thinking, it was better to sleep in a makeshift bed in the hallway than go to your room and have to return if you were suddenly needed. "I see you gave up your bed for another patient," Breckinridge would remark. "I don't have a bed," Mac replied. "Yes, I know," Breckinridge said.[2]

Mac was often on the receiving end of practical jokes, too according to Lucille Knechtly, who was secretary to the FNS staff for several years. As the story goes, one night Mac looked out the hospital window to see a man's bloody form draped across a mule. The victim was being led by someone who looked like he had just been in a fight. She quickly called for the doctor on duty and alerted the nurses. "We've got a gunshot case coming in," she said, running to the supply room for bandages and medications. Two of the hospital workmen carried in the casualty and transferred the man to a waiting bed. Mac set to work cutting clothes and removing several layers of grime while the other nurses stood around and watched. At one point she looked up, aghast at their lack of attention to a bleeding patient. "Well, don't just stand there!" she said. "This man needs help!" About that time, the injured party bolted upright and with a grimy sleeve, swiped the homemade tomato juice from his face. Then they all burst out laughing.[3] These lighter moments were what kept the nurses balanced, for the stark isolation of the mountains and the almost daily encounter with people in critical need took its toll.

Some of the nurses stayed only a short time, the reality of life as an FNS nurse at odds with their romantic, idealized notions of what it would be like. Some didn't care for the rigid control that Breckinridge exerted, a control she felt was necessary in order to maintain the integrity of the FNS. There were few social outlets for the nurses other than chapel services, community picnics, and the occasional square dance. Some nurses left because they didn't understand or appreciate the Kentucky mountaineers. During the first three decades of the FNS only a handful of nursing staff engaged in personal relationships with locals and there are fewer than half a dozen instances of FNS nurses dating or marrying an eastern Kentucky resident. It wasn't that Breckinridge disapproved, or that she had a prudish streak. Rather, from her standpoint it wasn't good business to jeopardize the credibility or reputation of the FNS by having her charges get involved with the very people whose lives they influenced and, in some cases, saved. The Frontier Nursing Service must be above reproach at all times, Breckinridge believed, or the entire organization that she had worked so hard to build could fall apart. In fact, only one FNS nurse, Primrose Bowling, born in 1928 in England, is reported to have married a local. The wedding, which took place in the 1950s—nearly twenty-five years after the FNS began —was sanctioned by Breckinridge and the ceremony held at Wendover.[4]

As a result of the insular nature of the organization, the FNS women were often forced to find ways to entertain themselves, by turning inward or to each other in circumstances that only another colleague could fully comprehend. One night after a hearty meal at Wendover, a nurse strolled down the pathway to the Garden House. As she passed an open window, she overheard noises that sounded suspiciously like strangling. "Someone's choking," she thought. She flew into action, running back to the Big House for the only tool she could find —a crochet hook. The victim, FNS nurse Anna May January, was indeed having trouble with something she swallowed, but when her peer approached her wielding the hook, all it did was frighten her into silence. "Be still. Don't swallow," the nurse instructed. "I'll be right back!" Again, she raced away, this time to the clinic where she grabbed another, more appropriate medical tool —

a pair of gallbladder forceps. Ensuring it wasn't a scalpel the nurse was holding, January willingly opened her mouth and allowed her colleague to probe. A few seconds later the stuck object emerged. "Hmmm..." the nurse said, turning it over in the light. "What is it?" January asked. "A bay leaf," said the nurse. "Bet that's the only time it ever met a forcep."[5]

Animals, highly treasured creatures on which the nurses lavished time, attention, and genuine affection, provided a daily source of comfort and entertainment. There were dogs, cats, cows, pigs, mules, geese, chickens, birds, and assorted other beasts and fowl. But it was the horses and mules that were particularly important, for the women literally depended upon them not only for transport, but for their safety and their lives. On average, there were up to forty head of horses in the Frontier Nursing Service throughout the 1930s and '40s. It was the blacksmith's job to shoe the animals, and also to put them out of their misery when the time came. "Just like an old car, we had to get rid of them," said one blacksmith. "We'd have two or three guys dig a grave, and I'd take the horse down, good-looking horses they were, and stand them beside the grave. Take a shotgun and shoot 'em right in the eye. They'd usually fall right in. That was something I never did like too much but it was part of life, part of my job."[6] His colleague, a talented farrier (one who shoes horses), said the blacksmith would follow this sad duty by drinking himself into a stupor. A courier usually found him, took him to the kitchen in the Big House, and sobered him up with pot after pot of coffee, all the while sympathizing with his plight.

Each animal had its own moniker, as did anything under the care and supervision of Breckinridge. She often chose names from Dickens characters: Puck or Chomondley. Confederate themes was another favorite. Traveler was named for General Lee's horse. Her motto was, "If you love it, you name it." That included everything from the trusty horses that led the nurses up and down the mountainsides to the well-fed chickens that roamed the paths at Wendover. (She even named a large beech tree at the Big House Brother Lawrence.) In the 1940s when jeeps eventually replaced the Tennessee Walkers, bumping and thumping along the rutted mountain roads, Breckinridge named each one of them too.

Among her favored horses was Babbette and a dappled gray mare named Tramp, which went blind and had to be put down; Teddy Bear, which liked to leap barred gates just for fun; and Nellie Gray, for which a river, however deep and wide, was "just a wet spot from here to the barn," Breckinridge said. Each nurse saddled and fed her own horse, especially in the first few years of the FNS when there were few extra hands to help with non-nursing chores. The horses were fed daily by seven A.M. in order to get what the neighbors called "a soon start." Breckinridge admitted that riding was difficult and often dangerous. "During the winter, when the cold spells come and streams freeze over," she said, "the horses, shod with ice nails, slip and stumble and often crash through with bleeding hocks. Sometimes a way must be made for them out to the rapids, where one commonly finds the fords, by a chivalrous mountaineer with his axe."[7] She went on to report that Edna Rockstroh, the first midwife to join the organization, swam the river atop her horse, Lady Jane, saddle bags and all, en route to visit a patient ready to deliver.

Travel and care of the horses took up more than 25 percent of a district nurses' workday. In time, FNS couriers would provide that service, unsaddling and rubbing the horses down upon the nurses' return to headquarters. Breckinridge would admonish the couriers to take special care of her horses "for they have to last as long I do." "No one loves his horse any better than we love ours," she continued. "We depend on the speed and surefootedness of these devoted creatures, not only for us but for those lives which the stork is bringing."[8] These intelligent animals even learned how to open stable doors and gate latches—sometimes letting other horses out as well. One, a beautiful black stallion named Tommy, not only opened doors but knew how to turn on a spigot. Unfortunately, since each nursing center had its own water pump and storage tank, an entire center could find itself without water. The only way to rein Tommy in when he misbehaved was to feed him sandwiches, preferably his favorite—peanut butter and jelly.

Though a few of the horses could be mean and hard to handle, most had a special affinity for children and would exhibit utmost patience around them. Breckinridge's gray mare, Babbette, had a stubborn mouth, a reputation for independence, and could be demanding of her rider. But whenever a child was mounted on her back, she seemed to know it was time to slow down to a gentle gait. Some of the horses learned that when a newborn cried immediately after delivery, it would soon be time to go home. One, a large horse named Commando that belonged to midwife Jane Rainey, would stick his head inside a cabin window and whinny joyfully whenever he heard the mewing sounds of a brand new infant.

But not all the staff shared Breckinridge's love and devotion to four-legged creatures. More than one midwife required riding lessons. The horse's name was Bobbin and the nurse, admittedly, was afraid of him. "With much huffing, panting, heaving, and tugging I finally got on him," she said. "But Bobbin didn't like my stretching act and tossed his head. My heart was suddenly in my throat. He danced around with all four feet like he wanted to take off. I begged to dismount. Very unceremoniously, I slid to the ground and heaved a sigh as I tried to hold my shaking knees still."[9] It took several weeks before she could mount the horse and ride without suffering a panic attack.

Tenacity was the Wendover mule, often getting loose and chasing newcomers up the hill behind the Big House and into the chicken lot, where she would roll them around in the dirt. New couriers were favorite targets, particularly if they ran off in the opposite direction. To up the ante, Tenacity would put her head down and charge, unwilling to stop the game until someone could get her in a bridle and lead her to the barn where she remained docile the remainder of the day. Agnes Lewis, Breckinridge's long-suffering records secretary, was terrified of the mule — and with good reason. "Tenacity really gave her a hard time," recalled secretary Lucille Knechtley. "She seemed to know Agnes was afraid of her and would go for her whenever she had the chance. I recall one Sunday afternoon that Tenacity escaped when she and the horses were brought from pasture. Just as we came out of the chapel after Evensong, down the hill came Tenacity — a courier with a bridle in hot pursuit. Tenacity sped past everyone until she spied Agnes. Down went her head and she lunged, causing poor Agnes to make a fast retreat through the chapel door."[10]

At the Big House, everyone had to go through Pig Alley as they made the sharp turn into Wendover. A brood sow named Edna, and her piglets, were the first ones to greet new arrivals beginning in 1926. Every subsequent sow through the years was also named Edna. Added to the litter was an abandoned piglet that one of the nurses found on a hillside and adopted. The nurse named it Bonzo and taught it parlor tricks, often to the amusement of Breckinridge and her guests. Lewis remembers assistant FNS director Dorothy Buck ("Bucket") often letting Bonzo stretch out in front of the fireplace in her cabin, near the Big House. Bucket spoiled the pig by feeding him dog food to the point that he would get angry whenever she withheld it. One night Lewis stopped by the cabin to see Bucket about an FNS matter. When the conversation was over Bonzo was blocking the door trying to get in — which only served to fuel Lewis' fear. "I'm not leaving with him out there," she told Bucket. "You'll have to get the night watchman to come over here and get him." And he did, often teasing Lewis about the incident. One visitor claimed that walking through Pig Alley he was assaulted by Bonzo and came to Breckinridge telling her he planned to sue for all the money he had in his pocket — a dollar and eighty-six cents. Lewis, realizing he was serious, wrote him a check for that exact amount.[11] With a sense of humor hinging on the wicked, Breckinridge liked to taunt her staff at dinnertime regarding the troublesome brood. "Is this the ham of Edna the fourth we're having tonight?" she would ask. Or, "Are those the chops from one of Edna's litters?"[12]

Peskier was the pet crow that was an incorrigible thief. Owned by the Wendover cook and her handyman husband, "Jim Crow" would fly past anyone outside reading their mail, snatch it, and take off. One courier had her check stolen by the bird while sitting on the Big House stoop. In addition, the Wendover kitchen staff was troubled by bats flying in from outside. Some of the cooks were so scared they took to wearing knotted scarves about their head so the bats would not get tangled in their hair. Others ran around the kitchen swatting frantically at the bats with a broom. Eventually, the creatures left the premises on their own.

The chickens lived in what Breckinridge referred to as residential flats on the hillside above the barn — little houses on stilts enclosed with wire mesh.

They got table scraps in exchange for producing eggs and meat. Cooks had to hide any food from Breckinridge they didn't want tossed to the chickens. Every day after lunch she would go to the kitchen to make their swill, throwing leftovers, peelings, sour milk, spoiled vegetables, and whatever else she could find into a large pan. Then she would plunge her bare hands in the mix while pronouncing it "the best hand lotion around." When a near-fatal disease struck the chickens while Breckinridge was on a fundraising tour, the FNS staff went into a meltdown. Every local remedy was tried including sticking a feather dipped in kerosene down the neck of each hen. With the help of the Department of Agriculture at the University of Kentucky, a cure was finally found that halted the sickness—and the terrible dread of telling Breckinridge her beloved chickens were gone.[13]

In her room at the Big House, she kept anatomical sketches of horses and a turn-of-the-century dog-eared text on veterinarian techniques. And she had her favorite pets among her virtual animal farm. One was a special hen she called the Universal Mother. Believing this bird had a gift for motherhood, she forbade anyone to kill it. Through the years, she adopted Biddy the red hen, Tom the yellow barn cat, and numerous geese, nicknaming one pair Dilly and Dally. She especially admired ganders, referring to them as "good husbands" since they tended to be faithful. "Too bad *you* aren't a gander," she told one errant spouse.[14]

Dogs and cats were allowed to roam the property at will, inside and out. Sometimes a secretary would have to climb inside the stone fireplace in the living room to retrieve lost kittens, emerging with soot from head to toe. Queen of the felines was Breckinridge's cat, Pitty Pat, which had run of the place, and shared a room with her mistress. Pitty Pat liked to aggravate nurses as they documented their cases and secretaries as they took dictation, curling up on their notebooks and pencils. The cat's favorite spot was on the fur rug before the fireplace in Breckinridge's room. If she was splayed out for a nap—as she often was—secretaries were warned, "Whatever you do, *don't* step on Pitty Pat!" When a horrible odor emanated from Breckinridge's room, the housekeeper turned Breckinridge's bed and pillows inside out to find that Pitty Pat had deposited a dead mouse between the mattress and the headboard. Breckinridge just laughed when she heard what it was. "At Wendover, animals always came first," explained Lucille Knechtly, who oddly enough was nicknamed "Thumper."[15]

If someone needed a temporary home for their pet, Breckinridge was quick to offer the Big House. Once, when Lewis learned that visiting cats were taking over the guest room she had so painstakingly decorated, she was reduced to standing in the hallway and wringing her hands. "What about those lovely drapes and the bedspreads I worked so hard to get?" she wailed to Breckinridge. "And what about that beautiful carpet!" "Never mind, Aggie dear," Breckinridge consoled with a smile. "The cats will love them."[16] The nurses' dogs often accompanied them on horseback rounds to visit patients. Brutie, a black cocker spaniel, was named for the Brutus Nursing Center and ran freely through the clinic and waiting room, playing with the children and bounding over the feet of patients. Betty Lester adopted a nondescript mutt someone had abandoned near Wendover, calling him Mr. Funny. He loved to follow all the horses but couldn't be counted on to return on his own.

When Lewis asked one of the secretaries if the dog could go with her on an outing to meet a group of couriers, the secretary was reluctant but said yes, as she wasn't going far. But the trip turned out more troublesome than she expected. "I came upon a shooting match in the woods," she said. "I knew Mr. Funny was gun shy and sure enough, as soon as a gun went off he disappeared into the hills. I called and called but couldn't find him. I didn't dare go back to Betty without him. When I met up with the couriers between Hyden and Hazard, they offered to help me look. We finally found him, scared and shaking, but unhurt. I dragged him out, mounted the saddled horse, and carried him on the pommel of the saddle."[17] All went well until they backtracked to the site of the shooting, where the dog promptly dived off the horse and went scampering into the woods. Another search ensued but no luck. When they finally arrived back at Wendover, Mr. Funny was sitting on the porch alongside Lester. "Where have you been so long?" she demanded. "Hunting *your* dog!" the secretary replied.[18] Every day at four P.M. at Wendover, staff, guests, and an assortment of collies, retrievers, cockers, and mutts would gather for tea in the living room. There, an occasional dog fight would break out, often when the place was teeming with important guests—many of whom would later write Breckinridge to thank her for their "unusual visit."

Cows had their place at Wendover too, and when they got into trouble, received the same care and attention the midwives gave to anyone or anything in need. Harriett, a Jersey heifer of which the nurses were particularly fond, suffered from an abscess following a bout of milk fever. On the Saturday that the abscess burst, two FNS midwives went to see about her and found the poor animal knee deep in a messy mix of gore. Another RN, Anna May January, was having breakfast at the Big House that morning. She came running with a huge roll of adhesive and together, the nurses began to wrap Harriet's middle, pulling it taut to control the hemorrhage. The cow's respirations were now labored as she mooed and swayed, unsteady on her feet. When the immediate emergency passed, the women asked Breckinridge if she had any textbooks on cows. She handed them one that explained normal temperature, pulse, and respirations of bovines. According to the book, Harriet's pulse and respirations were dangerously rapid. "We decided we would have to get help from Lexington," a nurse recalled. "But another problem presented itself. The telephone was down from a spring storm. Someone volunteered to ride into Hyden and find an exchange so we could put in a call to the University of Kentucky. They phoned back with orders for Harriet's care."

In the meantime, Harriet's stall was cleaned and scrubbed and a new bed of hay placed inside the barn. She was given all the water she could drink, along with a mash made from bran. Breckinridge was the only nurse among them who knew how to mix the concoction. But by working together, the team ensured that Harriet made a full recovery. At the end of six weeks, she was providing almost five gallons of milk a day and returned to pasture with the other Wendover cows. "And she was the most wonderful patient," raved one of the nurses who assisted in her care. "In fact, we think she loved all the attention."[19]

11

Ambitious Plans

By the mid 1930s, ten years after Breckinridge officially began the Frontier Nursing Service, the organization was showing impressive results. In a written summary of one thousand midwifery deliveries (data was reported by Breckinridge every one thousand births and compiled by the Metropolitan Life Insurance Company, which tabulated the findings), there was not a single maternal death. By contrast, within the U.S. the maternal death rate was five point two per one thousand live births (1930 figures) compared to Kentucky's statewide rate of five per one thousand live births.[1] Breckinridge, who kept meticulous records, was quick to point out in her reports this would be exceptional under the most favorable circumstances, much less in the conditions under which her nurses worked and the mothers delivered. Of course, many of the women were young and relatively healthy (almost half were under age twenty-five) but most had carried other children, putting them at greater risk. Of the thousand patients counted in this second round of record-keeping, more than one hundred seventy-five had delivered eight or more children.

The United States Children's Bureau recommended a first visit to a clinic or physician be conducted at or before the fifth month gestation. Yet only 21 percent of the eastern Kentucky women registered with the FNS *before* their sixth month. Length of labor reported by the mothers varied wildly since few homes had clocks and still fewer people owned a watch. Labor was reported as lasting from less than an hour to almost three days in length. Only sixty-six of the one thousand women delivered at Hyden Hospital. The rest delivered at their homes with a doctor attending in about 50 percent of the cases. For those remaining, the nurse-midwife handled the delivery and postpartum care.

The most common complication was bleeding, followed by rupture of the perineum. About 14 percent were extended breech — or malpresentation as it was called — which resulted in four stillbirths. There were two cases of eclampsia (occurrence of seizures in a pregnant woman), one of edema (swelling), one of urine retention, seven of persistent vomiting, and eight of high blood pressure. Infant deaths were higher than maternal deaths within the FNS, but that

97

was also true nationwide. The fetus was carried full term by all but forty-one of the one thousand women reported by the FNS in 1935. Of the forty-one premature deliveries, only nine stillbirths resulted. Among the remaining full term deliveries, there were an additional fourteen stillbirths for a total of twenty-three. This compared with thirty-one stillbirths for each one thousand deliveries in the rural white U.S. population.[2]

All in all, the Frontier Nursing Service was gaining credibility and a reputation for well-organized, high quality care. A Medical Advisory Committee was now operating in Lexington, a hundred sixty-five miles from Hyden, which provided oversight for the FNS organization. The committee, composed of physicians and specialists, authorized the medical routines for the nurses, similar to standing orders for public health nurses. Frontier Nurses followed this routine in their field work and the Medical Advisory Committee assumed the responsibility for their doing so.

The midwifery supervisor was housed at Wendover, but more often than not she was in the saddle, along with the outpost nurses. She was on call for all abnormal cases, which she attended alone or with the FNS medical director. Her duties also involved visiting all primiparas (first-time mothers-to-be), referring them for medical exam, and maintaining a card file on all active midwife cases, about a hundred on average. She would post them as they registered and close them out a month after delivery. Such a file ensured knowing what cases the FNS carried, how many were due, and what difficulties might occur. Once the case was closed it was sent to the Central Office at Wendover where it was carefully checked for accuracy.

There was also an FNS hospital superintendent at Hyden who supervised five fulltime nurses, ordered and distributed medical supplies, and managed eighteen patient beds. Yet seldom were there only eighteen beds occupied at any given time. Since no other hospital existed in the territory, and since it was unheard of to refuse medical attention to a patient, the wards could easily fill to overflowing. A few nurses were known to give up their own quarters in order to house patients needing care. In addition, public health nurses worked closely with the FNS and when funds were available, a public health supervisor was hired. During the Depression, however, when money was tight, many of the public health duties were taken over by the assistant FNS director.

Ernest Poole, a New York writer and friend of Breckinridge, came to visit in 1932, gathering material for his forthcoming book, *Nurses on Horseback*, which would provide the first in-depth look — and highly favorable view — of the Frontier Nursing Service. He wrote descriptively of his nights spent at Wendover, and occasionally at a local cabin.

> I stayed with a young school teacher and her family. She spent three years at a settlement school on the edge of the hills, learning cooking, sewing, and how to keep a house. She came back with ideas of what could be done to mountain cabins. The night I stayed, she and her husband slept with their two children and

gave me their room. It was square, with brown log walls and a sandstone
fireplace in which chunky logs burned softly through the night. There was a
clean plank floor, a couple of chairs, a bureau, a washstand, and a double bed. It
was one of the most comfortable beds a tired rider ever slept in.[3]

What he liked most, he added, was listening to the padded thud of horses'
hoofs on the dirt road alongside the cabin. He learned the comfort of the bed
came from a straw mattress atop the springs, several handmade quilts, and
another three-inch thick mattress made from feathers. And he marveled at how
clean and fresh the woman kept her home, herself, and her children. "When
people in dirty, noisy cities ask what's the use in trying to help 'those lousy
mountaineers,' I remember that cabin, those soft, low voices, that young
mother's friendly smile, and the light in her bright, resolute eyes," Poole wrote.[4]
By the end of May 1934, the FNS had paid more than 160,000 home visits,
received another 115,000 patients at clinics, and delivered over two thousand
pregnant patients with just forty-eight stillbirths. A total of 68,800 vaccinations
had been provided against typhoid, diphtheria, pneumonia, and smallpox. At
the close of the fiscal year, the FNS was carrying slightly more than eleven hundred families. "In regard to our plans for the future," wrote Mary Willeford,
assistant FNS director and a Ph.D., "we have two specific aims. The first is to
complete our planned demonstration area of a thousand square miles, of which
we now cover over seven hundred. Our second aim is to use our territory as a
training field for the preparation of nurses as midwives for other isolated sections of the country. There are other sections in America, not only in the Appalachian Highland region, but elsewhere in our country where graduate nurses
trained as midwives are needed in maternal and infant care."[5]

Mary Breckinridge had already sown those seeds in talks with Ernest Poole
two years earlier. "These people in the mountains are worth all that we can
give," she told the writer. "And in spite of all we've done so far, I feel we've just
begun. We are frequently asked to supply nurse-midwives to other communities. So this first experiment leads to the extension of such work. In the Ozarks,
the Allegany's, and the Rockies, on islands, and lonely strips of coastland, and
on the plains, nearly fifteen million of our fellowmen and women are living
pioneer lives. And these are the people who need our aid."[6] She was on a roll,
knowing full well she would be quoted in Poole's account. "We have heard too
much from modern writers of this nation that it has left its youth behind and
is now on the road to decay. The vigor of a nation is born again in its children,
and most of all in the country districts. Fully eighty percent, I am told, of the
men who direct our great corporations come from rural regions" (a figure dis-
puted by some). "Remember," she concluded, "that maternity is a woman's
battlefield. It is more dangerous even than war, but for her there will be no trum-
pets or drums. Off on the lonely farmstead where the true heart of America
beats, the young mother faces her agony that the hope of our nation may come
into life."[7] In other words, the Frontier Nursing Service, a private collabora-

tion financed almost entirely by voluntary contributions and subscriptions, spearheaded by one middle-aged woman, was poised to spread its wings and became a national and perhaps even an international nonprofit organization that would put nurse-midwives in every rural setting where medical services and facilities were lacking.

In Arkansas, one nurse was reportedly available for every 100,000 of the population. The newspapers had recently printed a tragic story in Idaho involving a critically ill patient with the nearest doctor a hundred miles away — by dog team. Private philanthropy must blaze the trails in health as in education, was the Breckinridge credo. If a man's house burns, his neighbors build him another; if parents die, neighbors bring up the children as their own. "Good American stock," as she was fond of saying, translated to self-sustaining people, importing nothing, and maintaining themselves in the hardy livelihood to which they are bred. Was there no better way to spend money than in protecting motherhood and the infants of such a race, Breckinridge asked? She and her brigade of nurses—"new pioneers on old frontiers" as she described them — could surely do it. She had a point, as usual. But it was still an outlandishly ambitious plan, even for the indomitable, irrepressible Mary Breckinridge. And it would prove more difficult than even she could fathom.

12

Suspended Dreams

No one will ever know if Breckinridge would have expanded her Frontier Nursing Service across national and international boundaries. Financial troubles during the Depression certainly hampered her efforts. A survey was conducted into northern Arkansas and southern Missouri by the St. Louis Committee of the FNS, but officers and trustees decided against expanding the service when funding failed to materialize. That alone would probably not have stopped Breckinridge. What did stop her was that only a short time after writer Ernest Poole left her side, she took the fateful tumble off her horse and broke her back. Once she got past the initial crushing pain, her routine shifted only slightly. She still rose early each day. Usually up by four-thirty A.M., she would pad down to the kitchen in her dressing gown and catch up on news with the night watchman. There was a battery-operated radio in the house but Breckinridge grew so impatient with its constant static, she refused to go near it. (Eventually, she would have one in her room but required help in learning how to turn it on.)

In the kitchen, there was always a small pitcher of hot milk and a pot of coffee waiting. She would take a tray back to her room where she would line up folders on the bed that contained work assignments for the day, organizing them according to who was scheduled to do what. Around eight, her assistant Agnes Lewis would come in, along with Betty Lester and one or two other nurses. There, they discussed current reports and upcoming events. One of those events was a scheduled hearing in Hazard, Kentucky, over a civil suit filed against the FNS for nonpayment of a horse. The animal's owner was an odd character, everyone agreed, and when he decided to "law" the FNS, the organization's attorney could not keep it out of court. The dispute centered around the horse coming to Wendover on a trial basis, where it was shod, kept two weeks, and found unsuitable. Breckinridge had the animal returned, explaining she could not pay the original amount agreed upon. The owner then sued, contending in addition to nonpayment the horse was returned with no shoes. "It was the only time I ever knew Mrs. Breckinridge to be nervous about anything," said Lewis. "She had never been in court and neither had any of her family."[1]

On the day of the hearing Breckinridge appeared in court with her back brace in place. Not only was it more comfortable standing, she explained, but she was accustomed to speaking upright in public. Lewis was there, watching her boss and mentor display her typical brand of chutzpah. "She turned to the judge with those big blue eyes of her and asked if he minded that she stand, as she had a broken back. Now, that was true. A straight chair was very hard for her, but that wasn't the only reason. She stood there in her back brace, stated her case, and we saw the twinkle in the judge's eye. And she won her case without one little difficulty in the whole wide world."[2]

As the FNS group left the courthouse, a Hazard attorney was heard to remark, "She's the best damn lawyer we have in Kentucky."[3] A dramatic speaker under the best of conditions, Breckinridge utilized anything she could to win her audience. "If it was wintertime, she would play up the weather," said Lewis, "the floods, the landslides, the breakdown in pumps; anything that would wring your heart. If it were summer, it was the lack of water while running the hospital, all that sort of thing. She could make it very graphic."[4] In addition, she was a prodigious writer, using her time in bed to compose letters, articles, and reports for the *Quarterly Bulletin*, the FNS voice in print that remains the official FNS publication today. Most of the articles she wrote and that magazines published were designed to raise awareness— and funds—for the FNS.

One of the more creative fundraising events was a cruise benefit held by the FNS aboard the *Britannic* on February 26, 1932. The ship set sail from New York en route to the West Indies with several of Breckinridge's cousins aboard and the U.S. Marines circling seaplanes overhead in a tribute to the FNS-supportive passengers. While docked in Havana, the ship's guests and crew were treated like royalty, with a band, refreshments, and dancing on the tennis courts as the sun set over the Panama Canal. The FNS cleared less than $6000 from the trip even with reduced ship rates, but considering the Depression was still underway, it was not a bad take. It allowed the organization to keep its New York, Boston, and Chicago executive committees active and led to the decision to hold another cruise the following year.

In the spring of 1933, an entire ship was chartered, the S.S. *Belgenland*, for up to a thousand paying passengers on a tour through the Caribbean. Marketed to the wealthy parents of debutantes needing a break from their social whirl, it cost the FNS $60,000 for the fifteen-day tour —funds they expected to earn back plus a $20,000 profit. Emboldened by the prospect of success, Breckinridge invited Will Rogers, a well-known American cowboy-humorist, philosopher, and motion picture star to accompany her guests on the trip. Getting Rogers on board would be a major public relations coup for the FNS. He graciously declined but agreed to write a public article about the cruise and sent Breckinridge a memorable personal letter, one she kept for posterity:

Well, if it ain't Mary Breckinridge. I have read more about you than I have Mahatma Gandhi. I can't be a midwife but I sure could hold the nurse's horse. Now about this pilgrimage you are making to the West Indies on behalf of better babies in Kentucky — that's a round about way to deliver babies and I can't go cause you can't do nothing when you are in the movies but stay home and make faces at the world. But when I get some time I want to make it to that virgin country of yours. So give me a good mule, and a good nurse, and I am ready to go into the mountains.[5]

With so many young people scheduled aboard the cruise, activities were geared to their tastes, from offering the best moving pictures of the day, to inclusion of handsome young men from Yale, Harvard, and Princeton to serve as dance partners for the girls. About two weeks prior to the event, the American banking system held a bank moratorium capping the nine thousand bank failures that had occurred between 1930 and 1933. Donors who had booked a cruise panicked and began to cancel. In short order, cancellations exceeded the bookings. Always good in a crisis, Breckinridge approached the shipping line about how to proceed. Through her negotiation efforts, the cruise remained on schedule, albeit with fewer passengers aboard, and the FNS managed to break even. After that, shipping companies besieged them each year to charter an FNS ship. "But by then we were dead broke," Breckinridge said. "So that ended our attempt to float our budget by means of floating a ship."[6]

She returned to the printed word to get her messages across, venturing into slightly more controversial territory. For example, in a 1930s article, titled "Is Birth Control the Answer?," Breckinridge let readers know for the first time where she stood on the question of contraceptives. She began by saying she rarely addressed an audience from which at least one person did not ask: "What about birth control for the mountain people?" She referred to their enquiry as "the get-rich-quick proposition" and took great pains to explain to readers the economic realities of eastern Kentucky and the compelling need for the Frontier Nursing Service. Her digression ended by agreeing the birth rate in her region was too high (46.0 per 1,000) compared to a nationwide average of 21.9 during an approximate fourteen-year period.[7]

Women were married by their teens, she said, some as young as fourteen, but that was true in most rural areas, not just eastern Kentucky, and were often left alone to tend home and childrearing while the fathers made a living. But would birth control solve the problem? No, she contended. Yet she also stated she was against existing legislation that restricted birth control information. "I am against all legislation which aims at invading the private habits of individuals," she explained. "[But] when birth control information is allowed, under proper medical direction, the deeper economic laws under which old Nature operates will continue to determine the principles of population."[8]

She re-phrased the question to ask if birth control would provide a solution for the acute conditions as they currently stood in eastern Kentucky. Then she spelled out five reasons why the answer was still no. First, there was cost. "A program introducing these methods in a remote rural area would be as costly a method of tackling the problem as could be devised," she said. Second, there was religious prejudice against birth control methods. "The fundamentalist habit of mind which accepts conditions and attributes them to a Divine agency, is characteristic of certain religious groups in the mountains, notably the Holy Rollers. Such groups do not, of course, represent the leading citizens. But they contribute powerfully to mold local public opinion." Third, she went on, was the inherent value placed on large families in the Appalachian region in terms of working the land. And she provided an example. "When the foddering season comes in, it's all hands on the job to get the fodder up before the rain sets in. The young child must leave school to help or go without milk through winter because the cow didn't have fodder enough." Furthermore, she added, in isolated regions family life was unusually strong and parents were typically devoted to their children, even when there were ten or twelve under one roof. "I myself wanted eight," she revealed.[9]

Her fourth reason involved the difficulties of using birth control in one and two-room cabins where large families lived together in close proximity. And fifth, she contended that the Southern mountains were a feeder for cities—"a nursery for the finest flower of the old American stock." This was a sticking point for her and one she would emphasize time and again—that rural Kentucky served as a starting point for some of the country's best people. "We cannot cherish too eagerly this segment of the early stock which built up our nation," she said. By focusing on this one positive, she believed it helped counter many of the stereotypes so common to the Appalachian region. Plus, despite its overtures of nativism, it served her fund-raising purposes. But the abiding reason she opposed birth control in eastern Kentucky, she concluded, was that it simply would not work for the majority. Even the most far-reaching and costly birth control campaign would be negligible, she maintained.[10] And so, within the Frontier Nursing Service framework, a large-scale birth control campaign was never conducted. That was true of all nurse-midwifery schools or services in the early to mid–twentieth century. By the 1950s, however, the FNS would take a giant leap forward by participating in one of the first clinical studies of birth control pills when a pharmaceutical corporation and the Worchester Foundation for Experimental Biology chose the FNS as a trial site for its oral contraceptive, Enovid.[11]

When Breckinridge wasn't defending her views or producing fund-raising articles, she was traveling to New York, Cincinnati, Cleveland, Ohio, and Washington, D.C., in an effort to keeps donations rolling in. Among the guests during a speech she gave at a wealthy benefactor's home in Cleveland in 1935 was Dr. Roger Egeberg, who had been practicing in Cleveland since 1930. He later volunteered with the FNS Committee as assistant secretary, then during World War II went on to serve as General MacArthur's private physician and aide-de-camp. That day in his neighbor's comfortably furnished living room, he listened closely as Breckinridge launched into her description of the eastern Kentucky region. He had been told she had something of a mannish quality about her, with her short, cropped hair, lack of makeup, and moon-shaped face. But instead, to him she seemed "a woman with a great deal of charm and force, and if the phrase isn't too hackneyed, someone with a vision."

"First, she told us about the difficulty of transportation, then the isolation of the families, and the general poverty that existed. She made a point that many of the people were originally from the British Isles, settled in the region, and never left. She explained there was sickness, both from coal mining and a high mortality rate in childbirth, with neonatal mortality afterward. She showed pictures of people on mules, and how babies were delivered way up in the 'hollers'; and how volunteers were trained." Egeberg said that following Breckinridge's speech, he sat there thinking, "By god, if I were a little bit younger, I'd like to go there myself and work!"[12] It was exactly the type of electrifying response Breckinridge was after — that and the prompt opening of wallets. Egeberg said he was worried the group might not be able to do enough to assist the financially strapped but deserving FNS. "You have to remember it was the bottom of the Depression and there were many people in Cleveland who had been millionaires the previous year, but were certainly not millionaires now. So it was a hard time to get money anywhere. They did, however, respond to her well."[13] Egeberg was taken with the concept of the FNS, and Breckinridge herself, but he wasn't sure the idea of midwives in general was an easy sell, even forty-four years later in a 1979 taped interview for a FNS oral history project.

> I think the idea of midwives in America is one that takes a continuing amount of education. They [the FNS] have set an excellent example of what can be done. But you know, the head of Ob/Gyn at Columbia, when asked if he would like a midwife in his office, said, "Hell, no." So, I think midwifery in this country has reflected the insecurity of doctors, who always seem to feel they are not going to have enough patients. It has to be a matter of education, of undoing habits, and doing things according to our culture. I think they are making progress but I don't know that it's as fast as it deserves to go.[14]

While Breckinridge conducted her speechmaking rounds and wrote letters to the staff at Wendover reporting her progress—from the Cosmopolitan Club in New York she relayed that a New York doctor was searching for a dummy pelvis to donate to the FNS—the nurses she left behind continued their daily rounds. She also shared with her staff and her many constituents that she was considering an operation on her back. The surgery would take place at the Massachusetts General Hospital, performed by a team of specialists including an orthopedist and a neurologist. In April 1938, she wrote an open letter (one of many through the years) explaining her decision: "There is no need to go into technical details. Most of you know that I have been suffering increasing pain and disability in the site of the old fracture during the past two years. I hoped to defer this for several years, for when is it ever convenient for a busy person to spend three months in a plaster cast?"

She referred to her almost chronic pain as "a useful teacher," but added it was hampering her efforts to get back to the work of the Frontier Nursing Service.

> As we say in the mountains, I shall be glad to get shut of it. There is one more thing to be said. Some of you will want to send me books and flowers. Please don't. The hospital has a marvelous library, so I shall have no need for books.
>
> As for flowers, my room is tiny and has only a bedside stand, so there isn't room for more than about three violets. These will be brought to me, I know, by New England friends with gardens. What I beg of you to do is relieve the only strain on my mind — the financial strain for the work I love so much, and send a wee extra check to our treasurer in Lexington. Send it with a card that says "Here is my book for Mary Breckinridge," or "These are my flowers."
>
> But if you are vacationing in New England after the first of July and pass through Boston, stop off and see me. That will bring me joy, and you will always find me "at home!"[15]

That fall, while Breckinridge recovered from her surgery, her staff stepped in help with outreach efforts and public relations, producing articles for nursing journals and women's magazines to draw attention to the FNS. Vanda Summers, R.N., wrote one such piece on the content of the midwifery saddlebags for the *American Journal of Nursing*.

"They each weigh about forty-two pounds when packed, with detachable linings of strong white material. All supplies are kept in little white cotton bags. In these bags, we have everything needed for a home delivery." She went on to explain that the work area in the log cabins was normally a table or wooden box "made clean with the aid of newspapers and white paper napkins on which is placed the 'set-up.' We carry five kidney basins, which fit one into the other and take up very little space. A large rubber sheet is carried for the bed. Rubber apron, cotton apron, cap and gown, sterile rubber gloves, Lysol, alcohol, olive oil, hypodermic syringe and catheter, clamps and scissors, are some of the main things we use."[16]

The nurses distinguished a midwifery bag from a general nursing bag through a color coded system. The general saddlebags, used in public health nursing, were lined with layers of multi-color hues; green for post-partum supplies, blue for urinalysis, yellow for drugs, and the sterile dressing bag a red-and-white stripe. Through these public relations efforts, others were finally beginning to realize the organization's widespread impact, not just on a national scale, but worldwide. One nurse received a letter addressed to her in care of the FNS from Kenya, Africa. Across the envelope, an astute African postal official had written the words: *Try Kentucky, U.S.A.* For the majority of nurses, however, insulated deep inside the Appalachian Mountains anyplace outside Kentucky was as distant as another planet.

No one felt this displacement more than the on-duty Frontier nurse in her day-to-day encounters with the elements and the local FNS clients, captured in these compiled FNS *Quarterly Bulletin* nurse-midwife accounts:

> On a raw, foggy morning in March, late 1930s the Frontier nurse ate her breakfast quickly and bundled up in a sweater, coat, fur-lined boots and gloves. A full day of rounds was ahead.
>
> She trundled off to the barn toting a bottle-laden saddle bag weighing nearly thirty pounds. With freezing hands, minus the gloves, she struggled with the rigid leather and iron buckles necessary to prepare her horse for the daily rounds. On days like this, riding was no longer a pleasure but a duty, especially with ice-coated roads that alternated between slick and slicker.

The first call was a one-room cabin perched on a clay-red cliff. Its back squatted low against a row of pines and inside, shadows danced across the windowless walls. The nurse made her way carefully over large, loose rocks to reach the front door.

> "How's Jasper today?" she called out. Two children and a mother huddled inside.
>
> "Poorly. He's punishin' terrible. But the baby — hit's pure wonderful how well hit's doin. But come in. Come on in and warm yourself."

The child was a rambunctious four-year-old already displaying a thirst for knowledge. She liked being read to by anyone who would sit by the fire with her. Further up the creek was another cabin, the next stop for the Frontier nurse. Here, a proud grandmother was cooing over her daughter's firstborn, swaddled in a percale gown and coarse gray blanket. The grandmother was grateful for the help her daughter, June, received from these "brought-up" women — the trained nurse-midwives.

> "June says this is the easiest she ever heard tell of a first one comin," she told the nurse. "You know how to make a body feel more comfortable. Elmer, bring the nurse a chair and show her that risin' on your leg."
>
> "Bring him into the clinic Wednesday morning if it isn't better," the nurse instructed after examining the infected leg. "It's also Trader Day so bring some eggs or milk and get yourself a nice, warm dress in exchange. There are some lovely things that people sent us after the last tide."

She left with an admonition about washing all diapers and cleaning hands. "And how are them twins you cotched up the branch last month?" the grandmother asked. The nurse smiled. "Getting fat as little pigs."

Wending her way back down the trail, she headed to the nearest nursing center for lunch. Travel time and just two home visits took an entire morning. The afternoon would be spent at the clinic, with patients gathered round the fire in the waiting room. They would talk of weather, road conditions, and changes in the river level as in — "my old man says it rose two feet since ten o'clock." A heavy pregnant woman received an exam; a tiny baby weighed and checked for developmental milestones; an older child pale from fever, treated for infected ears.[17] By 1939, with twenty-eight nurses on staff, deliveries averaged one every twenty-four hours. When deliveries were normal, the nurse-midwife carried on alone. When abnormalities were anticipated, the expectant mother was moved to the Hyden Hospital. That is, if time allowed. If things went wrong at the eleventh hour, the medical director was contacted and traveled on horseback to the woman's home. Though state roads were beginning to appear throughout the eastern Kentucky region, fully seventy-five percent of the FNS work was still carried forward on horseback.[18]

Alone on a midwife case, district nurse supervisor May Green recognized a "shoulder presentation" of the fetus. The husband was sent by horse to deliver a note to the nearest nursing center: Call the doctor and ask him to come right away. Green made her patient as comfortable as possible, encouraged her to relax, and gave her a sedative. Then she sat by the bed and waited for there was little else to do. It would take two hours for the husband to return. When he did, he reported that the doctor and another nurse, Dorothy Buck, were on their way. The fire was tended and a fresh pot of water put on to boil. Soon the mother's labor pains hardened and were coming at a faster rate. Minutes began to seem like hours. Green, attempting to hide her rising anxiety, wondered if she would have to take action before the doctor arrived. How long was it safe to wait?

Finally, she heard the welcome sound of hoofbeats nearing the cabin. "I'm so glad you're here," she told the arriving doctor and the nurse. Instruments were dropped in boiling water; the bedridden patient was prepped; the doctor scrubbed, capped, and gowned. A wobbly table was moved near the bed and sterile instruments placed upon it for easy relay. Green stood near her patient's head with a mask and a can of ether. Two neighbor women had arrived and offered to help. They were put to work supporting the patient's legs. Buck held a flashlight for the doctor. To ease the patient into a deep sleep, the fire was extinguished and the chimney lamps snuffed out. Buck's flashlight snapped on. With mask in place and the ether administered, the woman was soon mercifully unconscious. Her husband, who had left the room and was sitting on the porch, could only marvel at the wonders going on inside his home. The baby came, with some difficulty at first, but then presented full form, lusty and full of life. A few days later, after careful follow-up and nursing care, the new mother was sitting up in bed with her infant in her arms. She was talking to the neighbors who had stopped by to visit and admire the baby. "I had *two* doctor women and a doctor man," she boasted. "And they helped me, 'cause I had been like to die."[19]

The Frontier Nursing Service was now publishing its own booklets as yet another fundraising method. In one, titled *You're Wanted on Cutshin,* the story of a nurse named Marjorie illustrated the role that rural nurses played, not just in deliveries, but in public health services. The idea behind it was to establish a school to train graduate nurses in remotely rural techniques and midwifery in order to meet the growing demands of organizations wanting to model programs after the FNS. Graduate physicians were also included in the plan, who in turn, could train nurses for various positions in remote rural parts of the country. In the booklet, the young nurse, Marjorie, and the father were on their way to the delivery. The scene opened like a bad novel:

> It was a pitch black night, with an east wind blowing and a flurry of snow in the air. We walked fast and the father chatted gaily, carrying the bags easily. They hoped it would be a girl. From the bridge on the Middle Fork River we turned left and soon reached a few logs bridging a creek that sounded like a giant Niagara. In a few minutes we were at a backyard where I was told there lived an awfully mean dog. It came flying towards us, growing ferociously. I hastily muttered something—what I hoped would be the dog's password—and it allowed us to continue on our way along the river bank.

Bogged down in mud, Marjorie and her companion were soon using hands and feet to keep from rolling down the rain-slicked hillside. It was a sixty-foot drop to the river with a path not more than a few inches wide.

> When we had nearly reached the mouth of Owl's Nest Creek, I heard a thud and suddenly missing my guide I wildly shone my flashlight around. To my horror, I found my beloved saddlebags vanishing over the cliff edge, and a pair of hands fumbling in the mud. It took me a few seconds to decide which to save—the man or the bags. During those few seconds, he scrambled up unaided, much to my relief.

A mule was waiting for the pair at Owl's Nest, its owner handing the reins to Marjorie with an apology. "We didn't rightly know if you would ride a scary mule," he said. "The saddle is fixed with string and hardly good for a woman." As it turned out, the mule was just what they needed to maneuver around fallen tree trunks and slick boulders.

> When at last we caught sight of a light flickering in the far distance, said Marjorie, I thought my eyes were deceiving me. But as we slid and slithered nearer, we plainly heard a lusty yell from the new arrival. I staggered into the cabin; a dim light, a fire burning low, a white-faced anxious woman on a tumbled bed, and somewhere amongst the tangled bedclothes—an eight pound baby girl.

Marjorie examined the mother and the baby, leaving them "clean and happy in the peaceful little cabin." "With a sinking heart, I faced the return journey."[20]

Mary Breckinridge had wanted a graduate school as early as 1935. "It was my fault that it had been so long deferred," she said in a rare admission. "Despite my liking for small beginnings, I wanted the school to start on an established basis, in Lexington, affiliated with the University of Kentucky. Our plan called for the graduate nurse students to get most of their field work with the FNS in the mountains. A University school in Lexington did not come about because

I failed after several attempts to get it financed."[21] By the fall of 1939, there was no other option but to start the graduate program at Hyden Hospital, staffed by locals, where the program remains to this day.

Establishing the graduate school was an absolute necessity. In fact, it was a survival strategy on the part of Mary Breckinridge, who had started the FNS enlisting a staff composed almost entirely of British public health nurses. Without the graduate school in place, the FNS might very well have folded at this point. The program began in November 1939 as a six-month course designed on a scale similar to the Central Midwives Boards of Great Britain which included prenatal, delivery, and after delivery care. The pupil, upon successful graduation, was expected to recognize and give first aid treatment in abnormal cases. She was also given a certificate of registration which entitled her to practice midwifery. Federal scholarships were available for graduate nurse students from southern and western states who agreed to return to their "frontier regions." Through an affiliation with Johns Hopkins Hospital, the graduate school accepted four senior cadets each spring to teach them remote rural nursing. Eventually, the school's quarters were opened to doctors, nurses, and social workers from all over the world who wanted to come, observe, and study, "as long as they are genuinely interested in rural work," said Breckinridge.[22]

For the English-born women who had first come to America to work as FNS nurse-midwives and were part of the organization's startup and growth, a more pressing crisis was pending, one that did not involve new recruits, rural patients, or public health needs. It involved their homeland. Between 1939 and 1940, eleven of the twenty-eight British nurses on staff announced they were returning to the Mother Country. "They are giving the same gallant service to the homeland that they have given to us," said Breckinridge, "and under far greater danger."[23] It was a call to action in a world that would never be quite the same.

13

War Comes to the Mountains

World War II impacted the Frontier Nursing Service and eastern Kentucky as much as other every other part of America. Triggered by Hitler's armies marching into Poland on September 1, 1939, it arrived at the FNS in the form of unease among the British nurses who knew England had pledged its support if Poland were attacked; in the form of young men, many of them crack shots, suddenly aware they might be called away to battle; of ration talk that was all too reminiscent of the recent Depression; and in the form of a nerve-wracking fear that the Frontier Nursing Service, in view of its steady hunger for an influx of cash, might not survive a world distracted by something much bigger than itself.

Some said the war, which lasted from 1939 to 1945, was unavoidable, deriving from a combustible mix of policies that brought Communism, Fascism, Nazism, and western democracies into direct conflict. It split a majority of the world's nations into two opposing camps the Allies and the Axis, and resulted in the deaths of more than sixty million people before ending in an Allied victory. Under Adolf Hitler, Germany, and Italy, to a lesser extent, began flexing their collective muscles as early as 1933, pursuing increasingly aggressive foreign policies and demands. England and France tried to defuse the growing hostilities with diplomacy, while the U.S. basically took a hands-off approach until attacked by Japan in 1941. Once Germany captured Denmark and Norway, then France and the Low Countries, Great Britain was its next target.

That meant the women of the FNS, most of whom were British, were deeply affected. For nurse-midwives like Betty Lester, going home to England in no way minimized their loyalty and devotion to the Frontier Nursing Service. But they were torn between their love for the FNS and their desire to get back to England to serve during the war. "A few of us Britishers stayed around long enough to help train nurses for the Graduate School," Lester said. "We started with two, and gradually more and more American nurses came down to be midwives."[1]

Lester was particularly hesitant about leaving the FNS. Though she was

English by birth, somewhere along the way Kentucky had become her home. She thought her services could be better utilized by staying put in her adopted land. But she and a few of the other nurses were nudged to leave by Ann "Mac" MacKinnon, superintendent of the Hyden Hospital who had served in World War I. Mac received a medal during the first war, yet still wanted in the thick of things. She said that she, too, would volunteer for the European war. Upon her arrival in London, she was put in charge of an ambulance train that evacuated the wounded.

Before taking their leave from the FNS, the nurses got together for a final round of fun. For many, it was the first time they had been anywhere in months, other than straddling a horse on a rough mountain trail. And they were very excited. The big event was a trip by car to see a movie. Never mind that it was a hundred twenty-five miles away in Lexington. It was the blockbuster film everyone was talking about: *Gone with the Wind*. Breckinridge had already seen it in New York and gave the nurses permission to travel in shifts for the event. An official road had finally opened out of Leslie County. "We had radios," said Lester, "but there really wasn't much social life. We could visit people at the different districts, of course, or have guests come down. I think that's why Mrs. Breckinridge built the outposts as she did, to give the nurses as much comfort and home life as possible."[2]

There was tea at four each day; shared meals with generous servings of home-cooked food from fried chicken and mashed potatoes to mile-high pies and fresh baked breads; plus a few holiday parties. But most relief came from whatever the nurses could conjure up themselves. Breckinridge herself loved playing bridge in the evenings, though she had little patience with those who were not adept at the game. As a result, many of the nurses either gave in quickly and let her win, or made themselves scarce when she came looking for players. Sometimes the staff resorted to playing practical jokes. One American nurse-midwife convinced a secretary that a dangerous convict had escaped and was running loose in the Wendover neighborhood. Shortly after, the secretary turned in for the night and discovered when she lit the lamp in her room, the outline of what appeared to be a man's body in her bed. First she froze, and then she gingerly poked at the lifeless form. An eiderdown quilt had been shaped and placed under the covers. She would have to find a way to get even. "We also made up funny little skits," said Lester, "especially round the Fourth of July. It would be the British against the Americans, or the other way around. We would see who could win out with the best performance. Then we would sing the two national anthems and each group try to outdo the other with the most noise. It was silly things like that, but it was fun. Then it was back to work, taking care of our horses, and all that it required. Our horses were really our first consideration."[3]

As state roads began to thread their way into Leslie County, the occasional cars, primarily second-hand models, were spotted here and there. Breckinridge purchased a 1929 truck, then later an old station wagon for the FNS. The few nurses who could afford the cost and upkeep bought a vehicle for their own use. Lester had one she named Samanthy, a 1930s bright yellow Ford with running boards. Breckinridge railed against the coming war and what it was doing to the FNS, believing that as a general rule war was barbaric and destroyed everything while creating nothing. But this one, she had to admit, was different. She did not agree that America could continue to stand back and simply watch events unfold. "Like all democracies, we pay the penalty for our lack of forethought," she said. "We could have prevented the war. We didn't. We could have helped the Allies win and put a scare into Italy that might have kept her out. We didn't. Two choices are now open to us; we can unite with our sister democracies to ensure an everlasting peace, or we can wait until war and revolution are so universal that children unborn may not live to see the end."[4]

Faced with one of her most daunting challenges since the FNS began, she now began to seek ways to raise more funds by taking advantage of the uneasy times. One way to accomplish that was to compare the loss of men in war to women in childbirth. Numerous articles began to appear under her byline in newspapers, magazines, bulletins, newsletters and any other form of communication that could serve as a platform to advance the FNS. "The young woman has a battlefield of her own," she wrote, "and that is childbirth. Here the hazards for Americans throughout our years as a nation have been greater than the hazards of war, and with higher casualties. Death and mutilation — mutilation and death — that is the lot of thousands of women throughout the generations."[5] Since maternal deaths were not recorded in the U.S. for all forty-eight states until 1933, Breckinridge could not get a firm grip on statistics to support her claims, but she calculated an estimated maternal mortality from the Department of Commerce's Bureau of Census to arrive at this figure: Between 1871 and 1940, more than 900,000 women died on their own "field of battle."[6] Thus, she concluded, she could ill afford to have the FNS fall by the wayside for lack of trained nurses who were going off to war.

Betty Lester sailed from New York in 1940 on a large ship named the *Georgia*. The government contended that since it was such a big vessel, no convoy was necessary crossing the Atlantic even though it was wartime. But there was plenty of speculation about German submarines. Upon landing, Lester learned that German subs had indeed spotted and chased the ship, firing a few torpedoes that fortuitously missed. Once in London, she volunteered for civil defense. When authorities learned of her expertise as a nurse-midwife, she was recruited to go west into the countryside and take on night duty in a hospital at Berkshire Downs. Her reaction was that it was the same old routine that caused her to leave England in the first place. Not quite. Almost daily, German bombers flew in waves over the villages on their way to more vital bombing sites. Lester and the other nurses stood outside and watched them zoom past, knowing full well that casualties would soon be pouring in.

In a joint letter written to the FNS staff back in Wendover on Easter Monday, 1941, Lester and another nurse, Peggy Tinline, made light of the wartime atmosphere in England, adding that they both "missed the hills of Kentucky." "We're at my sister's house for tea and naturally the hills are on our minds," she wrote. "Things are getting a bit serious but we'll come out all right. The war will be over someday. We have already starting planning how to rebuild London and where people are going to live. Peggy has marvelous ideas of coming to work in airplanes and arriving by parachute. But we haven't yet figured how to get the people back in them."[7] Within a few months Lester was transferred to London, in Kensington. Her duties were still midwifery and her shift was still at night. This time, the transition saved her life. They were called buzz bombs, and were Hitler's latest invention. The forerunner of today's cruise missiles, these V-1 guided incendiaries had a fuselage constructed mainly of welded sheet steel with wings built of plywood. The simple jet engine pulsed fifty times per second, resulting in a characteristic buzzing that gave rise to its name. It was also referred to as a doodlebug, after an Australian insect. And it was deadly enough to strike fear in the heart of anyone who heard its distinctive sound. "The first big planes would come over and drop five or six bombs," Lester recalled. "You could hear them, one, then another, until you knew you were safe. But the buzz bombs were worse. You could see them coming; you could hear them. All at once they would stop. The engines would die down and you just waited, not knowing where they were going to hit next."[8]

After dark hundreds of people moved underground to the shelters, gathering round the three-tiered bunks chattering and talking about anything but what was happening overhead, what they knew but seldom said out loud: homes, buildings, and people could vanish overnight. "At night, you lived, more or less, in the underground. And then you came up in the daytime to clear away the rubble," said Lester. Keeping fear at bay became an art form. Black humor was the norm. Jokes poking fun at daily catastrophes made the rounds; relayed from one person to another: "Yesterday I heard these new buzz bombs meant the end of world is soon coming. I told my friend, who has three children under the ages of seven, and whose maid had just quit. And her only answer was: Good!" "If you had to go anywhere on the train or the bus, everyone would be talking quite cheerfully about where the bombs hit last night," said Lester. "They were not about to let Hitler get the best of them."[9]

During one of Lester's night shifts in London in June 1944, just as she was sending her staff to the dining room for a break, a bomb alert sounded. There was a sudden flash followed by a huge explosion and a blast of air. As the walls shook and the ceiling began to collapse, Lester recalled that everything seemed to suck inward, then out, as though God himself had taken a breath and exhaled. She heard a thousand tinkles of shattering glass, then utter silence. The hospital had been hit and every window broken. Somehow the electricity remained on. Lester, who was standing at the foot of a patient's bed, quickly made rounds, running through the ward with her white, soot-flecked nursing cap askew. Most of the post-natal women were upright in bed, terrified that another bomb would strike any moment.

Lester also remembers the scene in the hospital as she ran from bed to bed, checking on her patients. "Why are all of you doing sitting up?" she called out. "Lie back down and try to relax. Everything's going to be all right!" One of the mothers spoke up. "Sister, we can't lie down. Our beds are full of broken glass." A woman in another bed screamed. "My baby! Where's my baby?" Lester rushed to her side, searching the crib that had landed upside down from the explosion. It was empty. As the women searched frantically, a student nurse appeared carrying a bundle. "I took the baby to the nursery to change him," she explained.[10]

Though some of the nurses were bloodied, with black-tinged faces from the blast, no one in the ward was seriously hurt. Lester suffered only an inch-long gash on her shoulder. As the night wore on, doctors and nurses from other parts of the hospital stopped in, asking if everyone was all right. About daybreak someone approached Lester. "Sister, have you seen your room?" "No," Lester said, "I haven't been out of the ward. Why?" "Well, you don't have a room. One of those buzz bombs hit the nurses' quarters and sheared off a corner of the building. Five were killed. It's terrible."[11] As the news sunk in Lester realized had she not been working the night shift, she would have been right there, along with the nurses who were dead. She had, in fact, been off that night, but swapped her schedule at the last minute. She also learned the real target of the strike was General Dwight D. Eisenhower, whose quarters were less than a mile away.

Later, combing the debris that was once her room, all she could find was one shoe. Everything else was gone. She had to borrow used clothes from her niece. The odd shoe would eventually be recovered and she would take the pair with her on her return to Kentucky, a visual reminder of the London blitz. She would also take memories, seared into her brain, of D-Day "with Americans and armor everywhere" in the streets of London; the rescue of British troops at Dunkirk using anything that sailed, from trawlers to sailboats, when France fell to the Germans; a glimpse of Winston Churchill chomping a cigar as he crossed the street from the Houses of Parliament to Westminster Abbey.

Meanwhile, the work she left behind in eastern Kentucky continued, because it had to. At Wendover, the FNS administrative staff had just completed the tabulation of another thousand maternity records covering the period May 1, 1937, to April 30, 1940. Only one maternal death was reported, an improvement over the last thousand. In total, the FNS had delivered more than four thousand mothers with five maternal deaths, two from prior cardiac conditions. And its education program continued to improve as well. Early registration for prenatal care was up, with 92 percent of the women registering in the first trimester. Testing for syphilis was now common and infant mortality rates were slightly below the state average.[12] Children in nearly all the schools had been vaccinated against smallpox, diphtheria, and typhoid fever, thanks in part to the state health agencies and universities that worked in harmony with the FNS.

The FNS outpost centers, when visited by outside physicians, were commended for "thorough organization, accuracy of records, histories, and methods." The service was now so widely known that nurses from as far away as Australia, Jerusalem, and India were sending in applications. The State Board of Health and the Kentucky Dental Association began working with the FNS to provide free or reduced cost dental work to school age children and expectant or nursing mothers within the FNS districts. The charge to patients: whatever they could pay up to fifty cents a filling or free work if they could not pay. Subsidized by the FNS and the state dental association, it was a service for which money had not yet been appropriated in the FNS budget. So donors were hit up who understood the importance of dental care and believed in preventive work. It was an impressive showing for an organization less than twenty years old in a world at war.

Statewide, the war was beginning to boost local economies by establishing jobs and providing military allotments for inductees. Diversified war materials, from aircraft parts to shells and casings, were under production. Kentucky workers assembled big naval guns, and sent sixty thousand employees across the river to Indiana to make gunpowder, ammunition bags, submarine chasers, and prefab houses. A thirty million dollar government plant was built in Kentucky to make TNT. Three distilleries for which the state was already famous (think Kentucky bourbon) were re-equipped for production of one hundred ninety-proof alcohol as a solvent for powder-manufacturing purposes. Yet there were still huge pockets of poverty in the Leslie County region, where an estimated one of every thirteen men was serving time in the military. One child appeared at a clinic in Flat Creek hugging a piece of old blanket tied in the middle with string. A rock fastened to one end formed a face. It was her doll, she explained.

Among the Hyden Hospital needs listed in 1941 were beds and bassinets for children who were treated free (adults were charged a dollar a day); furnishings for the men's wards; money for outside improvements; a laundry and storage room with equipment; and—classified as an "urgent" need—a fine cow, preferably a Holstein, for the babies. At one point the hospital was so full of young patients that children were moved to the veranda ward, their beds lined up against the hospital's stone exterior walls. Patients sat on chairs and the nurses wondered where they would all sleep. The nursing staff wrote letters and daily reports, most of which were sent to Breckinridge. "We have ten children today, four of which are burn cases. The courageous and brave manner in which these children suffer is enough to break a person's heart. One little boy was cutting wood and a piece hit him in the eye. The doctor thought the sight had been destroyed entirely, but this morning the boy could see the light and you have no idea how happy he was." Another nurse wrote of a small child who just wanted to go home. "We do have some darling youngsters here. One is a pretty little boy with a huge knee about twice its normal size. He cried the first three nights he was in the hospital and asked me to get the mule and take him home. I told him I could not ride a mule and he said, 'Well, if you put me on the mule I can go home alone.' He is four years old." A mother brought her baby in weighing just thirteen pounds, though the child was more than a year old. "The baby has not the slightest idea what food is and how to eat it. It tries to suck everything that is put into its mouth. Therefore it is quite difficult to get nourishment in. Its ears and eyes are infected too, not surprising."

Burn cases, some of which occurred in homes where the father was serving overseas and the mother left to tend to outside chores, were particularly hard on everyone involved. "Well, another dear little girl, age six, was burned to death," a nurse wrote Breckinridge. "They brought her to the hospital Saturday evening and she died Sunday morning. She was washing dishes when her clothes ignited, and of course she was in the room alone and could not help herself. Can you imagine — this is the eighth burn case I have seen in the short period I've been here."[13] Breckinridge fully realized that the women and children of the FNS region were making their own forms of sacrifice for the war. "The lot of the rural mother has been rendered easier in one way and harder in every other way by the war," she reported in a 1944 published article. "It is easier because the men who have gone off to war have made allotments for their families. This means there is more cash money than ever before. On the other hand, the lot of the rural mother is harder because the burden of the land now falls on the mother and her children where formerly the man shouldered the hardest part."[14]

The war; the uncertain future of the FNS; the money troubles; many of her beloved nurses in England now at risk; it was enough to speed the aging process in anyone, even the indomitable Breckinridge. Just past sixty, she showed few signs of slowing down, though her staff was beginning to take on an increasing number of responsibilities. Keeping creditors at bay and dealing with a potential disaster at Wendover, were among the things that would require particular finesse, even as the bombs fell on Pearl Harbor that quiet Sunday morning, December 7, 1941.

14

Money and Other Troubles

There is no documented account of who was doing what at the Big House the day Pearl Harbor was attacked and the U.S. was forced into a war on both sides of the world. Most likely, the women were wrapped around a radio, as was most of America, waiting for any tidbit of news that would ease the nation's shock. But Agnes Lewis, as records and financial secretary, let few things deter her from duty. Juggling the FNS accounts remained at the top of her to-do list, war or no war. "The end of the month came," she said, "and we didn't have money to pay the bills. All during the war it seems I spent most of my time writing to firms and saying, 'I enclose our check. This is all we can pay but we'll pay more when we can.' It was a nuisance, keeping up with it, but it kept the accounts open. And I never failed to write that letter."[1]

A local FNS executive committee wanted to close some of the outpost centers. Breckinridge said absolutely not. What would happen to the buildings? On a deeper level, it went against the grain for Breckinridge to give up on anything. Everyone involved with the FNS would just have to stop whining and tighten their belts, she said. If a facility required maintenance or an office supply was needed, Breckinridge would veto the purchase unless it was critical, even at the Hyden Hospital. "She expected our doctor and nurses to know how to get along with the minimum," said Lewis. "She wanted no fancy gadgets around, not even the new incubators that were just coming out. You brought immature babies through with hot water bottles and lamps. And they were just fine."

One day at Wendover, an FNS supporter was having lunch with the staff and it began to rain hard. With the roof leaking, water first dripped onto the guest and then created a steady stream at the end of the walnut dining room table. Breckinridge called for the cook to bring a bucket. The guest glanced up at the waterlogged ceiling and asked when they might get the roof fixed. "Well, we can't," said Breckinridge. "We don't have the money." Not long after the committee member left, a check arrived in the form of a donation for repairs at the Big House.[2]

In late 1941, a flu epidemic hit bringing nearly the entire Wendover staff to its knees with the exception of Breckinridge, Dorothy Buck, and Lewis. Most of the flu sufferers ended up in the hospital, leaving the three women alone to handle FNS responsibilities. More serious was a Wendover fire that started on January 8, 1942. It took place in the Garden House, a two-story, eight room structure with four rooms upstairs, four down. It was part quarters for the administration staff and a few of the couriers, part storage, and located just a few yards from the Big House. Winter temperatures had dipped to near zero that day with snow coating the ground. The dinner bell rang at noon in the Big House and the staff was just sitting down to eat, absent Breckinridge, who had managed to get to Cincinnati for a much-needed fundraiser. Agnes Lewis described what happened. "Someone ran in and said the Garden House is on fire! We all got up and rushed out, Lucille Hodges, our bookkeeper, ahead of us. She reached her office and pried a window open just enough to pull her type-writer out and a few of her books. I don't believe anything other than that was saved. It was a wooden building with a bin of coal in the basement. The social secretary had collected clothes and they were all piled in the basement for a grab sale."[3]

Word began to spread up and down the creek that Wendover was ablaze. In twenty-five minutes the Garden House was half gone. Just up the creek, less than a mile from the Big House, a young man home from the Navy was visit-ing his family. As fate would have it, he had manned a fire hose on board a ship and came running when he heard the news. Taking charge, he formed a brigade and kept the damage from spreading to the barn, the chicken houses, and the Big House itself. The water pipes up the hill, suddenly overburdened, burst and would require repair before water was restored on the property. And when it was over, nothing other than the typewriter and a few assorted items could be saved. The cause of the blaze was never fully determined but several possi-bilities were raised: frequent requests to add more fuel to the coal furnace by cold-natured employees; a cigarette tossed into the registry; and a box of woolen clothes cleaned with flammable liquids sitting nearby all added to the equation. "Those of us who lived in the Garden House lost all we had," said Lewis. "But that was of no consequence compared to the FNS records and work-ing items we lost."[4]

That same afternoon the staff sent a telegram to Breckinridge. "In less than twenty-four hours we had a reply," said Lewis. "She expressed her sym-pathy at being away and ended it with a request that I send her plans for a new Garden House." The response hit the mild-mannered Lewis the wrong way. She then did something almost unheard of for her and the entire FNS staff. She dis-obeyed an order. "We hadn't gotten the pipes thawed yet and the pumps run-ning," she said. "And we were getting practically no sleep, with no place for people to work, and everyone still disturbed about the fire. I took the telegram to Bucket [Dorothy Buck] and told her to tell Mrs. Breckinridge that when the water pipes are repaired and the pumps are running, and we know that the fire is really put out, I'll think about plans for the Garden House. But not until then."[5]

When the unusual response reached Breckinridge, she immediately contacted the FNS medical director, Dr. Kooser, asking him to provide Lewis with medication to help calm her down, for the poor child was no doubt having a breakdown. Kooser, in turn, was somewhat put out that Breckinridge appeared not to trust him to take care of her staff while she was away. "It was just all the tension that everyone was under," Lewis explained. "About four days later I took my secretary — I had a secretary by then — and one of the volunteers who was very good at drawing outlines and we did a rough sketch for a new Garden House."[6]

With the war on, and a shortage of building materials, they had to hurry in order to get the proper permits before supplies ran out. "Later," said Lewis, "people would ask why we didn't put in a shower, why didn't we do this, why not that? And I said never mind, we did well to get anything during the war. Just be grateful for what we have."

By September, nine months after the fire, the reconstructed Garden House was complete, "fresh and clean," said Lewis, for the new occupants. She requested a vacation so that she could recoup from the stress-filled year. In truth, she wanted to get away before the staff — and the animals they encouraged to romp inside — messed up the place. *That* she couldn't stand to witness. "Sure enough," she fumed, "when I came back there were marks here and yonder where the dogs had been on the paint, left their footprints in muddy rooms, and all that sort of thing."[7]

Before long, the hillside behind the Garden House and the Big House began to inch forward, rocks and boulders loosened from the summer rains. In the basement of the new Garden House, a crack was forming in the foundation. Lewis, alarmed, asked Breckinridge if she would come take a look while on her way to the chicken coop. "What's the trouble, my child?" she asked. "I think we need a proper engineer to advise us about this," Lewis said, pointing out the problem. "Then get one," said Breckinridge and went on her way to feed her chickens.[8] Lewis contacted an engineering firm in Louisville, which first told her they were too busy handling war work to deal with her shifting hillside. They did, however, finally send an advisor to Wendover who determined that a retaining wall should be built to support the hillside behind the Garden House and prevent more landslides. Twenty-five hundred dollars— money the FNS could ill afford — and a beautiful new stone wall later, the problem returned once the winter rains began. The new retaining wall cracked and bulged like an overfed beast. "The engineer had no sooner returned to Louisville than the hill began to slide again," said Lewis. Another engineer, this one from the Ford Motor Company on Red Bird River, was called in. He agreed to come as a courtesy to the FNS. Having lived in the area for years, he was familiar with the tricky nature of mountain slides and came up with a four-point plan that included extensive drain ditches, steel rails cemented into the cliff, a redesign of the retaining wall, and elimination of water pockets, all of which eventually worked.[9]

Secretary to Agnes Lewis was Lucille Hodges (later Knechtly), who came to the FNS in 1942 and soon developed the odd nickname of "Thumper." Prior to arriving at Wendover, she worked for the General Electric Company in Cincinnati, Ohio, but grew tired of the city. Hearing of the Frontier Nursing Service, she placed a call to Wendover where she learned the organization was interviewing for a secretary. Lewis told her to come on down. "I was living with my cousin," Hodges said, "and went home that night to tell her I was going to Kentucky in two weeks. She thought I was crazy, and so did my employer."[10] She took the bus to Lexington, spent the night at a hotel, and caught another bus into Hazard. Helen Browne, who would someday take over the role of FNS director, and a courier named Marian Lewis, met the prospective employee. "I remember we went to a restaurant called Don's, in Hazard, and ordered a steak. Helen and Marian asked for a bag to take the bones home to the dogs. Having never seen anyone do that, I thought it was the strangest thing. But within six weeks I was doing the same thing."

Once the trio arrived in Hyden, they were provided a car for the brief ride to the FNS headquarters. By then it was dark and Hodges was told the Big House did not yet have electricity. The deeper into the woods they drove, the more convinced she became that they would never be seen or heard from again. "The women pointed to the hills and said 'There it is!' All I could see was a bunch of trees. We had to use a flashlight to get out of the car and they motioned up the hill to something called the Upper Shelf. I thought that meant I would be sleeping on a big shelf. That was my introduction to Wendover."[11] The Upper Shelf, she learned, was a four-room cottage with a front porch nestled among a thick patch of rhododendron just above the Big House. This was where some of the nurses slept, congregated, or slipped away if they wanted a few moments alone. With a fireplace in every room (the only source of heat) and exactly one-hundred-and-one steep steps to the front door, it was a perfect haven for the work-weary staff. On many a cold winter night, girls would fill the small rooms, pile up on the beds, the chairs, or on the floor, popping corn in the fireplace, roasting chestnuts, or mixing a fresh batch of chocolate in the fudge pot over the open flames.

Following her interview, Hodges got the job. As with other employees, she was required to sign a contract that she would stay at least a year. And like Lewis, for whom she was working, she was miserably unhappy at first. "They stuck me in an office doing figures and I never liked accounting or ordering things, that type of work. I never got out to a center. I never got to see any of the frontier nursing work. I hated it. I had a cousin with the Indian Bureau in Alaska and that winter he came home around Christmas, recruiting secretaries

to go to Alaska. I said yes I would go with him. I even took a Civil Service test."
But December was a busy month, she added, for secretaries and midwives. "I
had to get Mrs. Breckinridge ready to go East for her many speaking engagements. And it seemed as though everyone tried to get their babies delivered
before Christmas. We also had to plan for the children's holiday. The party at
Wendover and the six outposts was the only Christmas many of the children
had."[12]

She and an FNS nurse were assigned the task of driving into Hyden to one
of the few retail stores, a five-and-dime, to buy trinkets for the event. The
nurse-midwife spied a large stuffed panda bear, announcing that was something
she always wanted. So she bought it for herself. "When we got back to the
mouth of Muncy Creek, the river was up," said Hodges. "So we had to leave
the jeep in a neighbor's yard and carry all our purchases, including this huge
panda, across the swinging bridge more than a mile to Wendover." Just as
Hodges' contracted year was coming to an end and she was ready to make her
getaway, she came down with appendicitis and ended up in Hyden Hospital.
"It was so crowded they put me in the midwifery ward. I finally got to meet
some of the nurses. They were all friendly and so helpful." As Hodges watched
the FNS women at work, her outlook slowly shifted. These women were doing
important, much-needed work, and if she stayed, she could be a part of it. "I
never went to Alaska," she said. "Instead, I became Mrs. Breckinridge's secretary."[13]

She stayed for fourteen years. She would then go on to become a public
school teacher and the author of an entertaining booklet titled *Where Else But
Here?* that recounted her days at the FNS. Soon after deciding to continue at
Wendover, she came by her unusual nickname. "We had a courier named Helen
("Pebble") Stone who tapped at my office window one day and announced,
'We're going to call you Thumper.' I think it was because they saw me thumping away on the typewriter so often. A lot of people never knew my real name.
So everyone called me Thumper."[14] As secretary to Breckinridge, she was privy
to most of the FNS correspondence, including wartime letters from the British
nurses who had volunteered their services elsewhere. Among them were several missives from Betty Lester.

"The news this morning was good," Lester wrote in May, 1943. "Resistance
in North Africa ceased last night. This brings one phase of the war to an end
and now we wait for the next phase to begin. I am on a week's vacation staying on a farm in Kent and having marvelous weather. It's quiet and I am thoroughly enjoying the rest and peace. All hospitals are short of staff and I was
beginning to feel the strain."[15] And later that same year, she wrote New Year's
greetings to the staff, expressing regret over the recent loss of her yellow Ford
convertible, Samantha, which she learned had finally petered out beyond repair.
"I can't believe Samantha is no more. I had such fun running around in her —
getting drowned out in the Middle Fork River, stuck in the mud, chugging up

creeks, taking myself and Barrie [her collie dog] off to commune with the hills; going into town and finding people sitting on the running board waiting for a ride home. It seems impossible that little yellow car won't be there to greet me home."

A fellow FNS nurse, Nora Kelly, wrote from her corner room in the nurses' quarters at the Mother's Hospital in London, in December 1943, where her daily cross to bear was wartime shortages and bureaucratic snafus. "I am in the throes of trying to get equipment for a department in war time. We can't get some things and others we get too much. For a start, how about twelve mirrors? Are they for mothers, babies, or nurses? But there are no babies' baths, not one to be had! It's funny when you are in the mood to see the joke. In the meantime, all the beds are booked and I feel rather overwhelmed. But what can I do when I hear such pathetic stories? People went everywhere for hospital beds before coming here." Then, not wanting to end on a negative note: "Also, we had a flock of pigeons flying about and if I put out a few crumbs, they come get them, even though our helper complains bitterly about the mess they make. I am in a corner room with two windows. Over the chimney pots I can look out and see the trees on Clapham Common, and the birds this time are seagulls."[16]

At the bombed out London hospital where several of Betty Lester's peers were killed, most of the facility was no longer fit for patients or staff so Lester was transferred again, this time to a hospital in Chelsea where she remained until 1945 when the war ended. But her thoughts—and her heart—were more and more often wending their way back to the hills of Kentucky and the patients she felt still needed her care.

Seven miles from Wendover, a sixteen-year-old pregnant girl named Easter was about to give birth to her first child. The nurse-midwife on duty at the Big House was Ethel Broughall, who had just settled down with a magazine. She was scanning an ad that displayed a cheerful baby creeping toward a metal can of baby powder. Reading the caption she had to smile: "Ready or not, here I come." That's just like us, she thought. Then she heard a knock at the gate. Within the next few moments she was mounting her horse, Pinafore, and was on her way to the head of Rocky Fork. "For the previous three weeks, the baby had been in breech position," she said, "and all attempts to turn it had been unsuccessful. We planned for her to go to the hospital closer to her due date. But now she was in labor."[17]

Broughall arrived at the cabin about nine-thirty that night to find the mother, only a young teen, moaning and writhing in pain. "My examination determined the breech position remained the same so we began to prepare for the trip to the hospital. The first four miles from the house was a narrow horse trail. A stretcher was hurriedly but well-constructed of saplings, rope, and quilts. We sent for neighbor men to carry it and a messenger sent to awaken the driver of the nearest truck. He was to meet us at the end of the trail."

With the war on, there was not only a shortage of food and gasoline, but fewer strong men capable of bearing a patient down a rough mountain path. Normally eight men were mustered to carry a stretcher, four at time, taking turns so one group could rest while the other carried. The armed forces had taken the youngest and most physically able, including Easter's husband. Nonetheless, three older men showed up near midnight following a long day in the fields, and Easter's mother-in-law agreed to pinch hit as the fourth stretcher bearer. A female neighbor carried a carbide lamp to light the way, while the FNS nurse brought up the rear. "After what seemed like endless miles of stumbling over rocks, wading creek beds, and reassuring Easter who was in ever-increasing discomfort," said Broughall, "we reached the truck."[18] However, the little group found the half-ton vehicle too small to accommodate either the stretcher or the bed, so they had devise a place for Easter to lie prone on the floor of the truck atop a pile of quilts. A spare tire was chained to the back, taking up more precious room. "We took turns in what space was available," said Broughall, "and for the remaining miles I knelt on the floor beside her, watching her progress by moonlight as my flashlight had failed me." She worried they might not reach the hospital in time.

About a mile from the hospital door, the baby decided to come. Broughall rapped frantically on the window signaling the driver to stop. "As efficiently as I could," she said, "on the bed of a pickup truck already overcrowded, I set up for delivery. And by the bright illumination of the moon, I delivered 'bottoms up' a six-and-a-half pound girl with none of the dreaded complications occurring." She said later that throughout the entire ordeal, the magazine ad kept running through her head, "Ready or not, here I come."[19]

Across the ridge, at the Caroline Butler Atwood Center in Flat Creek, a patient arrived to have sawdust removed from his eye; another had a crushed finger from a sawmill accident; and a seven-year-old boy fell out of a tree sustaining a wrist injury. His mother told the nurse, "It looks right quare."

In England, Lester was penning her final letter that year. "This will arrive sometime in the New Year so here's wishing you all the nice things you wish for yourself," she wrote. "For me," she added wistfully, "my only wish is a speedy return to Wendover.[20]

15

Coming Home

With the European war's end in May 1945, Lester had to badger the American authorities in order to return to Kentucky. They told her she had no priority for a re-entry visa. And she had no idea how to get one. Then she thought of Breckinridge, who had access to important people in Washington, D.C. If anyone could pull a few strings, she could. Furthermore, Breckinridge needed as many nurses as possible and, Lester knew, would welcome her back. While she continued working in Chelsea she instructed her sister, Nan, to stay alert for a letter from her former boss. Nan wasn't keen on the idea that her sister wanted to return to America, much less to the remote Appalachian Mountains, but realized it was futile to try and persuade her otherwise.

In Leslie County, a new FNS nurse had just arrived from "up North" to work at Hyden Hospital and was forming her own opinions about the region. Jean Bradley, R.N., remembered the bus ride from Hazard into Hyden the prior winter, the winding river that snaked its way into the mountains, diamond-studded icicles glistening like sharpened knives against the dull gray boulders. She had a sense that she was traveling back in time. The bus lurched to a halt in front of the drugstore in Hyden. As Bradley looked around, the tiny town appeared "like an ancient etching, the courthouse and buildings clustered about it white and still."[1] Someone with an FNS insignia emblazoned on her sleeve was scanning the passengers as they exited. "Are you Jean-something-or-other?" the FNS courier asked. "Yes." "I'm supposed to take you up the hill." "I realized we were in a valley completely surrounded by hills," said Bradley, "and to me they all looked alike. Gray, rocky cliffs covered with leafless trees. An occasional pine gave a spot of the green to the otherwise dull landscape"[2] At the hospital on the hill above Hyden, Bradley marveled at the mazelike passages and flights of stairs inside the old stone building. In the children's ward, she was introduced to a four-year-old whose prized possession was a pink hair bow. The child offered up the treasure as a gift, then changed her mind. Instead, she explained, she would just tell everyone she loved them. "The whole place had a spirit of friendliness and informality that put this newcomer at ease in these strange surroundings," said Bradley. During her first few weeks at the FNS, she crossed her first swinging bridge en route to Wendover, had tea with a group of nurses in the Big House, and in an effort to see more of Leslie County, accompanied the medical director on rounds. "The roads were smooth in spots and very rough in others," she recalled. "Dirt had been dumped in huge piles for use in repairs. At the schoolhouse we parked the car and waded across the shallow part of the river. It was covered with about ten inches of ice. The doctor traipsed across and I followed, gingerly picking my way. We had come to check on an elderly couple. This was an easy call. While Dr. Fraser talked with his patients I warmed my feet at the unprotected open fire grate, typical of these houses. And I wondered how children kept from getting burned too close to the fire."[3]

A call came next from Beech Fork Clinic, where the patient was expecting her twelfth child, *none* born with the assistance of the Frontier Nursing Service. The mother's general condition was poor but the delivery went as planned. What seemed remarkable, said the visiting nurse, was how cold the rooms were and the patient's gratitude that, unlike her other deliveries, she wasn't given hot pepper tea as part of her post-partum recovery. Meanwhile, Breckinridge spent a good part of 1944 and 1945 in "a string of engagements" in New York, including a speech to the Ladies Emergency Society, lecturing a class in nursing and health at Columbia University, and speaking before a group of her former colleagues at St. Luke's Hospital. She met with what she considered "one of the outstanding nurses in obstetrics in the world," who was head of the Maternity Consultation Service and like Breckinridge, had suffered a severe injury. "When I see her," said Breckinridge, "I feel I should never even mention my broken back. She has had a broken neck for twenty years and wears a metal collar. She has to put her hand on someone's arm before she can walk — yet her life is one of the most active and useful in America."[4]

Breckinridge had tea with some of the former couriers, dined with several friends and family members, then traveled on to Boston and finally to Washington, D.C., by night train. The business at hand was putting plans in motion for the annual spring benefit with scheduled guest speaker, Cornelia Otis Skinner, an American actress and writer known for her wit and social commentary. Then it was on to Baltimore where she got stranded in a train station. A senior student at Johns Hopkins Hospital was scheduled to meet her but the station was packed and the young girl could not find Breckinridge in the crowd. "I sat down on my luggage in the train shed and waited comfortably for twenty minutes before I laid eyes on a porter," Breckinridge said. "How can anyone be sure of meeting any train in the stations today?" *What a far cry from the quiet comfort of the mountains surrounding Wendover,* she thought.[5] She was rescued by a train porter, placed in a taxi, and sent on her way to Johns Hopkins where she spoke to a group of students that same evening. Several hospital cadets were scheduled to come to the FNS as part of their training and she wanted to meet them before they arrived in eastern Kentucky.

Following a short holiday in the Shenandoah Valley —*taken* from Virginia during the Civil War and *given over* to West Virginia as she, as a diehard Confederate, liked to point out — Breckinridge returned to Hyden. It was pouring rain near the Big House and the swirling Middle Fork River was at high tide. "There to meet me, at the foot of the swinging bridge, was my flea-bitten gray mare, Babbette," she recounted. "It's good to get the feel of a horse against my knees again. While others struggled with my luggage in the driving rain, Babbette and I rode to Wendover as we have done so many times through the years. I was home, finally, from beyond the mountains."[6]

Thousands of miles away, across the Atlantic Ocean, someone else was just as anxious to return. In England, Betty Lester was packing what remained of her meager belongings. Most of her possessions had been lost in the London bombing. Due to war rationing there were few clothing or household items available to buy. On January 9, 1946, she set sail by way of Canada. The voyage across the Atlantic was awful, she recalled. The small ship held six people to a cabin and shortly after leaving England encountered a hurricane at sea. Lester was seasick nearly the entire trip. She arrived in St. John's, New Brunswick, on Sunday, January 20, to temperatures just below six degrees — the polar opposite of her maiden voyage to America in July 1928 when New York City was undergoing a heat wave. "I went on to Montreal the next night by train," she said. "In the Montreal station I had a breakfast consisting of orange juice, two eggs, bacon, toast, marmalade, and coffee. I choked when I saw it, as such a breakfast was unknown to me for so long a time, and I wished my people in England could have been with me."[7]

She then caught a train to New York, where Breckinridge had arranged for a Red Cross representative to meet her at Grand Central Station, a standing agreement that exemplified the strong working relationship between the two agencies. The Red Cross official hailed a cab for Lester and sent her to a local hostel for an overnight stay. The next morning, she received word that Breckinridge was back in New York, staying at the Cosmopolitan Club. The two women met up for lunch that day, greeting each other warmly. There was much news to catch up. One of the FNS nurses had come down with what was thought to be the flu but never quite recovered. Sent to Lexington for chest X-rays and further testing, she learned she had undulant fever, an infectious disease transmitted from animals to humans, often from drinking contaminated milk. It was the first case of its kind in the history of the Frontier Nursing Service and her case was chronic. "We had to dispose of some of our cows," Breckinridge told Lester. "Every Monday for three weeks Jean Hollins [head courier] had the sad task of rounding them up and taking them to Lexington for testing. Then the barns were scrubbed and disinfected. We've had new feed boxes made for all the cow stalls." She went to say when the tests came back positive, they were "sunk." They lost nine cows in all. "You can't keep house in the mountains without cows," she said, "as there is no other milk supply." She pleaded for help from donors, many of whom provided new heifers, all of which Breckinridge promptly named. Among them: Radiant Nancy, Radiant Remus Queen, and Remus Lily.

"Now," she went on. "I have something even more important to tell you." Her serious look made Lester draw back. "What is it?" she asked. Maybe Breckinridge had decided she didn't need her services after all. "Well, when you get back to Leslie County no one will believe it's you." "Why not?" Lester asked. "Because you're dead. You were killed in the war in three different ways. First, we heard your ship was torpedoed and everyone lost at sea. Then we heard you were on an ambulance train and it had been bombed. Finally, we heard that the hospital where you were stationed was totally destroyed. But here you are. Now won't they be surprised?" "Yes, especially when I'm resurrected," Lester responded.[8] She shared her survivor tale about the lone pair of shoes she retrieved from the bomb blast, telling Breckinridge she brought them with her for good luck. It was the type of delightful story Breckinridge loved and would relay many times throughout the next few years.

Lucille Hodges accompanied Breckinridge on the New York trip to carry on with duties related to speeches and fundraising. Greeting Lester on her return from the war was an extra incentive to go, for Hodges had heard nothing but positive things about the English nurse and looked forward to meeting her. Since Lester now had so few personal belongings, Breckinridge instructed the secretary to take her shopping. "But I don't know where to find anything," she told her boss. "And the only stores I've heard about are Macy's and Bloomingdale's." In truth, Hodges didn't know where the two renowned department stores were either. She was hoping they were right down the street. "Just go, child," said Breckinridge. "Well," Hodges admitted, "this is how stupid I was. I told Betty I would meet her at Macy's in the ladies room. I didn't know the place had fifteen floors, each with their own bathroom. So when I got there, I had to start at the bottom and look in every single room until I found her. I ended up being forty-five minutes late. But she and I became pretty good friends throughout that trip."[9] Lester, grateful for Breckinridge's generosity, remarked how nice it was not to count clothing coupons as she did in London during the war.

Newly outfitted, she returned to Wendover by bus, stopping off in Manchester en route to Hyden, still thirty-five miles away. Standing on the bus station platform were several drivers, one of whom gave her a startled, searching look. She thought about what Breckinridge had told her. "Howdy," she said, remembering the common Southern greeting. "Do I know you?" the driver said. "Yes, Daniel, you do. I took care of your wife when all three of your children were born." The man blanched. Then he grabbed her shoulders and enveloped her in a tight bear hug. "But I never thought I'd see you again, Miss Lester. Everyone said that you had been killed in the war! I'm so glad you've come back to us." "Me too," said Lester, laughing.[10]

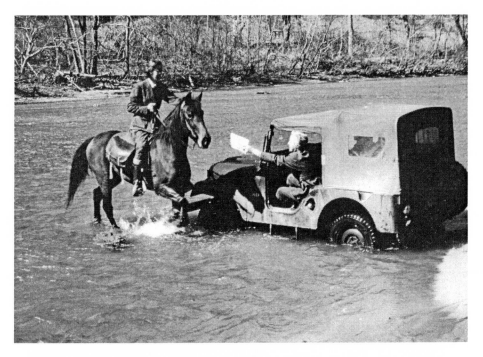

FNS nurse-midwife P. Anne Cundle on her horse, Sweet, meets FNS nurse-midwife Betty Lester in Middle Fork River to retrieve a message. Jeeps became a more practical form of transportation within the FNS following World War II. Undated photograph taken in the 1950s (courtesy Special Collections and Digital Programs, University of Kentucky Libraries and the Frontier Nursing Service, Inc.).

Janie, one of the new Jeeps recently acquired by the FNS, with a courier at the wheel, met Lester at the mouth of Muncie's Creek. As they drove through Hyden, she noted few major changes in her six year absence. "The town itself had not changed much, except there were more cars parked on both sides of the street and fewer horses and mules. There were still the same friendly greetings on every hand and more animals than cars downtown. But at the hospital what a lot to see: the doctor's clinic; the out-patient department; X-ray; and the midwives' quarters. And there were several new nurses."[11] Had she made note of it, she would have also realized the ratio of British to American nurses was now almost totally reversed.

Lester and the courier headed to the Big House, the jeep bouncing through potholes on the narrow, twisted road. "We crossed the Middle Fork River, and came up through the mud and darkness to Wendover," she said. "We were greeted by Bucket, Agnes, and Lucille, along with lots of new people, and of course the dogs. We had dinner and I went to bed, tired out but so glad to be back." She slept for twenty-four hours straight.[12] The next day Lester walked down the stone-lined path to the Victory Shrine Chapel just below the house, stepped in quietly, and gave thanks for her safe return. Despite her dramatic wartime experiences, she often said later that one of the most exciting moments of her life was receiving word that she could return to Kentucky.

Her first outpost visit was to Bull Creek, where she was stationed shortly after her arrival in 1928. Local people who knew she had returned from the war approached her shyly are first, some to shake her hand, others to reach out and put their arms around her. "Some looked at me with tears in their eyes and said, 'I sure am proud to see you back.'"[13] At Beech Fork, she marveled over the new Hyden-Harlan road which was just getting built when she left in 1940. She stopped by to visit families at Turkey Branch and Leatherwood Creek, sitting on their porches or at their humble tables sharing whatever they had to spare. She borrowed a horse to follow the well-worn trails she had traveled in the past. And as she rode across the misty mountaintops and gazed at the distant ridge-line views, she realized why she had come to love this place so well.

She noted the families and that they all had good gardens, with seeds provided by Social Service. Some of the boys she knew as children were now soldiers and sailors, stationed at far-flung places all over the world. She heard the memorable cases and various escapades relayed by the FNS nurses and staff she had left behind. Among them: A new cadet nurse was preparing to step into the tub at Wendover before supper when she heard someone call her name. A delivery was coming due just across the river from the Big House. Despite the few cars in the region, horses were still very much in use, so she and another midwife saddled up for the trek across the river. The new nurse recalled the brief but arduous trip. "Flood waters had left great quantities of sand in the ford in front of the patient's house, so we had to ford the river at the mouth of Muncie Creek, and go back up the river on the other side. Since the path was more sandy than usual, the horses hesitated to go over it. Time was short, so we dismounted and led them. When we were halfway to the house, something compelled me to turn around and see how the saddle bags were riding."

To her shock, the bags containing all their medical supplies were gone. "Bertha went on to the patient's house while I hitched Cameron to the nearest tree and stumbled back along the path searching for the bags. My legs could hardly carry me fast enough. I wished I might trip over them, anything to find them in a hurry and reach the house before the baby made its grand entrance."[14] On the verge of panic, she spotted a familiar looking brown heap on the path ahead. It was the saddle bags. "I slung them over my shoulder and literally raced back to Cameron. The dear old horse must have sensed my predicament because he hadn't slipped his bridle as he customarily did." She hurried to the house and was met at the door by Bertha, who convinced her at first the baby had already arrived. "Then I saw a smile breaking through. There was no kerosene for the lamp so we stumbled around in comparative darkness to save our two flashlights for the main event. The corner fireplace which heated the room supplied an occasional flicker of light when it was stoked with coal. Two hours passed and at last we 'caught' a fine baby girl. We bathed it in warm oil, measured and weighed her."

After the mother and baby were tucked in for the night, the other children woke up. One, a young boy, walked up to the nurses and spoke in the darkness. "I know what you brought," he whispered. "You brought a baby in your saddle pockets. I seen hit's diaper in that bag we carried."[15] The young mother had a normal post-partum period. But the two nurses who cared for them not only got razzed for losing their saddlebags, they had to cross the river in a boat on their next two visits, whereupon the boat tipped, they were dunked, and caught in a sinkhole before their safe return to the Big House. "We decided to give up on boating," said the new cadet. "Although the walk was long and the saddlebags heavy, we made our subsequent visits on foot, the bags slung over our shoulders."[16] Lester no doubt laughed when told of the women's travails for she had been through similar experiences herself.

She also heard in depth of the water troubles at Hyden Hospital. Floods had occurred the previous spring, causing the hill on Thousandsticks Moun-

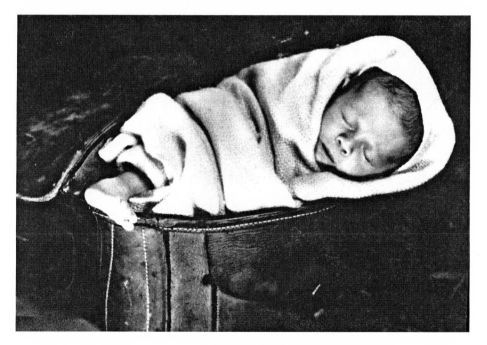

Children throughout the Frontier Nursing Service region thought that nurses brought their newborn siblings in saddlebags when they tended their mothers, hence the term "saddlebag babies." Infants and small children who needed specialized care were brought to the Hyden Hospital on horseback in the early days but most medical care was conducted in the homes (courtesy Frontier Nursing Service, Inc.).

tain to slip and break the water lines. For months, the pumps didn't work properly. Then one of the cows at the barn accidentally turned the water on, nearly draining the tank before the broken pump was discovered. None of this was known to the hospital staff. On an otherwise cheerful Monday morning, several of the FNS nurses were in the dining room when someone interrupted their breakfast to inform them the basement was flooded. "Since it was not deep enough to get into the fire box," nurse Florence Samson recalled, "we relaxed and enjoyed our meal. That was the last rest we would have for two days. When one lives in mountain country, it is never safe to sit back and feel smug."[17]

A foot of water had flooded the lower main rooms and the drug room. A shipment of bandages lay on the floor, most of them waterlogged and ruined. The nurses set to work to correct the problem, rigging up a garden hose to serve as a siphon. It required constant monitoring to keep it unclogged. They donned rubber boots and began to empty the water a bucket at a time, then would run up the stairs to dump it in a drain. They bailed, rested, ran upstairs, emptied, ran back, and bailed some more, only to find that the water was not receding. In fact, it was rising higher. "This was bad," said Samson. "The drain was evidently working, but obviously in the wrong direction. A few local men arrived and found the drain did not carry the water outside. Instead, it was going into a deep hole in the far side of the basement. They discovered this unexpectedly by stepping *into* the hole and sinking waist deep. We thought this was a good time to stop for lunch."

Afterwards, they dutifully returned to the mess below. Someone detected an odd odor. "It smells like cod liver oil," a nurse remarked, wrinkling her nose. "It *is* cod liver oil," said Samson. She knew the feel, the smell, and the look of it. "No one enjoyed this," she added, "except Crickett, the hospital cat. But the poor thing couldn't find the source so he spent most of the day sitting on the basement steps sniffing, dodging our booted feet, and humming softly to himself." The men tried using the damaged pump but it continued to clog. Most of the day was spent taking it apart and cleaning it. "Bailing was more efficient," said Samson. "We soon began to bail in earnest."[18]

Staff from the hospital, just getting off from their regular shift, came by and offered to help. Two visitors from Wendover made the mistake of dropping in and found themselves recruited to the bucket brigade. One volunteer was so tall she kept hitting her head on the pipes. "I suppose after a time she grew numb, for she continued to bang her head, ducking, and passing buckets," said Samson.[19] They finally reached the deep hole in the corner where two of the nurses climbed in, dipped water, and passed the buckets along to be emptied. The job was finally finished late that evening. "After a session in the living room over cups of steaming coffee, we took our creaking bodies to bed," said Samson. "Someone had kindly given us bubble bath for Christmas and it was badly needed this night. For it helped remove the faint but continuing odor of cod liver oil."[20]

Twelve miles away, at the Confluence Center, a new secretary was straightening the twin beds in the red-and-white checked guestroom when a nurse-midwife named Bertha called her downstairs and asked if she wanted to ride along on a home delivery. The place was Devil's Jump, off Hell for Certain Creek.

A few minutes later we were on our horses. While we were saddling, Bertha handed me her stethoscope. It wasn't until we had gone about half a mile down the trail that I discovered I had dropped it. By the time I found it, I was a half-hour behind Bertha. At last I arrived and ran up the hill to the cabin, the stethoscope around my neck. But when I walked in, Bertha wasn't there. I asked the woman rocking by the fireplace where the nurse was and she just looked at me with a blank expression. Then I heard groans from the bed in the corner — the familiar "Lordy, Lordy"— that sent chills up my back. I couldn't deliver a baby![21]
Even more hopeless was the thought of going back over the mountain to look for Bertha, who had either lost her way, fallen from her horse, or was lying somewhere with a broken leg.[22]

The frightened secretary did the only thing she could. She boiled water. "That's what they do in the movies," she explained, "so I did that for a while. At last, when I had exhausted all my ideas, one kept coming. What were those "ten easy lessons" on delivering a baby that I had typed so many times for the midwifery students? Staring at the pan of boiling water, she remembered: "If the baby comes before the nurse arrives, make sure you wipe its eyes and mouth, wrap it warmly, and do nothing else until the nurse is there."

I felt better now. Everything would be all right. I was even a little disappointed when Bertha came rushing in a few minutes later. She had taken a wrong turn on the trail and had gone through more agony than I did, I am sure.
After the delivery, we ate breakfast and waved goodbye to the family with the new heir. It provided a laugh to all midwives and a lesson to all secretaries: When you are doing straight typing, pay close attention to all the words.[23]

It wasn't long before Betty Lester was back at work with her own FNS cases, including one that resulted in a dangerous postpartum hemorrhage. The baby had arrived minutes before Lester arrived at the patient's home, assisted by a local midwife, the patient's mother-in-law, and a sister. Both mother and child appeared in good condition and Lester was preparing to cut the umbilical cord when there was suddenly a rush of blood followed by a steady flow.
The local midwife attempted to place cold cloths on the woman's abdomen, the only method for control of bleeding that she knew. The mother-in-law sent her son, the patient's husband, running a mile up the creek to a man known for treating patients through "an absent cure." The patient's sister asked if she could assist Lester. "By now, my patient had no pulse, was cold, and without color," said Lester. "Her blood was dripping steadily from the rubber sheet onto the floor. Only once did she cry out, 'I feel numb. Oh god, help me.' I, too, was praying silently for help." With the nearest phone four miles away,

and the medical director another twenty miles away, Lester was on her own. Then she remembered that the closest neighbor, less than a mile from the house, owned a truck. "Fortunately, the sister could write so I had her take a message to the neighbor asking for help. I finally got the woman's bleeding under control and began treatment for shock—heat, rectal saline, coffee, and elevation of the foot of the bed. After I was sure the bleeding would not recur, I gave her a stimulant by hypodermic as authorized by the Medical Advisory Committee."[24]

To Lester's great relief, the patient began to rally and her color return. By the time the neighbor arrived in his truck, the woman's pulse was steady and once again strong. She called for water and Lester gave her sips while cautioning her to stay still and quiet. Three hours later, Lester was still by her bedside, checking the patient and writing her report for the doctor and the midwifery supervisory. "'Estimated blood loss,' Lester wrote, 'was forty-eight ounces.' What I could not report was that when the husband returned I asked out of curiosity what had happened at the place he visited where cures were made 'in absence.' He said the man told him to go home—for all would be over."[25]

To celebrate Lester's return to the mountains, a box supper was planned in her honor on a Saturday night at the Thousandsticks School in February 1946. One of the students at the FNS Graduate School learned of the event and approached Lester, asking if she could come along.

> I had heard enough about box suppers to know that each girl brought a fancy-wrapped box of food to attract the high bid of her chosen boy friend. After it was purchased, it was her romantic privilege to eat with him from the box. Betty said I could attend but I would have to prepare something. With our maid's help at the school, I fixed a sizeable box, using fancy wrap and red tape left over from Christmas. I included a can of beans. My classmates worried about how we would get it open, but we decided that someone would surely have a knife on hand.[26]

They started out in mid-afternoon, the student riding on horseback alongside Lester.

> We talked about the FNS work, about the things that had happened to Betty in England, and sometimes we didn't talk at all, just enjoying riding in silence. About four P.M. we arrived at Edith Wood's house to have supper and "take the night." Some of the most delightful smells greeted us—fried chicken and baked bread. There were vegetables, real butter and cream, a salad of crisp lettuce, strawberries Edith had canned from her garden, and fresh lemon pie. It was fun watching Betty, who couldn't get over the abundance of butter, milk, and eggs.
> While Betty and Charlie swapped stories, Edith and I fixed our boxes. We arrived at the school to find a number of people had gathered. There was a sound of thunder at the door and in came the young men of the neighborhood. They had been too bashful up till now to enter, and were standing around outside.[27]

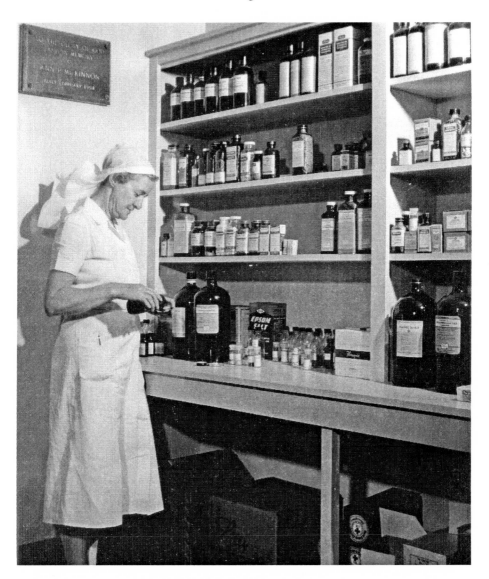

FNS British nurse-midwife Betty Lester at the Hyden Hospital pharmacy, circa 1940s (courtesy Special Collections and Digital Programs, University of Kentucky Libraries and the Frontier Nursing Service, Inc.).

When the time came for the boys to claim their bids, the young nurse found herself faced with a partner who was more interested in eating than having a conversation. "I searched my mind for some topics that I thought he'd like to talk about, and hit on one or two. Then someone called me from across the room and I excused myself." When the student nurse returned, the boy had taken off with their box supper and disappeared into the night. "I was glad he liked it, even if he was a little shy," she concluded.[28]

En route to Hyden by train from New York, was another young woman. Her goal was to become a nurse-midwife at the FNS. As fate would have it, her seatmate was also headed to the Frontier Nursing Service. The two girls hit it off and spent their time wondering what was ahead in eastern Kentucky. Neither had been to the region. In Lexington, they transferred to a bus, laughing at the driver who seemed to stop "at every telephone pole," chatting up people he knew. An occasional passenger boarded the bus with a crate of chickens in tow. At Campbell's drugstore in Hyden, the girls disembarked. It was a hot day in mid-afternoon. Like Betty Lester, who had first arrived in Hyden more than twenty years earlier, there was not a soul in sight to meet them. A jeep suddenly appeared on the horizon with a woman at the wheel, who came to a screeching halt in front of them. It was Jean Hollins, head of the courier service. She was here to pick up the new nurse and the young writer who planned to spend the next few weeks at Wendover. The writer's name was Elizabeth Hubbard Lansing, from New York City, and she would soon produce a well-received teenage novel based on the life and adventures of the unsung heroines of the FNS — the Frontier Nursing Service couriers.

16

Unsung Heroines

The remarkable young people who volunteered their time and energies to serve the FNS worked in conditions that were just as harsh as any the nurses encountered. They were the couriers of the Frontier Nursing Service, many of whom gave up their summers and in some cases, parts of their lives, to live and work in eastern Kentucky. Almost all women, they ranged in age from their mid-teens to their thirties and came from backgrounds as diverse as the regions from which they traveled. Most were from the areas in which there were FNS committees: New York, Boston, Washington, D.C., Pittsburgh, Cleveland, Cincinnati, Chicago, and Minneapolis. Junior couriers served a six week term; others stayed on as needed. A few lived at Wendover as FNS couriers for many years.

The younger girls were generally supported by wealthy or influential parents who gladly paid a small fee to cover their daughters' expenses, encouraging them to spend a voluntary summer with the FNS. By the 1940s, the option of serving as a courier was so popular there was a waiting list. When photos of FNS-delivered girl babies were posted in the *Quarterly Bulletin*, there were often references to "future FNS courier or nurse-midwife," only half in jest. One child, aged ten, produced an excellent detailed sketch of a horse's anatomy and sent it to Breckinridge with a note, asking her to share the pictures with the couriers. Upon receiving Breckinridge's thank-you, the little girl wrote back: "I am so glad the couriers liked the horse pictures I sent. And you sure have my permission to do anything you want with them. I was ten last December and I still have nine more years to wait to become a courier."[1]

The only formal requirement to become a courier was that one be an expert horsewoman, and by the 1940s, capable of driving a jeep. But in reality, what the couriers needed most was a high level of self-sufficiency and an ability to withstand the spartan environment. Experienced couriers contended that you had to be the type of person who exhibited common sense, initiative, and remained calm under pressure. Two of the FNS couriers were women pilots, either serving in the military or ferrying planes from factories to fields during

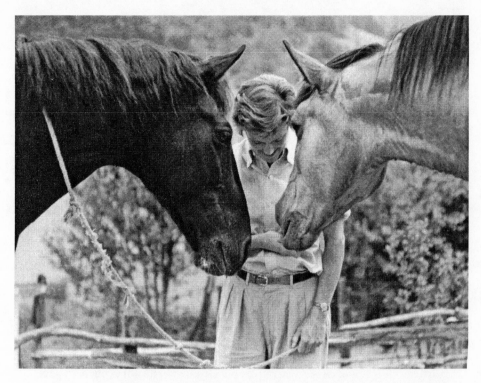

Couriers served a vital role in the Frontier Nursing Service, not only caring for the animals that belonged to the FNS, but also assisting with administrative and nursing-aide duties. This photograph of courier Freddy Holdship standing between Missy and Merry Legs was taken in the 1950s on the Wendover property (courtesy Frontier Nursing Service, Inc.).

World War II. Another was a social worker sent to Persia, Africa, Egypt, and Iraq with the Red Cross. One published a novel inspired by her visit to the FNS. Others were socially connected debutantes or secretaries, teachers, lab technicians, homemakers, artists, and government workers. Some went into nursing after observing the nurse-midwives in action. "I remember watching nurses by the light of their kerosene lamps," said one courier who served at the FNS during the 1930s. "Sometimes they would sit up until midnight checking little boxes of what they did during the day. They were very well-trained and very faithful about keeping those records."[2]

While the definition of a courier ranged from a messenger who carried mail for the Armed Services, to someone who assisted with transportation, the FNS couriers were the epitome of today's multi-taskers. Their duties included escorting guests, grooming and watering horses, painting interiors at outpost centers, handling the correspondence for fundraising appeals, stuffing envelopes, making tea for the staff, and as one courier put it, "serving at the beck and call of people when they needed us." A few even helped deliver babies or worked as nurses' aides.[3] Catherine Towbridge, a young woman from Chicago, heard Breckinridge speak at a luncheon on the FNS in the late 1920s. What impressed her was that Breckinridge held her audience captive throughout.

> We sat at a big, round table and I remember she was middle-aged, short, with straight gray hair and these enormous blue eyes, a very attractive-looking woman. She was wearing a simple dark dress with a set of beautiful blue beads. Her accent was southern but she had a strong voice. Her stories about the people in the mountains were mesmerizing — we had never heard about nurses on horseback. As we listened, I realized she knew a great deal about many subjects, from agriculture to business, and was able to talk at anyone's level.[4]

Towbridge arrived at Wendover in 1931 shortly after Breckinridge broke her back and recalls visiting her upstairs room to play bridge, indulging her love of the game. The only thing that worried Towbridge was that she did not have the skills required of an expert horsewoman. "Mrs. Breckinridge was eager to have someone from Chicago as a courier even though I was never a good horse-woman. However, I had done a lot of different volunteer work in the Chicago area. I was also older than most of the couriers. So they made a special arrangement for me, and gave me a very safe horse. I helped in the office and did whatever I could to be useful. It turned out to be a wonderful experience."

She got an insight into mountain life when she stayed overnight at a cabin with a Scottish nurse-midwife who had requested the help of a courier. "It was an isolated little valley where the family lived," said Towbridge, "and the labor was long. The nurse sent word by a little boy that she needed extra food and medical supplies, so I followed him back. When we got there, no one else was in the cabin except the mother and the nurse. The family all left to stay with neighbors." There were only two beds, both made from rough-hewn logs and stuffed with straw. As wind whistled through the cabin cracks, the courier and the nurse took turns sitting next to the fire to get warm. Towbridge recalls glancing at the walls lined with newspapers, and catching glimpses of news from her hometown. There was even a long article about people in the Chicago area that she knew. "It was so strange to come all the way to Kentucky and see it in this isolated cabin."[5]

Like all couriers, she was not allowed to travel alone at first on horseback. They had no uniforms those first few years — that would come later — and were considered "furriners" by the locals. "But once they knew we were working the Frontier Service, they welcomed us," she said. "The only danger was in winter, if icicles fell from overhanging cliffs and frightened your horse, you could go over a precipice. And yes, my parents worried. They wondered if I would be safe 'down there.'"[6] Towbridge stayed two months during that winter, mostly alone since the majority of couriers devoted only their summers. Upon her return to Chicago, she set to work establishing a chain of courier volunteers from Chicago, a venture never quite as successful as she hoped. "Most girls came from the east, not the mid-west," she said. "Maybe it was because they had to be horsewomen. But our committee always had an ear out for girls that would be interested, someone of a certain age who was free at certain times in her life, and wanted to do something worthwhile."[7]

Fitting that description was Jean Hollins from Long Island, New York. She arrived in the 1930s and stayed on at Wendover for more than thirty years, eventually becoming head courier. Learning there were no vets in the area, she took a course in animal husbandry at the University of Kentucky in Lexington, which only underscored her special affinity for animals. She could also be highly protective. When a junior courier brought in an overheated horse and let it drink before cooling down, Hollins displayed a rare flash of temper, telling the frightened young girl, "You just gave Rex the colic!" Breckinridge once sent Hollins and another young courier to Louisville with a pickup truck loaded with cow dung. The delivery site was the home of an FNS trustee who wanted it deposited on her rose beds. When they arrived, they discovered the socialite was holding a formal tea. They also knew they carried with them a pungent smell of manure. "That's all right," Hollins said to the junior courier. "I'll just put on my white gloves and we'll go right in."[8] She suffered from a chronically poor-fitting denture and once lost her false teeth in the mud as she dislodged herself from a jeep. Unperturbed, she reached down, fished them out, and stuck them in her pocket, much to the horror of her companion. But Hollins was nothing if not single-minded in her determination to do whatever was needed for the FNS.

When World War II resulted in so many of the British nurses returning to England, she took a nursing aid course in order to help out. Her golden retriever Lizzie by her side, she would hurry to Hyden Hospital and bathe patients, empty bedpans, or perform the mundane chores that freed the nurse-midwives to do other things. Arriving about the same time as Hollins was the first male courier — one of only three throughout the FNS history. Just a youth when he got to Wendover, Brooke Alexander was a second cousin of Breckinridge. "My Aunt Jane came to spend the winter with us when Breckie was four," Breckinridge wrote in her biography. "She brought with her a grandson, Brooke, so that the two children might each have companionship. Older than Breckie, he was better poised and more responsible, an imaginative, intelligent child, as dark as Breckie was fair." She went on to say that the two boys became so close "if one fell down and hurt himself, the other one grieved."[9] In time, Breckinridge asked Alexander if, when he married and had children, he would name his son "Breckie." And of course he said yes. (He would also have a daughter named Brooke.) "There was a very close relationship between my grandmother and Mary Breckinridge," said Alexander. "Her favorite name for Mary was 'Matron' and so I was trained to call her Aunt Matron." He arrived in Wendover as a teenager in 1926, where he volunteered to spend his summers for the next three years.

I made myself useful by running errands on horseback to outposts or the rail-road, or to Hyden. Going into Hazard was great because I could get a steak or buy an ice cream, rare treats unavailable at Wendover, or for that matter, in Leslie County.

"Amusingly enough," he continued, "I was also sworn in as assistant postmas-ter. This enabled me to ride into Hyden, pick up the mail bags, and bring them back to Wendover [designated as a fourth class post office].

That was a nice little bonanza for the FNS because the government subsidized each letter. The more letters that were mailed, the more money the post office made.[10]

By federal regulation, as postmaster, he was required to carry a pistol.

It was very heavy and it rubbed a blister on my hip. That was about the most I ever did with it, but I can remember riding past the mouth of Muncy Creek with the mail and hearing some pretty aggressive gunfire. It was probably a moon-shiner being rousted by federal agents, but I really don't know. Perhaps it was a feud or even a party.[11]

When a photography buff and friend of the FNS came to visit, the young Alexander served as his guide, receiving a complete set of early FNS photo-graphs as a thank-you gift. And the boy's humble first quarters—a tent—served as a repository for the Wendover dogs, where they and the many fleas they car-ried slept on top of his bed. A close friend, James Parton, joined him the sum-mer of 1929. As courier, the two boys set out to savor their summer adventure. Parton was sixteen and described himself as a "tousle-haired Tom Sawyer." He would later graduate from Harvard.

I had never been on a horse in my life. But when I got to Hazard there was Brooke on horseback, leading another horse. I shoved my duffle into a pair of saddle bags and climbed on. It was a twenty-two mile ride over the mountains to Wendover, fording several streams. The horse was a trotter and I didn't know what I was doing. At one point, while fording the stream, the girth slipped and I fell off. So did all the gear. We also got into quicksand. It was quite scary because we came close to losing our horses. The suction was so great it pulled the shoe off one of my horses' hooves.

He also said that by the time he got to Wendover, he was so sore he was unable to sit for three days.[12] The boys bunked in a primitive shed behind the Big House with wooden plank floors, thin walls, and screens for windows. Their primary job was to greet the British nurse-midwives as they arrived and escort them to Hyden Hospital or to whichever outpost center they were assigned. It was often a forty-mile ride round trip, with some of the English girls as unac-customed to riding as they were. Bringing them in, according to Parton, "took considerable effort." Other chores included cleaning the stalls, making sure there was hot water and clean towels for the nurses, and once even helping restrain a mother during delivery. In the evenings they played bridge by them-selves or with the nurses, or listened to the crackling radio known mostly for its poor reception. If the river was high, they'd take a swim — once encountering a group of local boys who harassed them and received a dunking for their trouble.

One night the two teenagers, ready to turn in at Wendover, were told they had a special assignment. Someone near Hell for Certain Creek had been bitten by a rattlesnake and needed serum. They must go now, and hurry, for there was no anti-venom at the outpost centers and none at the hospital. "But we had some at Wendover," said Parton, "so Brooke and I set off on our horses carrying the snake serum and galloping up and down the trails as fast as we could. I forgot there was a low-hanging branch and when I hit it I disappeared — clunk! — off the horse. Luckily, my feet didn't catch in the stirrups. I landed on my rump in the dirt."[13] The boys made it in time and for years enjoyed recounting their gallant "midnight ride."

About once a week the horses were taken to the north fork of the river where they were bathed and given a rubdown. Parton didn't normally mind the routine, but he did have trouble with an old mule named Bluey.

> I think he got his name because he constantly had saddle sores and needed a blue medicine. He was very stubborn, especially when fording the north fork. When the water was low, there were frequent sandbars and Bluey couldn't resist getting down to roll. You had to jump off of him fast, otherwise your legs would get caught and you'd be injured. Someone told us to put a pebble in his ear to keep him moving. Moving around was the only way he would shake out the stone.

Unlike Parton, Alexander had a special fondness for the diminutive mule. "He was simply a marvelous character," he said. "On a number of occasions I took the horses to the railroad and had to ride Bluey back, getting off and walking him in the steep places. It wasn't difficult because he was patient and would allow me to grab hold of his tail while he pulled me up the mountain."[14] It was Alexander and Parton who found Teddy Bear, Breckinridge's favorite horse (and the one on which she was frequently photographed) after the animal had fallen and critically injured itself. The teenagers considered Breckinridge an expert, elegant rider "absolutely devoted to Teddy [Bear]." "After their day's work, the horses often gathered down at the pasture gate, where they would graze and then return to the stables," Parton said. "One evening Teddy [Bear] didn't show up. Brooke and I went looking for him and found the poor thing upside-down on his back in a rock crevice, two feet deep alongside a huge maple tree. He was totally wedged." The boys ran to find help, coming across some neighboring mountaineers. "The locals were always cooperative in this type of situation," Parton recalled. "They said they couldn't cut down the tree because it was too close to the horse's side. Finally, they managed to grab its front legs and lash them together. They lashed the two hind legs, got a rope and a pulley, and we lifted the horse out."[15] If the men had not helped, the boys claimed they would not have known what to do. "We were just kids," Parton said. "The sad thing was that Teddy was so injured he did not survive."[16] The beloved horse died two days later; a blow to everyone at Wendover.

In 1933, the year Breckinridge decided to charter a ship as a special fundraising event for the FNS, she invited Parton and Alexander to serve on board as "assistant cruise directors." Both in college by then, Alexander cut three weeks of classes at Princeton and Parton did the same at Harvard in order to take what they considered a hard-earned FNS vacation. Ann Mulhauser, Mardi Perry, and Susan Putnam arrived as new couriers in the mid–1930s. They all remember the numerous animals on the property, particularly Breckinridge's annoying squad of geese, including Pete and Repeat. "She thought they were the nicest little goslings," Mulhauser said, "but I thought they were mean. I was scared to death of them because they kept coming after me." One complained the geese ran up and bit her in the fanny every time she got near them. Two of Breckinridge's favorites, Splash and Bottle, hung out at the barn where the couriers worked with the horses, and were generally loathed by the young women. "You'd fill a bucket with water for the horses," said one courier, "bring out a horse that was thirsty which had been shut in a stall for several hours, and a goose would have its nose in the bucket. So we'd have to throw the water out and fill it again. In the meantime, the horse was trampling all over us because it needed a drink."[17]

The girls recalled that Hyden in the midst of the Depression was totally cut off from civilization, "a drab and dreary spot," said Putnam. "Main Street was a small dirt road full of enormous holes. Pigs and cows and an occasional mule wandered up and down the streets. On either side were dilapidated wooden buildings. The courthouse was the social center, or so it seemed, for there was always a trial going on. Of course that was an excuse for all the locals to get together for fun." Putnam said she often felt uncomfortable riding through town "because the jailbirds would stare out at you. There was need, unfortunately, for these trials due to whiskey-making during Prohibition. Men would be caught at their stills by the sheriff and a feud would erupt. But whatever ill feelings the mountaineers might have toward government or each other, they had the greatest respect for Mrs. Breckinridge and her staff of nurses and helpers."[18] Therefore, it was generally safe for a nurse or a courier to go anywhere at any time of day or night. Still, she added, it was wiser to stay away from town on Saturday nights. Putnam, originally from Boston, recalls one of the oddest sights she encountered during her summer in the Cumberland Mountains.

My first solo job was taking an extra horse to one of the nurses living at the most distant center, off the usual circuit. I spent the night at Flat Creek and continued the next day over a completely strange route. The horse was lazy and nearly pulled my arms out trying to lead him. The country was flatter than usual and quite uninhabited. Only occasionally did I come across a cabin. It was hot, so most families sat on their porches and shouted a friendly "Howdy" as I went by.

Toward evening, on my return trip, a wild-looking mountaineer rode toward me. He was on a white mule, wore a big hat, and as he came closer I realized he had only one eye. The other was an empty socket. But he greeted me with the usual howdy and I felt all right about him. Then, after he passed me, I turned around to stare at him. And there, riding on each hip pocket, were the handles of huge six-shooter guns.[19]

By contrast, Breckinridge made a unanimously favorable impression on the young couriers. Some referred to her as "a great person, a great talker, never at a loss for words." Others said she had "a great mind," and made a stern, but reasonable employer. "There was a lot of respect and a little trepidation toward her," said a 1937 courier. "She didn't mind telling you off if you were wrong about your thinking. So you minded your P's and Q's. But she was always very fair." [20] The couriers felt they were treated well by the other staff, but at the same time knew their place in the FNS hierarchy. At the dining table in the Big House, which usually held twelve or more people on any given day, the couriers sat at the far end. Everyone had a designated place, with Breckinridge always seated at the head of the table.

There was no electricity at Wendover in 1935 and little indoor heat, so the couriers who stayed past summer had to endure the inconvenience of kerosene lamps and bitter cold winters. Most bunked in one of the outbuildings near the Big House. One courier recalls having to break the ice that formed in the pitchers every morning in order to wash her face and hands. Mary Wilson Neel was one of the couriers who periodically gave up her freedom for the FNS. Her fiancé told her the greatest competition he faced in winning her hand was her "other beau," the Frontier Nursing Service. Yet she would later call her tenure with the organization "the strongest chapter in my life." She became a courier in the late 1930s, served a term, and then returned home to Abingdon, Virginia.

I had only been home about three weeks when a courier friend and I received an emergency telegram from Mrs. Breckinridge saying that everyone at Wendover was down with the flu, and could we return. My friend Marian had a little Chevrolet convertible she shared with her sister. It had wooden floorboards, no rug, and no heater. We set out in February and drove the entire distance in one day.

When we arrived, we slept on cots in the office on the first floor of the Garden House. Everyone in the Big House was down, just decimated with flu, with no one to run errands or do anything. About half the population in Hyden was sick too. So we just started pitching in doing whatever we could.[21]

At night, the two exhausted couriers would hole up in their room, hoping they wouldn't get sick. According to FNS rules enforced by Breckinridge, the couriers were not allowed to drink anything stronger than sherry. "But," said Neel, "Marian had a little bottle that she kept hidden in the bottom drawer of the file cabinets and she will tell you to this day that the reason we did not get the flu was because we had a nip of whiskey before we went to sleep each night. Before that, I never drank whiskey in my life."[22] During her term as a courier she also recalls having to carry kerosene lamps, a constant fire hazard, from one room to another. "Even if you went into the next room for five minutes, you took it with you or blew it out. We were terrified of fire and, of course, the Garden House did later burn down. The bathroom was down two flights of stairs, one of which was an outside set of stairs, and down through the furnace room, all of which was a nightmare. So you didn't do this often in the wintertime."

With no two workdays alike, she said they never knew where they would be from one hour to the next. But the element of surprise was what appealed most to the couriers—that and a chance to work outside with animals. "We got up in the morning, put on our old blue jeans and went out to water the horses," said Neel. "You might think you were going to Brutus Center, to the hospital to work, or be cleaning tack in the barn. The chances were almost a hundred percent you'd be doing something different."[23] Senior couriers escorted the junior employees to the different nursing centers.

> You were terribly important that first time. Then you were expected to know how to get to those places and how long it was going to take you, how many creeks you had to cross. You wore comfortable clothes with a little FNS name tag in large letters which you sewed onto your sleeve. It really wasn't necessary because everybody recognized the FNS horses and the FNS girls. Kentucky women didn't ride horses in riding boots. They wore dresses and walked or rode on the back of a mule.[24]

As with other couriers, many of the local conditions took her by surprise. She had a singer's ear and was sensitive to certain speech patterns. Getting a handle on how people spoke required some effort. And the abject poverty was startling to Neel. "Everything from mittens to shoes was a hand-me-down. Sometimes a boy would say his brother couldn't come to school or go somewhere because he was wearing the shoes that day. His brother would come the next day, or the day after, when it was his turn to have the shoes."[25] "Everyone struggled, but they were not disgruntled," said a courier who worked for the FNS in the early 1940s. "Despite what they lacked, they were always very pleasant people with a wonderful sense of family. I remember attending a party one Saturday night and the only refreshment they served was water. That was all they had. Yet everyone had a good time."[26] Couriers learned to appreciate the strong sense of community and the steady willingness of neighbors helping neighbors. "When someone died, the women took care of the deceased's body," said Neel. "The neighboring men or members of the family made the pine coffin and carried it on their shoulders to the burying ground. There were no strangers involved in this, no money changed hands. And I thought that was quite significant; a big difference [in cultures] that I noticed immediately."[27]

On Election Day in Hyden, residents rode in from miles around on horses and mules. Entire families came to town for it was often the only time they had

a chance to socialize. Once, when an FNS mare became ill, the nurses and couriers discussed how best to treat the sick animal. Someone suggested a mash
made from alcohol might work. But they all knew Leslie County was dry.

> We were well aware of the fact there was moonshine around. But it was com-
> pletely taboo to discuss it. So I asked one of the nurses what we were going to
> do. She told me the "mountain grapevine" would take care of it. And so we
> began to spread the word about the sick mare. The next day I went down to the
> mailbox and there was a pint of white lightning. I made up a brown mash for
> the mare and twenty-four hours later, she was on her feet.[28]

Among the more unusual experiences Neel had with the FNS was one involving herding cows on a two-day trek down the river. The newly bred cows were
scheduled for delivery to Bowlington Center and the trip would require an
overnight stay. Neel and another young courier were assigned the job of transporting them.

> We were on horseback, with the Kentucky stitched-down saddles which did not
> have a horn. And these heifers had never been out of the pasture, or on a road,
> never been halter broken, or led anywhere. So we had to hold the horses' reins
> with one hand and the heifer with the other. On several occasions, we were fol-
> lowed by bulls which were loose and wandering through the countryside. They
> attacked our heifers in various undignified manners. And the mountain people
> did nothing to help us because they thought it was the funniest thing they had
> ever seen. We would go down the road and a path would go right or left. The
> heifer would veer in the opposite direction and we'd have to physically drag the
> thing back.

She later said it was the most exhausted she had ever been in her life, not
to mention the most fearful she was of failing at her job. Yet she grew to love
the mountain region. Each season brought its own sense of wonder. "I liked
going on rounds from one center to another. In winter, you could only ride for
a short time before your foot or leg would get frozen to the stirrup. You'd have
to get off and walk a bit; get back on. I was cold all the time. But the mountains were beautiful during that time and I loved it."[29] Like the nurse-midwives, the couriers turned to each other to break the isolation and counter the
hard physical conditions. One way to have fun was by playing practical jokes
on each other.

Helen "Pebble" Stone was a senior courier from Long Island. Her colleague, Marianne Harper, from Chicago, remembers her as a serious girl whose
primary goal was to keep the other couriers on task and in line. Stone would
later serve in the military as a courier-aviator ferrying airplanes; she had a no-
nonsense attitude that sometimes riled the younger couriers. "As a result, she
wasn't very popular with me and another junior courier," said Harper. "One
day she went off to an outpost center and returned to Wendover dusty and
tired. All she wanted was to get into a nice, hot bath."[30] The girls offered to fill
the tub for their coworker. Stone, surprised but pleased at this unusually kind

gesture, sat down to relax. A few minutes later the girls motioned her into the room where her bath was waiting — filled to the brim with live ducks from the chicken yard. "We also played simple board games and worked puzzles," said Mary Neel. "I did a lot of reading. Mrs. Breckinridge had many books, classics that were translated into French, Tolstoy, things like that. The evenings went by quickly and we were usually tired."[31] Every so often a square dance was held in the cabins closest to Wendover, drawing people from miles around. Three of the couriers were invited to a dance held on a Saturday night in the mid–1930s. Their only form of transportation for the three-mile trip was a mule which they took turns riding to the social. What one courier remembered most was not the mule that transported her, but the role of the hostess once they arrived.

> Quite a crowd of men and women had gathered and one man was tuning his guitar. He only played two notes the entire evening. But just as the dance began, the hostess came around and collected all the pistols for lockup. One man refused to give up his firearm because he had it in for another who had gone off with his girl. There was a slight altercation between the two, but nothing came of it. It was hotter than hinges that night, and we were pushed and pulled and shoved in all directions during the dance. After a while we caught on to the steps and were quite exhausted when we finally got back home.[32]

But in the end, it was Mary Breckinridge herself who left the most lasting impression on the girls.

> She was a great influence in my life and in my thinking. She had a spiritual quality and warmth of spirit that I have never met in another woman. She came to my house one day after I had my two small children. Employed at my home was a very dignified nurse of a mixed race, wearing a starched white uniform. Mary Breckinridge put her arm around the nurse and said, "Ethel, aren't these children lucky to have someone like you to love and take care of them?" Whereas my mother's friends would just come in and say, "How do you do?" But Mrs. Breckinridge would embrace you; make you feel like a better person.
> Now how many people greet strangers that way?[33]

Of the couriers, Breckinridge said they aroused more curiosity from outsiders than anything else related to the Frontier Nursing Service. Referring to them as "these young things," she said that by and large, they left her with the impression they were one step ahead of her own generation. "They have more initiative than we had," she declared. "They are less evasive, and in their frankness, they tend to see things whole. Although I would not say their courage is greater than ours, it has been tested in ways that lay beyond our remotest dreams. What they gave us," she added, "was the generous abandonment of their youth."[34]

17

A Day in the Life of a Courier

Courier Dorothy Caldwell arrived at Wendover in 1935 while the Depression was still underway. Her first impression of the region was that it was poor, with subsistence farming, no mining or logging industry as yet, but nonetheless a hardy, friendly community. "I loved the local people. I remember one in particular, a Mrs. Morgan, who worked a lot with Mrs. Breckinridge in the garden. Mrs. Morgan would share old mountain tales about herbs, flowers, and weeds. Keeping ahead of pigweed was a big problem. Her favorite expression was that the only way you could get ahead of pigweed was 'to die and leave it.'"[1]

Caldwell also remembers Breckinridge with her broken back propped up in bed amid "a block of pillows, coffee in hand," planning orders for the day and maintaining a grip on every ongoing activity. The couriers often made her tea — terrified it would turn out wrong — and listened while she entertained herself by attempting to shock her assistant Agnes Lewis. "Physically, Agnes was a tiny woman and very prim," said one courier, "and there were certain things she didn't like discussing. So Mrs. Breckinridge would try to get a rise by talking about the best way to make a fly trap with a little honey and manure, things like that. I always thought her very amusing, if somewhat a little off-color at times."[2]

The loyal, hardworking Lewis was in charge of the couriers during this decade. "It was always a very incongruous situation because Agnes didn't know beans about horses," said Caldwell, "or about frontier living. But she would undertake absolutely anything she was asked to do. And she accepted it very graciously, though she did an awful lot of worrying." As she learned the ropes, Caldwell said a few truths began to unwind: not all of the horses were Tennessee Walkers. And despite common beliefs, medicine bottles did not normally break in the saddlebag, for they were well-padded and packed. "For a novice rider, a Tennessee Walker horse was most comfortable," she said, "because you didn't have to do anything but sit there. But I never had one, and there were lots of us who didn't. None of the English nurses were familiar with them. Even so, some took to caring for their horses very well, as Mrs. Breckinridge tried to make them all responsible for their animals." Betty Lester, she says, as district nurse at Red Bird Center, was a good rider. "But then Betty was one of those people who did everything well."

She once accompanied Lester on a delivery where a local granny midwife was trying to assist the new mother. "She was called a granny midwife though she was just a girl herself," Caldwell said. "She was only about twenty-four and told us this was the first woman she had tried to deliver. But she had lots of experience in birthing pigs."[3] The delivery went as planned and Caldwell gained a new appreciation for the expertise of the "top-notch" nurse-midwives and the entire FNS organization.

Another misconception was that nurses and couriers were always getting lost. While that did happen on occasion, couriers had a map of the county that showed creeks, roads, and those areas where the creek *became* the road. In addition, said Caldwell, whenever a courier met someone on the trail, it was commonplace to ask if they were on the right road or path. "The locals were always helpful," she said. "And if you were near their house they most likely invited you in. You couldn't normally accept, because you were under pressure to get somewhere. But they were very friendly."[4]

A typical day in the life of a courier was poetically captured by Patricia Pettit during the 1940s through almost daily letters she wrote to her mother during her stay at the FNS. At first she found the steep Cumberland Mountains stifling, as though they were pressing in around her. Before long, however, she began to appreciate their stark beauty and felt protected by them, calling their timelessness "majestic." "I grew to love them," she said, "especially when there was clear, golden sunshine with a crisp breeze. I shall never forget those mountain nights with the stars luminous in the crystal air. It was absolutely silent except for the rush of the river. It was the most heavenly life: Wind, pines, brooks, clean rain, log fires, and all around the great, quiet mountains continually carrying your eyes upward."[5]

Up at seven for breakfast, she began her routine by grooming the horses, a chore she likened to "grooming bears, with furry-wooly coats a mile long." "The horses, an odd combination species, were sturdy and sure-footed. They ranged from plantation walkers to mountain bred gaited and had great long tails that dragged in the mud. We also cleaned tack — soaping the saddles and scraping the girths — washing out thick saddle blankets."[6] Lunch was always served at noon and might consist of fried chicken, hot vegetables, and fresh-baked biscuits. A "huge" supper was roast pork, browned potatoes, pickles, jams, carrots, fresh slaw, baked onions, and butterscotch pudding. Despite the intense physical labor and the almost daily horseback riding, Pettit gained fifteen pounds during her FNS stay.

She had packed the wrong shoes and complained that with all the mud which seemed to remain at Wendover between rains, what she needed most were rubber or even cowboy boots. "If you run into a pair of size seven and a half, with round toes, I sure could use them," she wrote her mother.[7] She liked riding the "funny little" flat bottom boat (a skiff) across the river at high tide; playing rummy or Chinese checkers at night with Yum-Yum the cat curled in her lap and Peter, the red-gold collie, at her feet; luxuriating in a hot bath; sitting around the fire reading while listening to *Pagliacci* play softly in the background on the antiquated Victrola.

Wendover was the ideal place to be alone, yet never lonely, she said. And she found it amazing and intriguing that livestock roamed the property at will. She wrote home:

> We never go down the road that we don't meet a couple of pigs and cows out for a stroll, whereas in Hyden any loose cow is put in jail and has to be bailed out with a dollar. The hospital cow spent a night in jail last week.
> But Wendover is perfect because while there are always plenty of people to chat with, it is possible to go your own way and have little or nothing to do with anyone. Everyone is so busy and occupied they never bother with you or intrude on your moods. It is a closely-knit community yet made up of separate individuals. Whenever we get to Wendover, we always have a warm welcome but not a cloying one.

Then she added a postscript to reassure her mother that she *did* have friends.

> If this letter makes no sense it is because Neville (another courier) is lying on top of her bed in pink pajamas, her hair in braids, horn-rimmed glasses propped upon her nose, sucking on a lollipop. She is reading a book called *The Human Mind* that amuses her, so she alternately reads out loud, then giggles, and has now decided she is going to analyze me.[8]

The highlight of any courier's stay at the FNS, however, was being asked to accompany a nurse-midwife on rounds or to attend a delivery. It could take up to a week to reach all the outlying FNS centers. "We visited two families who had pneumonia, Pettit wrote. "In one cabin the mother and baby were sick. The nurses bathed them both," the mother looking very young and pathetic. We took the blankets outside and shook them out, for they were full of bread and cracker crumbs, along with a few beans. Bed sheets were made from flour sacks."[9] On a scheduled visit to one of the post-partum mothers who had registered a dangerously high blood pressure reading, the FNS women found only the children at home, the stalwart woman having walked to the nearest store. Getting food for her children was a more critical need than having her high blood pressure checked.

Close to one of the outpost centers, a call came in that a mother was experiencing a difficult labor. The house had two rooms, fairly large by mountain standards, and was situated on a steep narrow path that ran alongside the creek. "The poor husband was in a state when we got there," Pettit said. "His mule had just died from an injury and he didn't know how he was going to feed his family without it. Polly (his wife) was sitting in a chair. It was dark and there was no light except for the fire. There were several things that didn't appear right about the birth, but Polly never uttered a sound throughout the whole thing, not even a moan when the pains came. The only way you could tell she was in pain was by her heavy breathing. When the baby was born, we thought it was dead. The nurse worked over it for forty-five minutes before it gave a real sign of life. By the time we left several hours later, the mother and the baby were both all right and Polly was asking for food. It was a lovely moonlit night and perfect for the ride back."[10] Making rounds with the nurse-midwives gave the couriers a taste of what the FNS was designed to do best — reaching people in need in the outermost regions of the mountains.

"We left Wendover about two and started up the river further into the mountains," Pettit reported following their trip. "The nurse rode Lassie, a black mare who is fine once you get on her but kicks like a mule when saddled. I rode Kelpie, a chubby little mahogany bay mare with an angelic disposition. We traveled through lovely pines, and a deep green river that breaks into foamy white rapids among huge gray rocks.[11] The 'road' crosses and re-crosses the river. Every few miles we passed cabins where thin, cold-looking children stared at us shyly. But the older people were all friendly. There are always a few pigs and a mule at these places. People ride the mules to go "outside" except when they are tide-bound, as they call it when the river rises." She also recalled passing a woman making soap, mixing the lye and fat in a huge iron-cast kettle while standing beneath a hemlock tree; going through main street Hyden en route to the hospital and watching "a million mountaineers laughing in front of the tiny courthouse."[12]

Outside the Hyden Hospital, FNS nurses were milling about in their riding clothes, admiring the newly constructed barn. Inside, the wards were full with patients including one who had walked in the night before and quietly put herself to bed. No one noticed her until the morning when during rounds, they found the formerly empty cot now occupied by an unknown woman. She said she had appendicitis. And upon examination, the staff learned she was right. She was moved to the Surgical Clinic. There was no anesthetist at the hospital so the superintendent volunteered to serve. They also needed type B blood for the patient. Word went out to the townspeople who voluntarily came up the hill to the clinic for type and cross-match. After more than thirty attempts to find a match, one of the doctors, a Type B, stepped up and raised his sleeve.

Courier Pettit's first outpost stop was Beech Fork Center, a white-framed house with a neat, four-stall barn nearby. She rubbed the horses down and settled them in stalls to rest while the nurse-midwife went inside the clinic. The nurse's role was to check in and discuss pending cases with the onsite staff. Like most of the outposts, Beech Fork had a home-like atmosphere — a large living room with stone fireplace, well-worn rugs and curtains at the window. "These nurses at the center," said Pettit, "were graduate midwives. The fact that it was still almost impossible to reach a doctor; the closest one our medical director at Hyden Hospital, made it necessary for them to be terribly well-trained."[13] The women stayed overnight at Beech Fork, enjoying a hot bath and a change of clothes taken from their saddlebags. Next day, they headed for the Red Bird Nursing Center. Before leaving, Pettit groomed the horses and found she had to tack a few nails into one of the horse's loose shoes. "We started up Bad Creek Trail, climbing a good deal of the time. We passed fewer cabins and rode a great deal in the creek beds. Everywhere were rocky creeks and slippery, mossy rocks. When we reached the Red Bird River, the country changed quite a bit — the valley broadened out and for the first time we could really see ahead. It was a pleasant change to be away from the weight of the mountains that seemed to overhang and enclose us."[14]

Flat Creek Center featured an open floor plan — large combo living room and dining room with the traditional stone fireplace plus a bay window, a design adopted for many of the outpost centers. There were also two guest rooms, one double room with beds, a clinic, a waiting room, a kitchen, and a maid's room. Tiger, the collie, met them at the door and Mary, the maid — "the envy of the FNS service," according to Pettit — cooked them a fine meal. A virtual domestic goddess, the maid also sewed slip covers for the chairs, designed and made quilts, milked the cow, and fed the horses.

> When we got there, a warm fire and tea were waiting for us. Benny, the nurse, who is young and English, was quite tired but very cordial. The day before, she had taken care of a patient who was carried by stretcher three miles to the Hyden Hospital. Just as she returned to Flat Creek, she was called for a delivery. Then a second, harassed father arrived on mule and begged that she come to his wife. The places were three miles apart. As her horse had been out all day, she walked, or as she says, ran from one cabin to another, and this was at night. She finally, she says, "caught" both babies.[15]

That night, sitting around the fireplace sipping hot coffee, the women talked about the current war news. Three of the FNS nurses had brothers stationed on battleships near the coast of Norway and worried about their safety throughout the war. There was talk of meat shortages and how tired they were of chicken, and conversely how satisfying it was to hear that women were now doing jobs formerly held by men — from driving trucks to loading heavy equipment. It turned cold the next morning, with snow falling in the higher elevations. Pettit spent the morning cleaning tack and grooming the horses, her hands going numb with the cold. At least she could sit by the fire for a couple of hours before they headed out to Red Bird Center. "It was a short and pleasant ride from Flat Creek," she reported, "though the dirt road had deep mud in places. When we got to the center it was early so we had plenty of time to prowl around. The house is built on the same plan as Flat Creek but is made from logs."[16]

They also visited the Brutus Nursing Center, stopping periodically to shift the weight in their saddlebags. They passed the strange, one-eyed man on a white mule who rode with them silently a while, and encountered a severe thunderstorm that left them drenched and chilly. At the center, the courier found an injured mule that needed tending. Its owner had used a hot, home-made compress that contained turpentine resulting in a huge blister on the animal's leg. A second medical opinion from the staff at Wendover was needed, so she tried using the phone to call Wendover. But there was no direct line. "It's maddening," she said. "I have to talk to Eva at Bowlington, then she talks to Hyden, and Hyden talks to Wendover, and their answers come back via Hyden and Eva!"[17]

The next day, after grooming the horses, Pettit and the nurse-midwife began their journey back to Wendover. It was a twenty-five mile ride which they covered in a little more than four hours. Throughout the strenuous trip, Pettit's admiration grew for the endurance displayed by the horses. "Just marvelous animals," she raved. "They travel miles and miles of rough country tirelessly. Kelpie and Lassie were still fresh and keen when we got in. It's amazing how quickly they cover the ground."[18]

Eighteen-year-old junior courier Mary Stewart, whose grandmother was an acquaintance of Mary Breckinridge, came to the FNS in June 1942 after making her debut in Cincinnati along with her close friend, Jean Sawyer. Stewart's mother told the girls it would be a good summer for them to do something worthwhile, like volunteer their time with the FNS. So the girls hitched a ride to Hyden with relatives en route to a vacation in North Carolina. It was ninety-five degrees when they arrived in Hyden. The first thing they would discover in the mountains was that few things happened in a hurry. As instructed, the girls waited for their ride to Wendover. "We sat there in the heat, waiting and waiting," said Stewart. "Finally this dusty old jeep approached us and stopped. The driver, a woman, helped us load our things. It was a long drive back in the hills, fording streams, going around the river in places where the water was too high to ford. I remember bumping and splashing through water and all of us getting wet. I looked at my friend and we both shook our heads. We'd never been anyplace like this before."[19]

When they arrived at the Big House, Breckinridge herself came downstairs to greet them according to Stewart. "She didn't seem terribly old to me at the time, but what did impress me was that she cared enough about us to come downstairs. We were hugged and kissed and told how much we were welcomed. There was a lot of friendliness and warmth among that early staff. Jean and I felt like we were their daughters."[20] The newly arrived teen couriers were told that among their first chores was to transport a week's worth of laundry — on horseback. Again, the girls looked at each other in surprise. "I had a pony in my youth," said Stewart, "but I really had not ridden much. My friend, Jean, knew a little something about horses." But neither knew much about laundry. The only way they could figure how to transport the cumbersome load of linen was wrap it in a sheet and secure it with a knot. "Of course it rained," Stewart said, "so out we go, miles down the road with this giant load in front. The rain made the clothing twice as heavy. Our job was to take it to the woman who did the FNS wash. She lived at the top of a slippery, muddy hill. I can remember getting off and leading the horse, wondering if I was going to make it. Directions were always so casual — 'Go up and there's a tree with a wonderful big branch that hangs over this stream and you take a right turn....[21] Anyway, I dragged this huge pile of laundry through the mud and up to the woman's door. How she ever got all that wash done, I'll never know."

On one of their rounds, Jean Sawyer suffered a severe asthma attack. Stewart ran to find an FNS nurse and begged her to give her friend an injection. But the nurse said she needed a doctor's permission to do so. Despite numerous attempts, the physician could not be reached. "The nurse was very capable," said Stewart, "and knew what she was doing. But there was a strict rule about giving medication without doctor approval. At the same time, people die if they don't get this type treatment when they need it."[22] As Sawyer's attack grew worse, the FNS nurse made a tough decision. "The nurse expressed a great deal of concern, but finally gave her the shot. She really put her career at risk by doing it. But I never heard a word of criticism from the doctor, or from Mrs. Breckinridge," said Stewart.

The girls became such reliable couriers that Breckinridge entrusted them to escort young patients to Cincinnati by train for treatment at the Ohio hospital. "We got on the train with this little child who was absolutely petrified, having never been on a train in her life," said Stewart. "And it was hotter than blazes; the train full of passengers. Trains were always full back then. We opened the windows to get some air and the coal dust blew right in. So we arrived in Cincinnati covered in black soot."[23] Cases like this, and couriers like Stewart and Sawyer, helped spread the work and the reputation of the Frontier Nursing Service, sometimes reaching the highest pinnacles of U.S. government.

As a White House party attended by a 1940s FNS courier, Mrs. Eleanor Roosevelt asked about specific cases involving children and the Frontier Nursing Service in general. She was a friend of Mrs. Breckinridge and appeared interested in the FNS, offering her name in the support of the organization. In fact, Eleanor Roosevelt led the list of Washington, D.C., sponsors for FNS fundraising events and often introduced Breckinridge when she spoke in the capital. She would then invite the FNS director to lunch or dinner at the White House, including a family meal with the president where he regaled her with stories of his horseback rides through the Cumberland Mountains.

Another, earlier prominent Washington connection was with Supreme Court Justice Louis Brandeis, the first Jewish Supreme Court Justice in U.S. history. Appointed by Woodrow Wilson in 1916, he served until 1939 and was a contributor to the progressive wing of the Democratic Party. He also supported competition, rather than monopoly in business. Brandeis' wife invited Breckinridge for tea whenever their paths would cross. With Kentucky ties in common (he was born in Louisville in 1856) Brandeis would sit and talk with Breckinridge, usually alone, as she marveled at his "vast and humane intellect that ranged all over the world."[24] That the First Family and the highest judicial official in the land had knowledge of and appreciated the Frontier Nursing Service was not only good business for the organization, but a major coup for Breckinridge and those who dedicated their work and their hearts in order to work alongside her.

18

Changing Times

Though horses would continue to be used through the early 1960s, the Frontier Nursing Service was turning to jeeps by the end of the war as an alternate form of transportation. The vehicles were obtained by an arrangement through FNS connections in Detroit where thousands of jeeps were manufactured for the U.S. Army. Breckinridge was quick to realize their practical value as newly constructed roads were beginning to make Leslie County more accessible to the outside world. The War Department agreed to lend the FNS a vehicle, and the Detroit Friends of the FNS drove it to Wendover in 1945 along with a mechanic to teach the couriers and nurses how to operate and maintain it. Like all FNS-acquired property, it soon had a name. It was dubbed Jane. Every week, Jane was thoroughly greased in order to ford and re-ford the Middle Fork River on its various treks in and out of Wendover. One of the first trips was transporting Breckinridge to Manchester in Clay County for a speaking engagement to thank the women there for donating handmade quilts used in baby layettes. Marion Lewis, an assistant to Breckinridge, was the driver. "Along the way, we met a road construction gang in another, larger jeep," said Breckinridge. "Marion said that at the sight of her 'big brother,' Jane quivered with thrills."[1]

Not everyone was enamored of the new form of transportation. Betty Lewis, for one — who had her fill of jeeps during the war in England — did not take kindly to the change. Horses did not stall out in the middle of the river or slide off an icy curve in the road; they responded when you talked to them; you couldn't pat a jeep and expect a grateful response; and most of all, how could you be a Frontier Nurse in a *jeep* of all things? After all, they were nurses on horseback — a romantic, adventurous image that would now be forever changed. Nonetheless, she admitted a nurse could carry more and go farther and faster in a vehicle. The FNS soon had six jeeps in its possession (including the fetching Leo, black with red trim and red leather seats) and had reduced its number of horses from forty to twenty-four, noting it was more expensive to feed the lesser number due to rising costs. Horses were still used at the Brutus outpost nursing center where there was no phone connection as yet, but patients could be transported from Brutus to the Hyden Hospital by jeep. Several horses also remained at Wendover.

Some of the nurses, couriers, and secretaries were experienced drivers; others were new to the wheel. Betty Lester learned to drive through trial and error in the 1930s, purchasing a bright yellow Model A Ford convertible she christened Samanthy that carried her and her friends from Maine to Florida. It was only after her return from England following the war that she learned the details of its demise: someone had borrowed it to fill his lighter from the gasoline tank and caught Samanthy on fire. As more jeeps were acquired by the FNS, arriving from the Willys Motor Company in Toledo, Ohio, they soon provided their own set of challenges for the staff. When administrative assistant Lucille Knechtly went to get her driver's license in Leslie County, her road test was in an FNS jeep — even though the examiner had never ridden in one. "During the driving test," recalled Knechtly, "he asked me what the two sticks on the floorboard were about. I told him it was for BAD roads only. Fortunately, he didn't pursue the subject."[2] Whenever the vehicles stalled in the river at high tide they had to be coaxed back to life. Head courier Jean Hollins once had Bounce on an errand in the early predawn hours when the vehicle died. Hollins removed her dry shirt, climbed out, waded through the water, and opened the hood to dry out the sparkplugs, re-dressing in the dark. It was also her thankless duty to ensure the other couriers could drive the cantankerous jeeps and perform basic vehicle maintenance. Hollins often remarked that with the advent of jeeps, she became gray-headed.[3]

Among the memorable adventures involving jeeps was a trip Betty Lester took with a three-month-old pig named Louise. A pure-bred Duroc raised at Wendover, the animal needed transportation to the Brutus nursing center at Breckinridge's request. What could be easier, she said later. The adventure was captured in a story published in the FNS *Quarterly Bulletin*: Louise was placed inside a crate in the back of the jeep and secured so she would not slide around over the bumpy road out of Wendover. All went well until she reached Hyden. An onlooker asked if one of her nursing jobs was toting pigs around. Lester, dressed in full FNS uniform, waved at him gaily. What she didn't notice was that Louise had her head squeezed between the bars in the crate. The pig had decided it was time to disembark.

Someone hollered at Lester, pointing to the back of the jeep. Lester slammed on the brakes and saw the squealing Louise run past and disappear down an embankment. She stopped the jeep and took off after her. The bank led down to the edge of the river, where Lester was cautiously approaching. By now Louise had stopped for a snack, munching on a patch of weeds. Lester reached out with both hands and grabbed the pig's tail. Louise spun and released a loud squeal. A trucker slowed down on the road above and Lester could see him pointing toward her, laughing at her predicament while Louise continued her high-pitched protest. Nurse and pig played tug of war. The most traveled road in Hyden and not a soul stops to help me, Lester thought. A coal miner walking home from work passed by. "Would you back up my jeep for me?" Lester yelled. "Aim it toward the pig!" He jumped into the vehicle, maneuvered it toward Lester, and climbed out, grabbing the animal's hind leg and one ear. Between them, the two adults managed to drop the still-squealing Louise into the crate, punching the bars into place. Lester had her dog's leash in the jeep and used it to better corral the pig. But she tried escaping again. "Oh no you don't!" cried Lester. She was amazed by the young animal's strength. She worried it would choke itself to death on the lease. Had the thing gone crazy in the heat? At this rate, she would never get to Brutus. Someone from the state highway maintenance garage stopped and asked if he could help. "Yeah," said Lester. "Wrap this crate with something to keep her from getting out." The man brought a roll of stout wire and secured the crate's bars. Louise, certain she was now stuck, settled down with her head between her front feet. "She slept the remainder of the trip to Brutus, with a disgruntled, disheveled Frontier nurse as her driver," Lester said.[4]

Like the horses, the jeeps had their own imposed personalities. Each acquired a name, of course, which served a practical as well as a whimsical purpose. Whenever a jeep went to the garage in Hyden, for example, the maintenance or repair was documented as service for Jane, Bounce, or Turveydrop (a Dickens character Breckinridge selected). In time, the nurses became almost as attached to their jeeps as they did to their horses. Jeeps were prominently featured in *The Road*, the third of three fundraising films produced for the Frontier Nursing Service. In the black-and-white film, an FNS nurse is shown driving past shacks with big-eyed children watching from the doorways; splashing through the river at low tide; bouncing along rutted muddy roads; and climbing the steep hill to Hyden Hospital, now a twenty-seven bed facility with two fulltime doctors on staff. Poetic in its narration, the film took a comprehensive approach to the needs and service of the FNS circa late 1960s, with an emphasis not just on midwifery but public health nursing as well.

The only visual of Breckinridge (who disliked having her picture taken) was a still photo mounted on her horse, a backdrop against a jeep crossing the river with reference to "the dream as she saw it, a road deep in the woods, high in the hills, where there is still so much to do."[5] Along with jeeps, a few other vehicles were now traversing the narrow gravel road that led to Wendover, including a mail truck that made deliveries from the fourth-class post office to the Big House, FNS headquarters.

Hazel Meyer arrived in 1943 as an official postmistress and quickly realized over 90 percent of the mail she handled was generated by and for the FNS. Revenues from the postal service went directly to the FNS. Yet she also processed mail for the district families who lived within a reasonable distance. "It was a mighty difficult job," she recalled, "learning who belonged to who because [it seemed] everyone's last name was either Adams or Morgan. A lad would come in and ask about mail for 'the Morgans.' So you proceeded to go through all the mail belonging to everyone with that surname, at which point he began to name everyone in his family. After doing that a few times, you knew this family very well."[6] She had been working in the post office several months and thought she finally knew everyone when an elderly woman walked in. "You're Mrs. So-and-so from way up on the right fork of Camp Creek," said Meyer, proud of her memory skills. The woman nodded as she reached for her mail. She glanced at it and politely handed it back to Meyer. "Nope, that's not me," she said. "That's my twin sister."[7]

High tides—heavy rains that swelled the river and spilled over into flooding—made the roads impassable and mail delivery difficult at best. But Meyer and her staff struggled mightily to follow the U.S. Postal Service creed—"neither rain, nor hail, nor sleet, nor snow"—to ensure proper delivery. One of the men working at Wendover obligingly carried mail for families that lived near him. He could not read but he devised his own delivery system: One family's mail went to his right shirt pocket; another in the back left pocket of his pants, etc. He never got confused and everyone got the mail that belonged to them. Meyer said when the truck couldn't get out due to high tide, mail and any telegrams were delivered by courier, and on occasion, her own form of delivery. "I never rode horseback much before I came to the mountains, but there were times when I had to ride with a bag of mail swung across each knee, and two across the back of the saddle. I always jumped at the chance to visit my mountain friends for a chat in front of their fire."

Beginning around March, many families ordered baby chicks from Kentucky hatcheries, so spring was always heralded at the post office with the incessant "peep, peep, peep" of the chicks' arrivals. "It was against postal regulations for us to feed or water them," said Meyer. "So when they arrived, we immediately had to make every effort to get word to their owners the chicks were here. One woman who worked in a laundry had ordered a hundred of them. The day they arrived she was home "ailin with a cold."[8] About 4:00 P.M. that day, Meyer mounted her horse, Calico, and set off on the four-mile ride up the creek to make the delivery. "Calico was a bit skittish that day, with the constant noise from the chicks. Then I heard the rumble of distant thunder and it began to rain. In my rush, I'd forgotten that the box holding the chicks was cardboard, and had visions of it bursting and hundreds of baby chicks taking to the hills in every direction. But I threw my coat over the box, and it held. The chicks arrived at their destination safely."[9]

Despite the poverty that still existed in the mid–1940s, the FNS staff found that people were, by and large, meticulously honest. One nurse-midwife recalled working at the Bull Creek clinic on a warm fall day. As she bustled about weighing babies, giving combined vaccinations for diphtheria and pertussis (whooping cough) and scheduling pre-natal visits, a man dressed in denim overalls walked in and asked to see the nurse. He was wearing a hat and carrying a kerchief in his pocket. "One eye was swollen and a tear trickled down his cheek," said the nurse-midwife. "He explained he had 'jarbed' a cornhusk in his eye and 'mighty nigh put it out.' I examined it closely but couldn't see anything but an inflamed cornea. A drop of argyrol (an antiseptic compound of protein and silver) seemed to sooth it and at his urgent request, I placed a patch over it. Then I urged him to see an eye doctor if it wasn't better the next day." But the man had no money, or as he explained "not nary a bit of change." "Then bring a nickel next time you are out this way," the FNS nurse replied. "Well," is all he said in response. The FNS nurse sent him home and promptly forgot about the incident.

Five months later she and another nurse were walking through snow en route to visit a friend. "We were on a strange creek many miles from the FNS boundary," she said. "As we passed a barn we noticed a group of men shoeing a mule. Suddenly one of the men got up and called out to me." "Ain't you the nurse what I owed that nickel to?" "No. I don't recognize you." "Yes ma'am, you are the very one. I don't forgit a face. If it warn't for you, I'd be about blind right now. Last fall, you fixed me up at your clinic, over the hill thar, and hit's plum well now. Here's your nickel."[10]

Running an FNS district nursing center in the 1940s was "a rich experience," several nurse-midwives recounted. Louise Mowbray, R.N., said she was often asked by outsiders what she did all day besides riding horseback over mountain trails and delivering babies.

> First there was the structure itself. It was usually sturdy-built, with cellar, attic, living room, kitchen, bedrooms, bath, dispensary, and clinic waiting room. Like all houses, it had to be kept up and since the nurse-midwife was the tenant, it was her responsibility. There were floors to be polished, rooms to be swept and dusted; beds to make; windows to wash.
> The clinic linoleum, over which numerable muddy boots tramp daily, required endless scrubbing. The oil lamps—there was no electric light as yet—needed trimming and filling. The kitchen range, which burned the soft coal that gave such wonderful heat but produced buckets of soot, needed cleaned daily. Otherwise, there would be no hot water or worse yet, the grates could burn out and collapse on the coldest day of winter.[11]

She went on to explain that "extra hands, even if only an untrained girl," were indispensable for these chores in order for the district nurse-midwife to devote most of her day to rounds and nursing duties. Usually, one or two local people were hired as housekeepers or cooks just as in the prior two decades of the FNS. But unlike the Big House, where there was now a full staff, the outpost nurse-midwives were often short-handed and sometimes had to perform the extra work themselves. "The nurse returned from her rounds," continued Mowbray, "after hours in the saddle with her horse as weary and muddy, or as hot and dusty, as she was. But the horse still had to be unsaddled, thoroughly groomed, and fed before the nurse could go from the barn to the house."

Among the outpost centers' greatest assets were the humble cow and a few chickens. "If the cow was cared for properly, it produced milk and butter. In exchange, it had to be fed and given gallons of water. And each morning and evening it had to be milked. The milk must be strained and put away. Two or three times a week, butter was churned. Chickens supplied eggs and fryers, but they too needed rounding up and shut in the chicken house, safe from marauding rats and hoot owls."[12] If the nurse was lucky, she had a barn boy who cleaned the stalls daily and laid fresh sawdust for bedding. In the winter, he shoveled snow from the paths and emptied furnace ashes. Otherwise, this duty fell to the nurse as well.

Daily food was needed for the household, for guests, and the working hands. Supplies required purchase from the tiny local store, or from a twenty-mile trip into Hyden for bacon, coffee, and ongoing staples. As in the early days of the FNS, the nurses still bartered their medical skills for whatever they needed: a bushel of apples, a hindquarter of lamb, help with plowing the garden or planting crops on the outpost acreage. Surplus fruits and vegetables were canned and stored against the times when food was scarce so help with the canning was always needed. She also maintained the center's fuel supplies: cords of wood for the fireplaces; tons of coal for the cooking stoves, delivered by hired helpers during the slack season between hoeing and harvesting. She planned her kerosene supply carefully so the huge drum of heating oil could be filled when the roads were open to truck travel. She ordered grain and salt blocks for the horses, and arranged for their haul over narrow roads from the nearest railroad some twenty miles away.

She supervised the local work hands who ensured the fencing was kept in repair, so neighboring pigs didn't enter and tear up the pasture; checked for needed water pipe repairs and leaky roofs; inspected the furnace grates and firebox for cracks; rebuilt stalls in the barn; whitewashed the house cellar; trimmed the trees and bushes throughout the property; and the list went on. Meanwhile, she was on call to deliver any babies, make rounds up the creek beds and over the mountain trails, and generally care for the health and welfare of the thousand or so residents who comprised her district. "The days were never long enough," said Mowbray. "And yet, one always looked forward to tomorrow."[13]

On April 12, 1945, Breckinridge heard the news by way of radio that President Franklin D. Roosevelt had died in Warm Springs, Georgia. In the next *Quarterly Bulletin*, she wrote a Memoriam in his honor, noting that his leadership "was accepted beyond the seven seas and the uttermost parts of the world." She recalled meeting him at the White House years earlier where she was invited to dine with the president and first lady. He had expressed genuine interest in the Cumberland Mountains, and the welfare of its people. And he told Breckinridge that in his youth, he had visited the region, riding the mountain trails on horseback. "He did not ask me a single political question," she recalled. "He was concerned, deeply concerned, over getting roads built, the development of forests, and the possible economic outlets."[14] FNS nurse-mid-wife instructor Nora Kelly, who had returned to London in 1940 as the eleventh British nurse to leave the FNS and volunteer her services during the war, wrote what a "stunning sense of shock" England suffered as a whole when they heard the news. "I cannot think what it must have been like for you in America. Every-one here thought how ill he looked at the Yalta conference, but I don't think we anticipated such a sudden death."[15]

As spring turned to summer and Breckinridge remembered President Roosevelt's interest in the FNS, another challenge was shaping up driven by economic disadvantage. Utilities taken for granted in urban parts of the coun-try were still lacking in many rural areas, especially the Appalachian region. In Frankfort, Kentucky, the Public Service Commission met in July 1945 to rec-oncile the cost of regional telephone service against the impoverishment within the isolated mountain communities. Breckinridge had a representative at the meeting, Minnie Grove, of Lexington, arguing for the need for more phone lines in Leslie County. On the opposing side was Otis Roberts, manager and part owner of the Leslie County phone company, whose father built the county's first phone system in 1906. In the end it would, of course, all come down to money. Grove spoke first, reminding the commission of the good work pro-vided by the FNS to "poor mothers in isolated mountain regions." One nurs-ing center, at Possum Bend, was connected to Hyden by a phone. Twelve miles away, at the Bowlingtown FNS center, was another line. But it was now in dis-repair. So Bowlingtown had no phone service. If there was a good road between the two centers, a courier could motor from Bowlingtown to Possum Bend, telephone Hyden for medical help, and return to Bowlingtown within half an hour. "But," she said, "only a trail connects the two centers, and it requires four hours on horseback. Suppose a mother in childbirth at the Bowlingtown cen-ter desperately needed a physician at Hyden. It would take four hours to get to the phone at Possum Bend, and four more hours for the doctor to arrive. That's much too long in cases of life and death."[16]

Breckinridge instructed Grove to tell the group she was willing to donate the cost of the phone wire if the Leslie County Telephone Company would restore the line between the two centers. It was Otis Roberts' turn to speak. He was all sympathy, he said, to the plight of the FNS and its difficult work con-ditions. "But the line built by my father was installed thirty-five years ago. The wire has disintegrated into rust. The trees the wire was nailed to have been logged away, and the poles have rotted out." Then he went on to explain his company's financial picture: a total of eighty-five subscribers provided a gross income of only two hundred twenty-five dollars a month. "I am in debt," he said, "and losing money every day of the year." He was actually trying to sell the company, he admitted, but so far had no takers. The agent for the Ashland Home Telephone Company in Hazard wouldn't even respond to his letter and Southern Bell sent an agent to look at the phone system but the man left and was never heard from again. "Even if Mrs. Breckinridge gave us the wire," he added, "there are not enough trees or fence posts to string it between Possum Bend and Bowlingtown because so many of the trees have been logged out."[17] He would have to buy a thousand dollar's worth of phone poles and pay labor costs of two thousand dollars to set them —funds his company did not have. "The Bowlingtown Center would provide only about thirty dollars a year in revenue," he concluded. "Thus it would take a hundred years to recover a capital outlay of three thousand dollars [at thirty dollars a year]." Repairs would impose an additional cost.[18]

As he saw it, Breckinridge and the FNS organization should tie in with the fire alarm system maintained by the National Forest Service. He suggested line construction that would take the Bowlingtown center through a personal switch to the home of a local resident, relay it by private line to Brutus center, on to Bullskin Creek, then by Forest Service line to Red Bird, and back to Hyden. One can only imagine the response by Breckinridge, who with her pragmatic nature, would undoubtedly shake her head in frustration, then almost immediately set about seeking alternate solutions. And that's exactly what she did. "We abandoned the idea of trying to re-establish phone connection," she wrote in the 1945 summer issue of the *Quarterly Bulletin.*

Among the ideas submitted to the FNS was to establish radio transmission between the Bowlingtown Nursing Center in Perry County and the Possum Bend Center at Confluence in Leslie County, a distance of some ten to twelve miles. Complications included a road that was part dirt and part overgrown trail, a river to ford, and a mountain to cross. Establishing direct communication between Bowlingtown and the Hyden Hospital made more sense but there was a range of steep mountains in between and the distance, twenty-four miles, even farther. Breckinridge corresponded with four manufacturing companies of radio transmission battery sets (there was no electricity at either nursing center) but the highly technical details were soon beyond her scope as well as that of the FNS staff. A request went out for help to determine the type of transmission needed. The FNS organization could then apply to the Federal Trade Commission for a license to operate radio communication. "One thing is clear in all of the letters," wrote Breckinridge, "and that is the interest each of these firms had in our problem and their desire to help us solve it. Once again, we are impressed by the kindness of people."[19] That's where the radio problem was left at summer's end. For in the day-to-day operation of the Frontier Nursing Service, there was always something else to worry about.

19

Social Services to the Rescue

Delia was not feeling well and the doctor thought her decayed teeth were causing her weakened condition. She lived on Camp Creek, about eight miles from a main road. The journey for help was more than she could bear — on foot through a stony, wet creek bed, five miles on the road to find a bus route, a twenty-mile ride to the dentist in Hazard, a long wait, and the return trip. It would take several trips to remove her twenty-two bad teeth and fit her with dentures. The cost was a whole different matter. Her husband had a steady job but with food and other expenses for their five children, there was little money left over at the end of the month. The total bill, she was told, would come to more than sixty dollars. We have to buy a new cow first, Delia told her husband. Then we have to buy seeds for spring planting. No, he argued back. You need to take care of this and the sooner the better.

She arranged for a neighbor to stay with her five children and then walked to a relative's home near Wendover where she "took" the night. Next morning, it was a relatively easy three-mile hike along a wagon road to the highway. She hitched a ride into Hazard and presented herself to the dentist. A ride home was arranged. He extracted ten of her bad teeth. On the ride back to Hyden, she was not only in pain, but got car sick, having seldom ridden in a motor vehicle. It was four in the afternoon when she arrived at the mouth of Camp Creek, still eight miles from home. But so anxious was she to return to her family, she decided to walk the last eight miles. It would take four more trips before she received her "store teeth." But when it was all over, she said she felt much better. Now if only they could pay the sixty dollar dental bill.

Jessie was crippled; the paralysis in her legs getting worse. For several years she had to rely upon a cane in order to walk. Now the cane was needed even when standing still. Along with this handicap, there were four children to look after — and she a divorced woman with no man to help her. The children were puny and poorly clad. They needed clothes and garden supplies so they could grow food. With winter coming, what would they do?

A letter arrived through the FNS that began: "I have got seven kids without any milk. Their father is old and feeble and the cow just died."[1]

All three of these cases came to the attention of the Frontier Nursing Service through the Social Services branch of the FNS. It was established as a national philanthropic project by Alpha Omicron Pi, a women's Greek fraternity founded at Columbia University in 1897. Its originators were determined to make a democratic, unostentatious society. (Among its notable alumnae: Margaret Bourke-White, internationally known photographer and journalist.) The social services project was endorsed by the fraternity in 1931 but did not begin receiving attention outside the FNS until the 1940s when the term "social services" was more commonly known and accepted. However, social work was a movement within the United States as early as 1905, designed to address the needs of the poor and immigrants. Early social workers were also advocates for housing and medical care, fair wages, and health and life-skills education. In addition, they worked to improve the experience of childbirth. So providing the dual services of nurse-midwifery and social work within the FNS was a logical move.[2]

In Leslie County, following home visits and investigation by Social Services into each family's situation, Delia, with the bad teeth, was provided funds to help cover her dental bill. Jessie, the crippled mother, allowed her children to attend a mountain boarding school with the help of a grant through Social Services. While there, they gained weight and were provided with new clothes. The family that wrote about its dead cow was given funds to help it obtain another animal — a cow suitable to forage steep mountainsides, exist on corn and fodder during lean months, and still give milk. In the meantime, a case of evaporated milk was delivered to the family. A half-brother offered to help by refunding Social Services for the cost of the cow, a few dollars a month until it was paid in full — typical of cases where assistance was provided until a family was back on its feet or a relative could take over.

The Social Services director was Betty Lester, whose return from England after World War II coincided with the departure of another FNS nurse-midwife. Lester's knowledge of the region, the people, and her own popularity among the locals helped her secure the position, one that she requested. It was a tough job, for social service needs were great among the many families still surviving on subsistence farming. But Lester appeared to be the right person at the right time. "I was not a trained social worker at all," she said, "but having worked so much on the District I knew about as much of social service work as anybody. I took handicapped children to clinics at Lexington or Cincinnati; provided food for hungry families or coal in the winter; money for seeds and potatoes in the spring." Most of her time was spent on the two-lane back roads in and out of Leslie County, driving a monstrous-sized (at least to her) nine-seater station wagon. The drive to Cincinnati alone was two hundred miles each way, requiring a two-day trip. One day a woman came to the clinic in

Hyden asking for any used clothing her children could wear. "I need something for Naked Betty," the woman said. *"Who?"* Lester asked. "Our baby Naked Betty. She's named for you, Miss Lester. That's what you told us to call her." Suddenly, Lester realized her mistake. So many families wanted to name their girl children after her, she must have jokingly told this family to refer to the infant as it appeared, just plain "naked."[3]

Overall FNS needs considered urgent in 1947 included: carloads of hay for the twenty-seven horses (costs had risen 300 percent over the past four years); gas and oil for the five jeeps, station wagon, a pickup truck and car totaling more than twenty-five hundred dollars for a year; nurses' summer uniforms (due to war shortages, cloth was hard to come by and the women had patched their uniforms until they were threadbare). One jacket and pair of riding breeches cost nearly twenty dollars. The Hyden Hospital needed a new sewage system estimated at three hundred dollars; electric wiring repairs which would run about five hundred dollars; and the ever-present miscellaneous needs, from rough lumber to hardware.

The year 1947 brought several important changes to the Frontier Nursing Service. February blew in with a series of snowstorms and near blizzard conditions, heralded by a wind that shrieked, whistled, howled and spun its way in and around the mountains throughout the entire month. The surrounding hills, dressed in snowy white gowns, glistened like jewels in the sunlight and the little town of Hyden lay nestled beneath them as pristine as a new Christmas card. From the courthouse a popular joke was making the rounds, according to an entry in an FNS *Quarterly Bulletin*: "Do you mean to tell me that you murdered that poor old lady for a paltry three dollars?" the judge demanded. "Well, judge, you know how it is. A paltry three dollars here and three dollars there — it soon adds up."

At the hospital atop Thousandsticks Mountain, there was now an obstetrical ward with two glassed-in heated verandas, a small general ward for sick children and emergency cases, a combination bath and utility room, and a delivery room doubling as a nursery for premature infants. Newborns were generally placed alongside their mothers to accommodate breast-feeding then returned to nearby small cribs. There were no glass-walled nurseries with separate cubicles. Among the sick children were several cases of pneumonia. Many lived in poorly heated homes and were susceptible to the lung ailment. Fortunately, a new drug, penicillin, was now available to combat the infection in which a child's fever could easily top a hundred and five degrees. Twenty-four hours later — after the administration of the miracle medicine, the kids were sitting up in bed playing. Ingenuity and adaptability were the hallmarks of good nursing care at Hyden Hospital during this decade. If a piece of equipment was not available a substitute was found; patients were taught to do for themselves; and when a crisis arose — as it did when severe weather caused the water pumps to quit — tubs and basins were filled from the reserve tanks in order to make do.

An experienced visiting nurse concluded that the Hyden Hospital staff, from the superintendent down to the youngest nursing student, worked together for the common good. "No one talked of unions or collective bargaining or overtime," she said. "These girls seemed to honor their profession above commercial value. Their devotion to duty, their cooperation, and their generosity was a never-failing source of inspiration to me."[4] Margaret M. Field, a staff nurse at the hospital, said it was the patients who deserved kudos — "the finest in the world" — she called them for they were "loyal, patient, cooperative, and appreciative." "One of the male relatives of a patient offered to shovel coal whenever necessary," she reported, "and he helped me lift an elderly woman. He also helped with the last rites when this same woman died at five o'clock one morning and there was no second nurse to assist in turning her. Everything was done in a spirit of quiet dignity and respect, the underlying motive being pure neighborliness."[5]

Another patient, a prenatal who required long-term hospital care, toured the general ward in the evenings to read and talk to the children, most of whom were lonely and homesick. Some had never been away from their parents. Other women patients adopted babies who were malnourished and required morning feedings at a time when the nurses were busiest. "Particularly outstanding is the spirit of sharing among the patients," said Field. "It may be only an orange or a stick of chewing gum, perhaps a whole chicken dinner brought in by someone's family. Whatever it is, they share with one another."[6] Volunteers within the FNS organization stepped up with gifts of supplies and services. A Breckinridge relative sent a set of sixty-three sheets for the hospital wards. The head of the Ritter Lumber Company in Hyden had the hospital's red truck, named Strongmore, refloored and painted. One of the FNS trustees sewed fifty pairs of baby booties, fifty little dresses, and seven baby blankets. Someone else donated a hundred sturdy baby chicks to Wendover. And a shipment of used eyeglasses, suitable for recycling, was sent from New Jersey, prompting one local recipient to exclaim, "Oh good, now I can see Spring coming!"[7]

Dr. Maurice O. Barney, a former Army captain and native of New England became the new medical director for the FNS in 1947, having heard much about the organization and its founder, Mary Breckinridge. He was one of a series of directors who served at the discretion of the FNS. One stayed only a few months; another stayed twelve years, leaving to join the Navy Medical Reserve Corps during World War II. Two of the interim directors were female, including the physician wife of a Presbyterian minister. One director was released from the U.S. Indian Bureau in order to serve the FNS. Sometimes finding a director who would stay proved a serious challenge. At one point Breckinridge said the effort to locate another medical director "involved me in correspondence a foot high with people all over the United States. There was no one left during the war except "elderly men."[8]

Only twenty-nine years old, Barney was among the youngest medical

directors to serve the FNS. As a result, the energetic physician and his win-
some family (a wife and three-year-old daughter) were a welcome change.
Brought up in Maine, Barney rode ponies from the time he was five, served in
the U.S. Army Medical Corps, and had firsthand knowledge of jeeps. A graduate of Bates College in Lewiston, Maine, he received his medical degree from
the Tufts College School of Medicine in Boston. The family was welcomed to
Hyden by the local FNS Committee, which held a dinner at the hospital in his
honor. All the members came bearing gifts: homemade canned goods, butter,
sausage meat, fresh vegetables, bread, soap, even a live chicken. What impressed
him most before he took the job was that here, in the furthermost region of
eastern Kentucky in the 1940s, medical help was available at such a low cost
that even the poorest residents could afford it. "Women are given the very best
prenatal and postpartum care and delivered, all for the sum of ten dollars; children are given medical care free. This organization stands on its own two feet,
refusing to be identified with any political group or religious sect. Visitors come
from all over the world to see what makes the organization tick and how it
operates. I wondered about that myself."[9] Privately, he also wondered if he was
entering a region of "good ole boys always fighting and feuding."

As with the nurses, learning the language and the local culture was the
first order of the day. One woman returning for a six week postpartum checkup
told the director's secretary, "My, you sure look natural." Another was asked
why she had not yet weaned her fourteen-month-old baby from breastfeeding.
"I can't wean him," the mother replied. "When I try, he throws rocks at me."[10]
"But these mountain folks I have met have been kind, honest people; even the
uneducated are innately polite and gentle," said Dr. Barney. "They live at a
slower pace than most in the U.S.; but they always take time to be kind to their
neighbors and friends. There is no keeping up with the Joneses here. But one
thing that does puzzle me is the little game they play to see who can build their
house in the most inaccessible place." Before long, he was referring to the FNS
women as "fearless Amazons who don the picturesque blue-gray riding habit
and courageously go out to their patients in jeeps, on horseback, and by foot,
any time of day or night, rain or shine, in boiling sun or ice and snow. I find
them a fine lot of women from the best nursing schools all over the U.S., Canada,
and England."[11]

Despite the FNS' efforts, there was still a shortage of medical care. During his two-year tenure, Dr. Barney made visits to the six outlying nursing centers, holding clinic at each. A separate clinic was held at the hospital three days
a week, in addition to emergency visits. On call twenty-four/seven, he was the
only physician within the FNS and the only male. What he encountered most
often was the recurring scourge of worms—hookworms, roundworms, and
pinworms—which had been greatly reduced but not eradicated by the efforts
of Breckinridge and her staff. "In some families every member had worms
except the nursing baby," said Dr. Barney. He also found a high incidence of

thyroid disorders, gall bladder disease due to fatty diets, and varicose veins in women from multiple births and "hard domestic labor, such as carrying coal, wood, or water." "The tuberculosis rate is high too, since many of these people live in crowded quarters; some cabins still do not have windows."[12]

Assisting the medical director were other doctors from Lexington or Louisville, volunteering to come to Hyden on their own time for surgical clinics, ob-gyn cases that required a consult, anesthesiology, or specialized care. Dr. Francis Massie, of Lexington, brought his entire staff along—intern, scrub nurse, and anesthetist—for three-day surgical clinics. Through the generosity of these physicians, dozens of Leslie County residents were provided with free medical and surgical attention. Whenever the visiting surgeons arrived, they were greeted enthusiastically by the locals who arrived at the hospital by jeep, wagon, mule, horseback, or on foot to see the "sargins" who would operate on them or their family member. Patients were screened and selected for their necessary surgery, resulting in a dozen or so operations over the next two to three days. One woman, during a particularly difficult labor, looked up at a visiting doctor and implored, "Please get me out of this shape, and pin a piece of grace on my soul."

And so, twice a year, spring and fall, the out-of-town physicians said they came to Hyden "to pin a piece of grace on the Frontier Nursing Service."[13] The doctors usually had dinner at Wendover on the first night of their clinic and it was generally the same meal: turkey hash, mustard greens, spoon bread, and green onions fresh from the garden. Breckinridge valued Dr. Massie's friendship and guidance in particular, and was one of the few people, according to her staff, to whom she would actually listen.

As spring turned to summer that 1947, the rains came, resulting in a devastating flash flood. It happened during the night of June 27 when torrential rain pounded the headwaters of both the Middle Fork River and the Red Bird River. Caught at their respective outpost centers with little or no communication, the FNS staff did not know how bad the damage was for several days. Battery operated radios mentioned only flash floods on the other side of the Cumberland Mountains. But in the upper Middle Fork region, several homes had washed away, along with schools, stores, and a post office. Hundreds of residents lost their possessions, including cows and chickens; thousands lost their gardens and crops. On the upper parts of the river so much soil had washed away that only bare rock remained. Good bottom land was covered with sand and muck that ranged from six inches to three feet deep.

Incredibly, no lives were lost. The American Red Cross arrived and like the U.S. Cavalry, saved the day with its efficient brand of disaster relief. Some of the Red Cross workers stayed at Wendover or at an FNS outpost center. Army tents were brought in for the newly homeless; mattresses and beds, food and clothing were distributed. Late hybrid seed corn and soybean seeds were provided free and the Red Cross made arrangements for the delivery of cow feed so that families would have milk the next winter. Even after the floodtide, rain continued hampering rescue efforts. The steady precipitation also made it difficult to get the "foul river water" washed from quilts and other bedding. Then nothing would dry out. The FNS Social Services Department, headed by Betty Lester, took Mason jars to families who managed to salvage a little of their garden produce. The Hyden School Board drew up plans to rebuild schools as quickly as possible and the Highway Department set to work repairing washed out roads and bridges. Almost all phone lines were down yet few residents expected a quick repair as phone communication was spotty even in perfect weather.

At the Big House in Wendover, it could have been worse. The two bridges leading to Wendover — the small foot bridge and the high swinging bridge over the Middle Fork River — were essential to contact with the outside world. The small bridge was washed away but the swinging bridge held, only its flooring battered. Seventeen members of the Alpha Omicron Pi national fraternity (which funded the FNS Social Services program) were scheduled to visit the FNS that same weekend. The plan was to arrive at the Red Bird Center for a picnic lunch, visit the Hyden Hospital, and then come to Wendover. The entourage made it in before the flood arrived but ended up swimming their horses across the swollen river and found they were unable to visit the flooded Red Bird region. They decided next to attempt the trip to Wendover. When they arrived, they found the bridges out. So it was on to Hyden Hospital. But they got no farther than the causeway at the entrance to the little town, where they were met by twelve feet of water, the route to the hospital completely blocked. At this point, recalling they had food for up to twenty people, they stopped and had a picnic on the causeway. It was hours before the water level diminished to the point where they could reach Hyden Hospital. There, they spent a restless night.

At most of the FNS outpost centers, the main buildings were too high above the river to be flooded but mudslides took out the fencing and good pasture land, causing several thousand dollars worth of damage. Outpost centers also suffered severely damaged roads, gardens, well houses, and water pumps. The chief courier at Wendover — "Pebble" Stone — reported that water was over the road below the Big House and there was all manner of things floating in the river — trees, logs, barrel staves, fifty-gallon drums, even parts of what appeared to be buildings. She grabbed her camera and took a few pictures until she spotted a huge floating tree headed straight toward her. She ran to avoid it, at one point finding herself waist deep in murky water. A rocking chair had lodged itself fifteen feet above her head in one of the trees.

Despite the flood, patients still needed tending and mothers-to-be were still on schedule to deliver their babies. Marjorie Wood, a student at the Frontier Graduate School of Midwifery in Hyden, was on call and received word that an overdue mother was "punishing," in the Beech Fork district. If the nurse-midwife could hurry, she was told, someone would come get her in a boat and transport her to the woman in labor. "A small crowd stood around as we swung into the boat, lifting the heavy midwifery bags," she recalled. "My guide was a shy, nice-looking guy who hardly spoke. After we landed safely, he took my bags and we walked to a truck waiting at the top of the road."[14] They raced toward Harlan, marveling at the power of the damage the flood had wrought. A small white house just off the road sat immersed in water up to its eaves. Bedding, dishes, chairs, and other household items were strewn carelessly along the highway. The young man told Wood he had started out that morning at nine to get her, and had to turn back twice. It was now mid-afternoon. They stopped at a muddy field and parked the truck. They would have to make the remainder of the trip on foot.

More determined than ever to make it to her patient in time, Wood grabbed her medical bags from the truck and they set off for the hike ahead. Her heavy boots sank into the mud. At one point, she had to hang onto to overhanging branches to keep from sliding down a hill. Her companion found himself hip-deep in mud that threatened to suck him downward like quicksand. "This is the worst mess I've ever been in," he said, laughing. It was an ironic statement considering he fought the Japanese in Guam. "When I get married, remind me to live on the highway."[15]

Along the way, they bet on whether the baby would be a girl or a boy. Since the woman had been in labor for several hours, there was a chance the infant was already born. "What great relief," said Wood, "when we finally walked through her door, half hour after leaving the truck, to see her calmly sitting on the bed." The baby was born late that night, a boy, added to the family of six, with no complications. After the delivery, Wood stepped outside for a breath of fresh air. Clouds covered the bright moon just over the mountains. The roar of the swollen creeks silenced the night sounds. Invited to stay over in one of the three double-beds available, she accepted, relieved she did not have to make the return trek in the dark.[16] Once the flood waters receded and repair work begun, routine returned to the Frontier Nursing Service.

Several international visitors arrived that fall at Wendover. Among them was Odette Pruent, a French nurse Breckinridge had worked with in France after the First World War. Pruent was surprised at the "charming" town of Hyden, and particularly the comfortable furnishings at Wendover. "Mrs. Breckinridge provides a warm, friendly atmosphere," she recounted. "I'll never forget Margaret, the jolly large laundry woman who arrives every morning perched on a horse and the faithful watchman Jinx, who symbolizes the mountaineers. I was introduced to the horses, chickens, cows, geese, the dogs and the cats. I was amazed to see not any fly or flea, for everything has been DDT-ed by Pebble (chief courier)."[17] Others came from India, Finland, Canada, and China, physicians and nurses who wanted to scope out the FNS organization, see actual medical cases, and meet the well-known woman who originated the concept of rural nurse-midwifery in America.

A Chinese woman physician, Yeh Shih Chin, who had devoted her life to maternal and child health in China, found Kentucky in 1947 "a unique world of its own, with lively, heroic nurses." "One came to take me along with her to attend a postpartum case," she reported during her visit. "I was surprised to see a complete change in her attire. She appeared in something like a Western cowboy outfit. But she handled the little jeep with agility and skill. We drove through tortuous terrain, then left the jeep and started climbing the mountain on foot. She picked up her saddlebags— weighing forty pounds— and climbed. Pretty soon I began to feel the strain of the steep climb and I noticed she, with her saddlebags, was panting too. She turned, smiled at me, and suggested we stop for a second." At the home of the second family they visited Dr. Chin noted the patient was "a very lovely young woman. She sat at the edge of her bed and answered every question in a low voice and shy manner. She reminded me of the Chinese women who lead a sheltered life and hardly cross the thresholds of their own gates. She was devoted to her new baby. Whenever it cried, she would pick it up and feed it, exactly as a young mother would do in China."[18]

When the Chinese doctor finally reached Wendover, it was tea time and Mary Breckinridge was downstairs in the Big House. Chin did not recognize her immediately. "She was a slightly hunch-back, white-haired lady whose apparel was well-worn. But she spoke about her work with such precision, clarity, and enthusiasm that it dawned on me this must be Mrs. Breckinridge. I considered it a privilege to be learning about the Service from its very source." "After supper," Dr. Chin said, "she lighted an oil lamp in the corner of the sitting room and invited me to sit with her to read newspapers and magazines. Outside, nature's orchestra was playing the harmony of the running river, croaking frogs, hooting owls, and chirping crickets. Inside, under the oil lamp, here I was, sitting beside the white-haired humanitarian."[19]

One visitor said that before meeting Breckinridge she was as nervous as child peeping through the fence post "breathlessly waiting to see his favorite baseball player." "I stood in the living room of her home at Wendover toying with how I would act and what I would say when I actually met her. Suddenly a charming, gracious lady came in the room and took my hand as though she were eager to meet *me*. It was Mary Breckinridge."[20]

Breckinridge had plenty on her mind that day, including the loss of four FNS trustees she considered personal friends (one through death; the others due to commitments that kept them from serving another term), and most pressing, the serious illness of her assistant director, Dorothy F. Buck, diagnosed that spring with ovarian cancer. The prognosis was not good. Following surgery in Lexington, Buck was brought back to Wendover where Breckinridge and the FNS staff had taken it upon themselves to care for her. She would be there for several months.

Dorothy Farrar Buck was born in Foxboro, Massachusetts, in 1895. Her father and grandfather were both Episcopalian ministers. Among her distinguished ancestors were doctors, teachers, judges, farmers, a few sea captains, ship owners, and a number of Revolutionary War soldiers. She did not consider herself well educated, though she graduated from Wellesley College in 1918 and obtained a master's degree in public health at Teacher's College, Columbia University, and Breckinridge's alma mater. Later, she would be one of the few American nurses who went to England at their own expense in order to train as a nurse-midwife. Like many of the career FNS nurses, she never married. A small woman with short brown hair and a pixie face, she first came to the FNS in 1928 as a floater (filling in wherever needed); the snow was so deep as she departed from the train in Krypton that the man who met her on a mule did not feel his animals should attempt to go any farther. She was dressed in the winter uniform of the FNS, which had been provided in Lexington. Told it would be the color of horizon blue, it was instead a dull grey and she donned it gleefully — "this Yankee in a Confederate grey uniform," she noted.[21] So — in weather so bad even the mules were banned from travel — she made the trek to the Possum Bend Nursing Center alone. It was to be her first station. En route she came across a figure wearing the recognizable FNS uniform who led her to the nursing center at Confluence. Many of the women arriving in the 1920s said the hardest part of joining the FNS was their initial trip into the region.

She stayed a week with the Possum Bend nurses, visiting patients on foot until her designated FNS horse, Remus, arrived. Within just a few days, she grew accustomed to hearing "Oh, nurse!" from cabin doors as she passed, people asking about her age, her marital status, and "the last year's corn crop in New York," where they thought the newcomer came from. She also found that Remus had a disconcerting habit of baring his teeth at strangers, but proved sure-footed and reliable. Bucket, however, accustomed to city sidewalks, said her first hours in the saddle, riding for "miles and miles and miles" resulted in wobbly legs, thudding heart, and a sore rump. The best she could hope for was that Remus would not want to take "his first bite of new nurse."[22] Bucket proved a highly capable nurse-midwife who could handle most any situation, including a case in which she saved a mother's life by reaching into the woman's uterus and retrieving the placenta after the woman suffered post-partum hemorrhage. During her twenty-one years with the FNS, she would rise through the ranks from a floater to district nurse-midwife at outpost centers, to supervisor. In the late 1930s she was made assistant director to Breckinridge, followed a few years later by first assistant director, and in the 1940s, dean of the Frontier Graduate School of Midwifery. Now in her cabin bedroom at Wendover, where she was convalescing from the first of two surgeries, she was already planning her return to work.

As Christmas 1947 approached it rained hard, putting a literal damper on plans for a large attendance at the Big House holiday party. The river was rising, making travel hazardous. Nonetheless, secretaries, couriers, maids, even the night watchman teamed up to decorate the recreation room, which served

as a drying room for laundry on weekdays. Its bare rock walls and iron sup-
ports were decked with red crepe paper streamers, silver tinsel, red Christmas
bells, and hemlock bows trimmed from the large tree that hovered in the corner of the room. They talked of Christmas the year before, when the holiday
was nearly ruined by a shooting that occurred in Hyden. A deputy sheriff, a
family man with nine children, was killed in the melee, and two young men,
sixteen and eighteen, were injured. The boys were transferred to Hazard Hospital on Christmas Day and a muted holiday celebration held at Hyden Hospital. Breckinridge and a few of the FNS nurses attended. By nine o'clock on
this year's Christmas Day, with rain clouds parting, almost half of the three-
hundred children and parents registered in the Wendover District found their
way across the swollen creeks and into Pig Alley. Breckinridge's annual Christmas event, a tradition she started in 1925 to gain the locals' trust, was something everyone looked forward to all year

Several of the children were scheduled to take part in the Nativity pageant, a tradition in which Breckinridge stood offstage and read the story aloud.
Special guest Santa was to appear after the play but somehow got confused on
the time and showed up fifteen minutes early just as the children were getting
into costume. Angels, shepherds, wise men, even the "baby Jesus" all burst into
giggles when Santa suddenly appeared before them. When the pageant was over,
the children lined up alphabetically by last name and waited on the first floor
of the Garden House for their names to be called. One little girl looked up at
the Social Services secretary and implored, "I hope Santa has a doll for me." "I
fervently hoped," said the secretary, "that she would be one of the lucky ones
who would find a doll in her Christmas bag, but I knew there had not been
enough to go around and that the nurses tried to give the dolls to the little girls
who had never owned one."[23] Yet the FNS staff also knew, having worked with
and for these mountain people over more than two decades, that whatever they
came by, they would no doubt share with others.

20

Spreading the FNS Story

Among the numerous strengths Mary Breckinridge exhibited were her marketing and public relations skills. Hardly a month went by in the late 1940s when an article did not appear about the Frontier Nursing Service, or some form of nursing material was not dedicated, at least in part, to Breckinridge and her endeavors. A booklet titled *Nursing as a Career,* by B. Ristori, was making its rounds, with acknowledgments to Breckinridge with whom the author worked in earlier years. The author, a nurse living in New Zealand, was now writing for prospective nurses, encouraging them to enter the profession and to keep in mind that nursing encompassed public health service as well.

No one knew the public health aspect better than the staff at Hyden Hospital where an occasional patient became more like a guest at a rest home. One elderly man, crippled, with no family and no money, was admitted to the hospital for erysipelas (an acute superficial skin infection). The nurses placed him in an area used for isolation, not because he was a danger to anyone, but because they knew he had no place to go once he got better. He stayed for weeks inside the glassed-in porch off the children's ward. When an FNS nurse went to tell him goodbye as she was going off duty, she found him propped up in bed grinning like a Cheshire cat. "How *are* you this morning?" she asked. "Fine," he answered. "I'm just lying here, being happy."[1]

Spring brought with it a tragedy at one of the Leslie County schools. During recess, a few of the students took shelter from a light rain under a large pine tree. Two local men, en route to a neighbor's house, had stopped to watch them play. The small group was huddled beneath the tree when lightning struck, killing the two men instantly along with a seven-year-old child. The remaining children were injured and taken to Hyden Hospital where they eventually recovered. That summer, electricity was finally installed at Wendover, where — according to Breckinridge — it was "as costly as wiring an Oriental compound." Running the line was tedious, labor-intensive, and nearly destroyed the terrain around the Big House, she added, referring to the power company crew as "the wreckers." Power lines had already reached the nursing center at Bowl-

ingtown, thanks in part to FNS friends and patients who raised a little over a
hundred dollars for the installation by holding "pie suppers and other enter-
tainments." Someone added to the fund in order to have a well drilled and electric pump installed — "a godsend to the nurses," said Breckinridge.[2]

Students of the Frontier Graduate School of Midwifery, nearing its tenth
year of operation, began referring to deliveries as "baby catching." Telephones
were now the common form of communicating that a woman in labor was
"punishing." But a horse was still the most practical form of transportation for
many of the FNS nurses. Helen Fedde was a Graduate School student at Frontier School of Midwifery in 1947 when a call came into the Midwife Quarters
at two in the morning, just as hazy moonlight streamed into her window. "It
was Doris and Elda's turn to go, so I lay in bed telling myself I was glad I could
stay here and sleep." She could hear her friends fumbling about in the dark,
mumbling to each other: "Wonder if it's cold. Do I need gloves? Where's my
watch? I can't get my tie clasp on" Fedde, unable to sleep, finally threw back
the covers and got up. The two nurse-midwives, one a student, the other a
supervisor, Doris Reid, were already at the stable, saddling up their horses. As
had happened in the past, the father had traipsed across the hills on foot to
accompany the nurses to his home. "I grabbed my flashlight and headed for the
barn," said Fedde. How could I sleep and miss all the excitement?"[3]

The troupe set off on one of the steepest, roughest trails they had ever
encountered, saddlebags tossed over each horse's middle. They could hear the
echo of barking dogs in the valley below, disturbed only the by clop, clop, clop
of the horses' hoofs. They reached the edge of Asher's Branch, lined by a rough,
rocky bank they could barely see in the dark. Reid led the way with a miner's
carbide light set atop her cap in an effort to cut through the darkness and the
fog. "Follow me," she instructed. "Keep your horse in the stream. Stand up in
your stirrups and hold onto to your horse's mane. Lean forward."[4] Once across
the stream, they climbed higher, topped the ridge, and began their perilous
descent. The horses skidded and slid down the steep ravine, nearly toppling
their riders. "Duck your head! Watch out for the low limb!" Reid yelled.

More barking dogs greeted them as they approached a small log cabin
where a soft yellow light offered up its cheery welcome at the window. It then
occurred to the student nurse: *What brave mothers to live in such remote places,
so far away from help.* The woman's husband, Marcus, arrived just behind them.
Amid protests and sleepy cries, he woke up the two children already in the
house and carried them off to a neighbor who had agreed to put them up for
the night. Later that morning, she would have fried chicken, biscuits, and coffee ready for the grown-ups, buttermilk and a thick molasses spread for the
youngsters. Just before daybreak, a good eight hours after the first signs of "the
terrible punishing," the young mother delivered a healthy baby boy, safe and
sound in the hands of the new graduate nurse-midwives.[5]

On a late winter evening just as dusk was gathering, another nurse at one of the FNS outposts received a handwritten note at the clinic door. Like most of the nurses, her story appeared too in issues of the FNS *Quarterly Bulletin.* "Ma says would you come and see Sam and John," she read. "They are both kind of puny. She thinks Sam has them worms with the pins on 'em." Realizing it was not an emergency, the nurse-midwife set out the next day. But it had snowed so hard the night before that it was much too slippery to risk taking the horse. So she decided to walk. Two miles from the clinic, all vegetation disappeared into the snow and the nurse found herself on hands and knees, attempting to grasp at whatever she could find to keep herself upright. "Halfway up the mountain, I found the going so rough that I could barely move in either direction. After about fifteen minutes of sitting put, I found the whole situation ridiculous. I wondered how my sock feet would work, took off my boots, and crept very slowly to the top of the mountain in that manner."

The other side of the ridge offered visible trees to hang onto, so she redonned her boots, dug her toes into the snow, and pretended she was on a downward ski slope. "Finally, I slid into my patient's front yard, which was a solid sheet of ice, landed on my rump, met the family pig having the same trouble I was, and together, we hit the porch about the same time." The cabin door creaked open. It was Edna, the mother who had written the note. "Shore bad time," she remarked calmly. "Shore is. I didn't think you'd make it. Come to the fire now and sit a spell." The nurse settled herself, sore rump and all, onto a large metal can the family used as a chair, and began to dry her socks by the fire. "Now Edna," she said later, after examining the children. "When John is over this illness, I want you to wean him." "I'm shore aiming to, nurse," Edna said, "next time the moon is full and the signs in my knees are right."[6]

Dozens of mainstream newspapers and magazines were now relaying stories like these about the women and the patients of the Frontier Nursing Service. Some were scientific pieces published previously in medical journals. Others offered a day-in-the-life glimpse of a nurse-midwife circa 1940s. All emphasized the rigors of the terrain and the weather; the stalwart nature of the locals; and the indomitable spirit of the courageous young women who battled the elements to reach their patients day or night. "The American press has been uniformly kind to the Frontier Nursing Service," said Breckinridge, especially, she added, in printing the names and photos of prominent sponsors and supporters of the organization. Of the feature stories in magazines spotlighting the FNS, even those of national prominence, Breckinridge was less enthusiastic. "They have been of little value to us. Not five hundred dollars in money for the support of our work has come to us from all the countless people who read them, and not a single person, equipped to help us, has joined us because of them. On the nuisance side, we get letters from old men who want to correspond, or from young women who want me to be their mothers."[7]

In Laura E. Ettinger's well-researched book *Nurse-Midwifery: Birth of a New American Profession* (2006) she raises interesting points about Breckinridge's "nativism" which pushed the "right" image of the Kentucky mountaineers through frequent references to their "true American heritage," and "great American stock." These were people who deserved improvements—a deliberate strategy used in the hopes that more well-off Americans would respond to this "worthy poor" by providing financial support. In other words, according to Ettinger, Breckinridge carefully crafted the use of eugenics and nativist beliefs to gain FNS support. She also encouraged the nearly mythical, romanticized image of the heroic Frontier Nurse-midwives through media attention that best served her purposes. As a result, constructed words, images, and selective outside attention *extended* stereotypes about the region and its people, while she sought donations and volunteers. Furthermore, Ettinger says, even as Breckinridge promoted this nativism, she was wrong about the "stock Americans" that lived there. They were not Anglo-Saxon as Breckinridge referenced, but typically Scot-Irish, who were as marginalized in their country of origin as they were here in the Appalachians.[8]

Nonetheless, Ettinger gives Breckinridge due credit for providing a solid solution to the problems of rural health care, adding that while reaction to the FNS by locals was mixed in the early years, most came to admire and respect the woman and the excellent care her nurses provided. Breckinridge *did* know how to say no to the press. When one metropolitan writer sent word that he wanted to come in and do a feature photographic essay, she told him the FNS was not interested. He wrote back: "And if I choose to come in and take photos of your nurses, what are you going to do about it?" An FNS trustee also happened to be the sheriff of Leslie County at the time. "Don't worry about it, Mrs. Breckinridge," he said. "We'll take care of him." The writer made the wise decision not to show up.[9]

Authors like Ernest Poole (who was a friend of Breckinridge) had produced a flattering portrait of the FNS in his 1932 book *Nurses on Horseback*, in addition to spin-off articles, and a young woman from New York, Elizabeth Hubbard Lansing (her mother knew Breckinridge's brother), was now set to write a teen novel called *Rider on the Mountains.* Its purpose was to capture the romantic flavor of courier life in the late 1940s. Lansing had read Poole's book and wrote to Breckinridge in 1948 asking permission to come to Wendover. Due to the family connection, Breckinridge said yes but almost immediately began fussing about the media's portrayal of the region. Lansing had also just borne her third child and said when she departed New York she was criticized for leaving the infant in a nurse's care. It was not an auspicious beginning for the young writer. "Right away, Mrs. Breckinridge started in about how dreadful these people were that came down and took pictures of 'her people' to make fun of them as though they were hillbillies; then how much she hated being photographed herself. One thing she disliked was that they took all her wrinkles out." "I worked eighty years for those wrinkles!" Breckinridge said, indignant.[10]

Yet when Breckinridge settled down, Lansing found her "a dear, both tough-minded and soft-hearted." She made up her mind right away not to be frightened of this formidable woman. "Children instantly caught her attention and she seemed to love them all. But she was not a person who suffered fools gladly. She was very forthright, dedicated, and a boiling hard worker. I never saw anyone work as hard as she did. One didn't argue with her, but occasionally I would answer her back. And she liked that. She liked it when people would speak up, not let her run over them."[11]

During her three-week visit, she stayed in the upstairs guest room just down the hall from Breckinridge. What she remembers most — besides the swinging bridge that terrified her and a bull belonging to Breckinridge that roared a welcome upon her arrival — were all the books inside the Big House. "As I toiled up the stairs with my suitcase, right in front of me was a huge bookcase filled with many of the same books we had at home. I remember the *Little Prudie* series, about Prudie and her sister, Susie. These were funny, old books that my grandmother owned. I used to read them as a child. And there were many others, a whole library, I think, that belonged to Mrs. Breckinridge." She awoke the next morning before daylight and was startled to see a shadowy figure in her room. "It was half-dark and I could scarcely focus. I thought *oh no, who is that*, when I realized it was Mrs. Breckinridge. She had gotten up early and come into my room to light the coal in my fireplace. I pretended I was asleep, but I thought how typical of her. She knew I would be cold when I woke up."[12]

After Lansing's novel was published in New York in 1949, Breckinridge had a comment or two about the book's characters. The story centered on a young woman who left her pious boyfriend behind while she volunteered to travel to eastern Kentucky to work as a courier for the FNS. Breckinridge called the male character "an awful stick, a real stuffed shirt." "And she was dead right," said Lansing, honored that Breckinridge actually read the book.[13] As Lansing's visit to Wendover ended, she noted the dogwoods were in bloom, the routine that never faltered at the Big House — tea at four; sherry before dinner; eat at six or six-thirty ("magnificent food, nothing fancy but lots of it") — and that there were always several people around.

Among them was Dorothy Buck. In a small cabin near the tiny chapel on the Wendover grounds, "Bucket" had returned in May 1948 and was preparing for her death. Felled by ovarian cancer, she had undergone two surgeries, the most recent at Hyden Hospital, and was told she had only a few months to live. Breckinridge would say later that she "turned her convalescence at Wendover into a glorious spring adventure." She also began turning her administrative responsibilities over to Helen Browne ("Brownie") until she grew too weak to make the daily walk to her office in the Garden House. On Thanksgiving Day 1948, unable to attend the holiday dinner underway in the Big House dining room, she was visited by the FNS nurses in her cabin room. To her long-time friend Ann MacKinnon ("Mac") who had returned from the war in England, she wrote a farewell note: "From an old nurse who is leaving to an old nurse who has come back."[14] Bucket told her colleagues that dying from cancer was not so bad, and that she was glad she had been given the truth about her prognosis, for it helped her appreciate her last days at Wendover, surrounded by the people, the mountains, and the organization that she had come to love over the past twenty years. She spent her last Christmas looking out the window watching snow land softly on the hills, listening to carols on her battery-operated radio, and catching a glimpse of a gorgeous red Kentucky cardinal as it swooped down and perched on her windowsill.

On New Year's Day 1949, Breckinridge and the staff took a cake with twenty-one candles to her bedside. She wasn't able to take food and couldn't keep many liquids down, but the symbolic appreciation from the FNS staff did not escape her. The nurses took turns handling her care, reading mail to her, telling her amusing stories of their daily encounters. "No such nursing, no such care, no such friendship could be found anywhere else in the world," she told them. Her last words to Breckinridge just before she died in her cabin on February 8, 1949, were, "I have such a feeling of peace; deep peace."[15] Bucket was laid to rest on Wendover property, part of a two-hundred fifty acre parcel — the first FNS nurse-midwife to lie there — that would become a designated place for any FNS staff who wanted to be buried there. Locust timber for a fence and gate was cut and donated by neighbors. More than twenty-five local men volunteered to help prepare the site. Neighbor women cooked and brought meals to the Big House. After the service, Breckinridge comforted her staff by telling them, "We know that her spirit is nearer to us than the grave we tend, because to us she gave the steadfast affection of her loyal heart."[16] The same, she knew, could be said of everyone involved in the Frontier Nursing Service.

21

A New Era

Response to Lansing's novel about the FNS couriers, published in 1949 shortly after Bucket's death, was generally favorable. A former FNS courier wrote a brief review for the *Frontier Nursing Service Quarterly Bulletin*, referring to it as "enjoyable reading for anyone interested in the life that goes on here, though it was definitely written for teen-age girls." A number of early couriers—some now scattered as far away as England and France—wrote to Breckinridge with their bits of "old courier" news. It was typical of former FNS staff to stay in touch, who felt they were leaving behind their family when they departed from the Frontier Nursing Service.

One was living in France with her husband where he wrote and she painted. Another was a case worker with the Department of Welfare in Virginia. Some sent remembrances of "Bucket" after her death, including one whose infant boy was Bucket's godson. "He is a year-old today and a bouncing boy with eight teeth. I'm the world's worst correspondent but I love getting letters from all of you."[1] A few of the junior couriers returned as seniors, including Kate Ireland who came to the FNS as a junior courier following a family tradition of supporting and working with the FNS. Her grandmother was a donor and her mother chairman of the Cleveland, Ohio, committee.

Kate Ireland would be at the forefront of a new era for the Frontier Nursing Service, one that with her take-charge personality she was more than capable of handling. A social peer of Mary Breckinridge, she was also one of the few people who respected Breckinridge but did not revere her. "One evening she and I got into the most awful political fight," said Ireland. "I was a dyed-in-the-wool Republican and she was what I considered a Jeffersonian Democrat. I was trying to convince her that there was no difference between her views and that of a more liberal Republican." The two women were going at it in such a heated manner that Agnes Lewis and Brownie had to physically separate them. They tried convincing Breckinridge to go upstairs to bed, and Ireland to come to supper. But neither would give an inch. "It was a good half-hour after the supper bell rang," said Ireland, "and when the Wendover supper bell rings, I mean, that's like the good Lord calling you to heaven."[2] Finally, the hard-headed duo called a truce. But Ireland says that was not the end of her "fun" with Breckinridge. During her tenure as an FNS courier, one of her duties was preparing tea each day for her boss. Not surprisingly, a power struggle ensued.

> Come hell or high water we always had tea. And as she [Breckinridge] got older, she used to want her tea earlier and earlier. I'm always late, so it was laughable for me to get the tea on the table at four o'clock. When she began to ask for it five, fifteen, then twenty minutes early, she would go in the kitchen and get it all set up for me to carry it in. This would just slay Brownie, Betty Lester, and Agnes.[3]
>
> "How could you have Mrs. Breckinridge doing that work for you?" they would ask.
>
> But it didn't bother me. I always said, "It's her tea. I'll do the carrying but she's already in the kitchen."

In the end, Ireland said both she and Breckinridge learned to laugh it off. "I revered her as one would honor a parent," said Ireland. "But I really had very little fear of her and I didn't mind disagreeing with her. Actually, we had an awfully lot of fun."[4] An ardent animal lover like Breckinridge, Ireland named all of her Labrador retrievers after her favorite drinks: Martini, Daiquiri, Gimlet, and Shasta.

FNS secretary Lucille Knechtly remembers a summer in the 1950s when Ireland brought her convertible and her pets down from Cleveland. "In the evenings we would load up all the dogs, five or six of them, and drive to the Hyden drug store. It was the one place we could get ice cream cones for dogs and people alike."[5] Though Ireland loved canines, she wasn't particularly fond of pigs.

One hot July day Ireland was given the chore of taking one of the Ednas to market in Lexington for Breckinridge. This pig was Edna, Duchess of Wendover, a Duroc sow that weighed in at over seven hundred pounds. Ireland, Hobert Cornett (an FNS employee), and a Wendover guest left the Big House in a truck, with Edna in the back. "We had to put the guest's baggage on a platform over Edna's head," Ireland recalled. "This definitely aggravated Edna who spent the first half-hour trying to dislodge the platform and remove all the luggage." A spare tire was tied with a heavy rope to the back of the truck's cab. "By the time we reached Manchester, Edna had severed the rope and was playing football with the tire. That was seven-hundred twenty-five pounds running around in the back of the truck."

As they were turning onto a main boulevard in Lexington, the distressed sow knocked the boards off the back of the tail gate, whereupon they went flying down the city street. Ireland and Cornett stopped, got out, and retrieved the boards. They would have to be nailed back to keep Edna in place. Ireland located a hammer and a wooden mallet. Cornett rounded up some nails. The hammer was for the boards; the mallet for Edna. "It may sound inhumane to hit a pig on the head with a mallet," she said, "but a big mad pig has to be controlled somehow. I hung on to the side boards trying to prevent Edna from raising the truck bed. But her weight being greater than mine, I found myself lifted three or four feet into the air. An amusing spectacle it must have been for the onlookers—except for those we were holding up in traffic."[6] Ireland said that after that debacle, she and Cornett didn't care if they never saw another pig. But their instructions were to pick up a "young Edna" from the University of Kentucky Agricultural Experiment Station and return to Wendover. "This new Edna, weighing in at only two-hundred sixty-five pounds, was so well-mannered and friendly that she renewed our faith in pigs. But we were still very happy when she was unloaded and in her own pen at Wendover." The long day ended when Ireland entered the Big House kitchen for a late night supper and found — what else — but *pork chops* for dinner.[7]

As 1950 unfolded a new decade, it marked the start of changes that were beginning to take place within the FNS. On a minor level, the nurse-midwives would soon be wearing navy blue skirts and white shirts as opposed to riding pants and vests. The pants were designed for practicality on a horse; the skirts for professionalism. More important, the organization was beginning to accept the fact that government assistance might be necessary in order to grow and thrive with the times. Fees were still unrealistically low through the late 1940s. So the five dollars per family for full medical care now began to rise. Despite Breckinridge's lifelong opposition to government aid (she felt there were too many hoops to jump through and too much red tape) the FNS had accepted federal dollars during World War II through the Emergency Maternal and Infant Care Program, whereby the FNS was reimbursed for its care of servicemen's wives.[8] More and more, government would intervene in the FNS throughout the 1950s and 60s; some by design, some by financial necessity. In time, it would change the entire face and structure of the Frontier Nursing Service. But that would be years in the making.

The year 1950 also marked the silver anniversary of the Frontier Nursing Service. Breckinridge and several members of her staff, including senior couriers Helen "Pebble" Stone and Freddy Holdship, were honored at the Louisville Country Club luncheon. The event was attended by a hundred fifty FNS trustees, members, and friends of the FNS. Breckinridge, dressed in a simple black-and-white print dress with a silver pendant draped about her neck, stood before the crowd and relayed statistics that emphasized the expanse of health care by the Frontier Nursing Service during the past quarter century. Though she was nearly seventy years old, her voice was strong; her smile and bright blue eyes as winning as ever. "We have delivered more than eight-thousand women in childbirth," she reported, "the greater part of them in their own rural homes, with ten deaths among those women, two due to heart conditions rather than maternal causes. In preventive health work, the service has given over a hundred seventy-thousand inoculations, and cared for more than twenty-one thousand children."[9] She went on to tell the audience of the three medical clinics held each week in Hyden, and how costs had risen through the years. Maternity patients now had to pay fifteen dollars (up from five dollars) whether the delivery was in the home or at the hospital; and each FNS hospital-patient cost the FNS an average of eight dollars and twenty-five cents per day. Children continued to receive free care. The FNS budget for 1950 topped a hundred seventy-thousand dollars, she said. Social work was still funded by an annual grant from the generous Alpha Omicron Pi national fraternity. And — to emphasize the far-reaching effects of the FNS — Breckinridge told the group that of the eighty-five graduates from the FNS Graduate School of Midwifery, established in 1939, many were working in Alaska, France, India, China, Japan, Siam, the Philippines, Africa, and South America.[10]

At Wendover, while Breckinridge was away, the FNS staff was holding a party at the Upper Shelf. Calling themselves the Upper Shelfers, they concocted an "official" report to Breckinridge in her absence. "Knowing how poorly you are kept up with the delectable news of the lousy staff at Wendover," someone wrote, "we thought it fitting and proper we write you this newsy bulletin." It was published in the next issue of the *Quarterly Bulletin*, containing all the details of their hi-jinks. Between fried hamburgers cooked over the open fireplace, a surprise birthday cake for one of the staff, and the swapping of strange but true job-related stories, the women had a rare, grand time.

"When you work in a clinic, you expect anything," a nurse-midwife shared with her peers. She told them what happened to her:

> I heard the clinic door open and a husky voice say, "He got shot with a .22 and we're afraid he won't make it." I rushed into the clinic waiting room, looking from one man to the other to see which one appeared most nearly "killed."
> Except for the woe-begone expression on their faces, I could find nothing wrong with them. Then one of them reached inside his jacket and pulled out a ... bird!
> "It's Hoot Owl," he said. "He got out of his cage this afternoon and somebody shot him, bad. You reckon anything can be done for him? We've had him a year and think a sight of him."[11]

"So," the nurse continued, "in spite of the fact I knew precious little about the anatomy of an owl, I could not refuse." She bandaged the bird as best she could and sent the men on their way. They promised to let her know how the owl progressed, but she never heard back.[12] Someone repeated a child's prayer they had heard that would soon appear in the *Frontier Nursing Service Quarterly Bulletin*: "God, please give things to the poor so they won't come ask for my things."

But things were changing and the women knew that as medical care evolved outside the hills of Kentucky, so too would their roles as nurse-midwives. Nationwide, hospitals were the setting for 88 percent of American births in 1950, a figure that would rise to more than 96 percent by 1960.[13] Although nurse-midwives continued to deliver in poor urban and rural settings, their practice was legally allowed only in New Mexico, Kentucky, and New York City. Furthermore, there were lingering stereotypes that still painted a picture of midwives as "kind, but uneducated birth attendants," which stunted the professional growth of these well-trained women. (By the 1970s, midwives attended less than 1 percent of births in the U.S.) In response, the nurses saw a need to organize. In 1955, the American College of Nurse Midwives (ACNM) was incorporated as the first midwifery professional organization.[14]

The upside to the FNS was that unlike midwives throughout the U.S. who were being marginalized within the health care profession, FNS nurse-midwives were not hindered by physicians or hospital-based nurses. And because they were serving an area in which few physicians had an interest in setting up practice, and didn't typically reach the middle class, they were somewhat shielded from medical establishment criticism (and competitive fear) of the midwifery profession. Nonetheless, more and more babies were being born at Hyden Hospital in Leslie County — nearly 53 percent from 1952 to 1954 compared to 12.3 percent in 1940. Some of the increase was the result of more women *outside* the FNS territory getting medical care, or requiring more specialized care. Thus, hospital beds were by and large saved for deliveries with complications, or for women who could not be confined at home due to distance and topography.[15]

Fewer home deliveries were also the result of fewer families. Breckinridge used U.S. Census figures to counter "the nonsense written about the size of mountain families," by pointing out that the number of people in a family within the FNS districts had dropped from 5.18 (in 1930) to 4.53 (in 1950). These numbers were within a fraction of a point compared with the national average, she added.[16] When FNS nurse-midwives did go out into the night — some on horseback, some by jeep — they found much better living conditions than in years past. Homes were bigger, nicer, with more amenities. Power and telephones were no longer the rare exception. Radios and newspapers were bringing more events from the outside world and introducing mainstream American culture to the Appalachian region. Food was generally plentiful and children did not go to school barefoot — or if they did it was duly noted and the home generally visited by the FNS Social Service department asking if assistance was needed. And in those larger families they still encountered, there were few of the outdated mountaineer stereotypes.

A student midwife, in one of her first cases, found herself on call late one night at Hyden Hospital. About midnight, in the Midwife Quarters, she heard another student on the telephone saying yes, they would come.

> I jumped out of bed when Edna relayed the message, and started floundering around in an effort to get the right wearing apparel. My mind was in a jumble of thoughts—*mountain riding, nighttime, horses, should I wear long underwear, would I get there in time?*
>
> As I dashed into the hospital I found a calm man sitting there, grinning. He

was attired in mining clothes, a cap complete with carbide light on the back of his head. That was the father, come to get us. You could tell he had worked all day but he was here for his family. My supervisor was putting last minute things together and stopped only long enough to ask if I had gloves.[17]

At the barn, the student was told the horse she would ride was Doc, who stood "seventeen hands high."

As we trotted off, I learned he likes to lead, not follow. We forded the Middle Fork of the Kentucky River, followed Owl's Nest creek and rode up a small mountain. The nightmare began when we were coming down the other side. We had to dismount, walk down the slope — slippery from wet leaves — leading the horses behind us. I was afraid of getting in Doc's way as I already had purple toes from placing my foot where another horse wanted to go[18]
At one point, Doc nudged me to hurry me along and I fell on my back. I thought he was going to bite me or trample right over me. But he stood and watched with amusement as I scrambled to my feet and started off again.

At the family's home, they hitched the horses and rushed inside, convinced the baby had preceded their arrival. "However," the student nurse reported, "we found a thirty-four year old woman lying quietly in bed, smiling as us. She told us her babies "never come fast." The house had three sections: a kitchen with a coal stove, a large table, a smaller table for milk and water pails; a room with a bed on which lay an older boy; and a middle room with three beds. Five children were sound asleep on one large bed, across the room from the mother. A neighbor bustled about, boiling containers of water in the open fireplace. The father went outside to retrieve more coal to keep the house warm and the oldest child, now awake, said she would herd the younger children into the other room when it was time for delivery. "At seven-thirty A.M. a cute little blonde-haired girl made her way into the world and was greeted by her very enthusiastic family. It seems hard to believe in this age of smaller families, a ninth child would receive such an ovation. But she was welcomed as though she was the first."[19]

As the FNS nurse-midwives monitored her mother, the oldest daughter told them she had breakfast prepared. It was a meal, and a gracious family the student nurse would never forget. "We found a table laden with fried eggs, fried chicken, the best biscuits I've ever eaten, and coffee. As we ate, the children gathered round, refusing to join us but grinning their welcome and their thanks for a new baby sister. I almost hated to leave. They seemed so glad to have us there."[20]

At Wendover, Agnes Lewis, now executive secretary of the FNS, was dealing with a new administrative headache. She had been through the ropes with contractors, building permits, water and sewage problems, a major fire that destroyed the Garden House, deaths and illnesses of nursing staff (as well as her own family) and a dressing-down or two from Breckinridge. The latest project under Lewis' charge was new construction for the Margaret Voorhies

Haggin Quarters for Nurses at the Hyden Hospital. (Haggin was the wife and widow of James Ben Haggin, a wealthy, successful horse breeder in Lexington. Mrs. Haggin funded the project.) It would serve as a dormitory for the graduate nurse-midwives with a kitchen and common living area, space badly needed for the growing number of graduates beginning in the late forties. Lewis— despite her twenty years of FNS experience — was still as angst-ridden as ever when it came to new projects which she had to oversee. "It was wonderful news that work on the quarters was to start," she said, "but it sent my spirits to the heights one minute, the depths of despondency the next. I knew that no contractor would take on a building at Hyden with all of the hazards that made it a gamble, unless he took it at a price that would be prohibitive for us."

Breckinridge had facilitated the building of the hospital more than twenty-five years earlier amid circumstances that would have stymied most people. "Since then," said Lewis," all of our buildings for Mrs. Breckinridge have been child's play in comparison. She knew every pitfall of building in these mountains." Lewis, with Breckinridge's help, approached those engineers and trustees who had been in the trenches with them through the years, putting four experienced men in charge of the Haggin Quarters construction. "It's going to be fun," Lewis predicted.[21] Famous last words. A dump truck went over the precipice at the hospital construction site. No one was hurt, but the vehicle required repair. Another truck caught fire. The high loader reared up *too high* and toppled the driver, breaking his arm. And that was in the first twenty-four hours on the job. Then the rains set in. "Natural springs began bubbling up out of the hillside," said Lewis. "It was a wet, muddy, slippery mess, which slowed everything down."[22] On the bright side, they now knew where the springs were located and therefore could intelligently lay drain tile to control them.

The excavation process, which should have taken three days, took three weeks to complete. Neighbors kindly offered to give them stone for the foundation. But the contracted mason said he could not afford to haul it to the site, for there was no road in place from the homes it was offered. "With stone all around us," said Lewis, "it was ironic that we had to end up having it hauled from an adjoining county." The foundation was set and walls went up, marking real progress for the nurses' quarters. Then disaster struck, as Lewis described in her own words. "We were having tea on Sunday afternoon at Wendover" she said, "and someone remarked that two men had been killed over the weekend in a shooting. It turned out that one of them was our contracted stonemason. On Monday morning, a skeleton crew of masons showed up for work, with guns by their sides. The carpenters, all unarmed, were tense as they worked alongside the masons. No one knew who had done the shooting so they were all 'studying' each other."[23]

By day's end, with Mrs. Breckinridge out of town and a decision pending on what to do about the potentially explosive work crew, Lewis called in an FNS trustee and his son, both long-term residents of Leslie County. "This was a matter for men, not women," she explained. "They decided to stop all work for a day until they could meet and come to terms with what happened. There were many conferences."[24] Despite their differences, the workers proved honorable, telling Lewis they never failed to meet a contract and "didn't aim to start now." By the end of the week the crisis had passed and work resumed.

Soon the roof was on, the plumbing and heating was installed, and interior walls set up. A mud slide followed, lodging huge boulders against the new construction. *Well, that's the end*, Lewis thought. "That was my first reaction," she said, "when the phone woke me before seven A.M. and I was told the bad news. The boulder came down in the middle of the night with mud and muck, smack against the back wall." A cup of strong coffee later, Lewis said things didn't look quite so grim. A crew of men calmly set about cleaning up the mess; the local coal company let its driver park a dump truck near the building so that rock and mud could be more easily removed. "This was done as a courtesy and at no charge to the Frontier Nursing Service," said Lewis. "The cost of the truck and driver alone would have been prohibitive for us."[25] This gesture alone was testament to the ties that bound the FNS and the local community in loyalty and kindness toward each other. If you gained trust and credibility, and needed help, someone would always be there.

When the building was nearly complete, simple furnishings were ordered: A metal bed for each room with comfortable mattress and springs but no headboard; an unpainted chest of drawers with a mirror above it; a combination desk-table; a gooseneck lamp; a bedside rug. The only feminine touch was a set of dotted Swiss curtains. The common lounge area was dedicated to the late Dorothy "Bucket." "She really cared about the comfort of the nurses in their off-duty hours," said Lewis, "and thought nothing much of her own comfort on or off-duty. We wanted it to be bright and cheerful, but informal. It should be a room that was lived in every day."

The walls were painted a pale green, she added, offset by the dark woodwork. A huge stone fireplace sat between two double windows that provided long range views of the Cumberland Mountains. An FNS trustee built a sturdy library table using a black walnut tree cut from the pasture at Wendover. The tree was cut so that electric lines could be installed at the Big House. "Mac [FNS nurse Ann MacKinnon] and I went to Lexington and picked out furniture, lamps, and odds and ends," said Lewis. "We could almost hear Bucket chuckling as we made our different selections."[26] As the Margaret Voorhies Haggin Quarters for Nurses was completed and furnished in the spring of 1950, Lewis said the pangs of construction began to recede with the joy of completion. So many people helped make it possible, she said, "their names are too numerous to mention. But their kindnesses we shall never forget."[27]

22

Brownie and Breckinridge

As the new nurses' quarters were being completed in 1950, the assistant director of the Frontier Nursing Service, Helen Edith Browne (known as "Brownie"), was preparing for a trip to the Fourth American Congress on Obstetrics and Gynecology in New York City. The first international meeting of specialists in ob-gyn held in the U.S., it drew doctors and nurses from all over the world. Breckinridge wanted Brownie to attend in an effort to promote the FNS among prestigious medical specialists, and to bring back any new knowledge she gleaned on midwifery techniques. She once called Brownie "the most brilliant teacher we ever had and the most lucid in imparting knowledge."[1]

Born in 1900 in the English village of Brushbrook, with a population of less than three hundred, Browne said she wanted to be a nurse from the time her mother became ill and nurses were constantly in and out of her home. She explained how she came to eastern Kentucky: "My mother had complications after my younger sister was born. In those days, in England, the midwife came and stayed for a month when the baby was born. This particular woman was very nice and we were quite fond of her. After she left, we had a series of other nurses, so this introduced me to the profession."[2] Her father, in banking, thought secretarial work in a bank was a better field for his spinster daughter, so he sent her to someone to learn shorthand. "I thought this was the worst thing in the world," said Browne. "I could not bear it. Looking back, I realize how stupid that was; I should have taken the time to learn it.[3]

With her mother's sympathetic help, Browne persuaded her father to let her enter nursing school instead. In 1930, she entered Bartholomew's Hospital School of Nursing, a three-year program, followed by entry into the same midwifery school that both Betty Lester and Mary Breckinridge had attended, British Mothers and Babies. It was considered one of the best midwifery training schools in England, said Browne. It was here that she handled the first of many birthing complications she would encounter as a nurse-midwife.

We had a case involving a Maltese woman who spoke very broken English. She had already lost two babies, though not with us. She was told that if she came to the British Hospital, they would save her baby. She went into labor and everything seemed to be going along normally.

I came in at six the next morning to relieve the night duty midwife and she said to me, "I don't know what's going on here." She was examining the mother and was feeling intestines or something. It turned out to be a ruptured uterus. We sent for the doctor and had to prepare for surgery. The baby just kind of floated out, and it didn't live. Some have been known to live if you can get them out in time, but I think this baby's heart had stopped before we even sent for the doctor.[4]

I remember the doctor was getting ready to stitch the mother up and I spoke up to say that I didn't think we had the placenta yet. It too, had separated and floated out of the uterus. So the doctor felt around and discovered the placenta had wrapped around the kidney. This was in the days before penicillin, so the woman developed a severe infection. She was terribly ill, but she finally made it.[5]

Browne learned of the Frontier Nursing Service, then in its first decade, while she was working private midwifery for a couple who lived outside of London. "They were kind of kooky people," recalled Browne, "who wanted a midwifery delivery at home. Everything went normally and I stayed on to help with the baby. The first week was very hard because the baby was expected to sleep with the midwife rather than the mother. She expected me to be in uniform when I took the baby to her, even if I had been up half the night. I brought the baby into the room, turned it over to the mother, and was told there was a call for me." It was another nurse who informed Browne that midwives were needed in eastern Kentucky. "*Kentucky*?" Browne replied. "What's that?" She knew little about America as a whole, much less some obscure region deep in its heart.

Once Browne completed her nursing commitments, she talked with the nurse who had notified her of the FNS, learning that not only were midwives needed, but they got to ride horseback in rural country. "It sounded very exciting," said Browne. "I told her to get me an application and a permission form to go."[6] Six weeks later, in July 1938, she arrived in New York City en route to Leslie County, exactly ten years after FNS nurse-midwife Betty Lester had first set foot in America. "I got to New York dressed in my traditional wool suit and it was very hot," said Browne. "My first impression was that when I stopped to get a cup of tea, it was brought in a cup with a lukewarm tea bag. And I was absolutely horrified. These Americans did not know how to make a decent cup of tea. Never heard of 'iced' tea, and when I did, I didn't consider it tea at all."[7]

Accompanied by a Red Cross nurse who met her in New York, Browne traveled by train to Lexington, then on to Hazard, just as Lester and other FNS nurse-midwives had done before her. And like the other nurses, she had trouble with the local dialect. At a stopover in Hazard, a waiter asked what she wanted for breakfast. She told him a bowl of "corn flakes." He brought her a bowl filled to the brim with corn cakes. By now, she said, Wendover seemed like "the end of the world." When the bus driver let her off on the narrow road into Hyden she was met by an FNS courier who handed her a pair of pants and told to put them on. "Right here in the middle of the *road?*" Browne asked. "It's all right," replied the courier. "You can go over there behind the bushes."[8]

At Wendover, every window in the Garden House was open, with curious FNS staff hanging onto the sills. "They were looking to see this new body from England," Browne recalled, "for they hadn't had a new nurse in quite some time. Dorothy Buck was among the first to show me around, and to recognize how tired I was. It was delightful to go to bed in the Big House." Breckinridge was away having back surgery, so Browne received her FNS initiation the next morning when she visited nursing outposts in heavy rain, in which she had to cross the swinging bridge and stay afloat on the river as her horse swam across. "I was petrified," she admitted.

A few weeks later Browne was back at Wendover when Breckinridge returned home. "The staff were all running around like ants," she said, "getting ready for her, making sure everything was just right. Then I came down with an awful sinus infection and had to be put to bed in the guest room down the hall from Mrs. Breckinridge. I remember her coming into my room, my first meeting with her, and she had a book in her hand. 'Can you read French, child?' she asked. "Then she handed me the book and said read it. So I read it, though I had to think rather carefully to get through it. In those days, we never argued with Mrs. Breckinridge. If she said something was to be done, it was done, come hell or high water. That was my first impression as a newcomer."[9] Her initial outpost was the Red Bird District, where she learned to attune her ear to the local dialect, even, in time, picking up certain speech patterns, as in saying "huh" either before or after a sentence. She called it "a dreadful habit." "It was one I found myself doing until one day Agnes Lewis said 'Brownie,' you must stop that. It's perfectly awful.'"

Only a year after her arrival, World War II broke out in Europe and thirteen of the British nurses returned home. Browne was not one of them. "I was then thirty-nine, and was feeling a bit hemmed in by the hills. I decided to take a vacation and go to Vancouver Island where my mother had some cousins. The round-trip ticket from Lexington to Vancouver was two hundred dollars, including four nights on the train. While there, I thought about going back to school, but I really couldn't leave the FNS."[10] She returned to the FNS that same year and worked at the Bull Creek District, then Flat Creek, and on to the hospital at Hyden to handle the clinical duties at the newly formed Frontier Graduate School. Her contact with Breckinridge during this period was sporadic. "I would see her about once a week when she came over to have tea with the students. She also liked to have the nurses come to Wendover to talk with her."

Browne noted that despite receiving the same training at the British Mothers and Babies Hospital where she was certified, Breckinridge "never caught a baby in Kentucky." "She was far too busy running the FNS organization. She tried to deliver a baby on several occasions when she went out to the districts, especially if the midwives were out when a call came in. I remember once, when a courier was with her, she said 'Child, get the delivery bags, we'll at least start out.'"[11] The courier had to remind Breckinridge, who was then in her seventies, that she could no longer see very well. "That's all right," said Breckinridge, according to Browne. "I can at least give the mother my support."[12]

Browne became Hyden Hospital superintendent following Ann Mackinnon's departure for England during World War II. In 1947, she moved to Wendover in order to work with Dorothy Buck, whose role she would inherit upon Buck's death. It was "Bucket," in fact, who, learning of her own poor prognosis from cancer, chose Browne to succeed her. "Bucket was worried, "said Browne," very worried about how difficult I might find it to work for Mrs. Breckinridge. She told me 'Mrs. Breckinridge is a very demanding person.' And I said, well, I will give it a try."[13] The two strong-willed women, Breckinridge and Browne, had already disagreed on a couple of nursing procedures while Browne was hospital superintendent. One incident involved the length of time new mothers should be up and about following delivery. Breckinridge used stinging sarcasm to get her point across when she dropped by the hospital to check in. "Brownie," she told me, 'I really don't mind you getting them out of bed if you would just make them walk on all fours. Nature didn't intend man to stand up so soon.' Of course, it's been proven since then that getting the mothers up fairly soon made for a more satisfactory recovery," said Browne.[14]

As Dorothy Buck lay dying at Wendover, she turned many of her administrative duties over to Browne, telling her she needed to start with one of the toughest parts of the job — rejecting nurses who wanted to join the FNS. Browne said the hardest letter she had to write was to a young American-born Japanese nurse just after the war had ended when racial tensions were still high. "She had excellent references. I took her file to Mrs. Breckinridge, explaining the woman had been interned here in America due to her heritage, and I just wasn't sure what to do. Mrs. Breckinridge said she would take it up with the Hyden committee. And she did. When the case was presented to them, an old man stood up and voiced his feelings. He said, 'We've just been fighting those yellow-skinned people. She'll be blamed for anything that happens to a patient under her care.' And he was absolutely right. So I wrote to the girl and told her exactly what happened. And I got a very nice letter back. She said she had been turned down by so many people, but never given a reason, and she was grateful to know why."[15]

By 1950, when Browne attended the international conference, she had taken over the duties of assistant to the director. (Eventually, she would become director of the Frontier Nursing Service). As right hand to Breckinridge, many of the directorship duties fell to her when Breckinridge began her autobiography, *Wide Neighborhoods*, published in 1952. The book would take her nearly two years to complete, using Agnes Lewis and Browne as her readers, a chore which proved difficult at times. "She wrote a chapter a week and we were to read it on the weekend and review it for her on Monday morning," Browne recalled. "Sometimes it was on bits of scrap paper and we'd turn it this way and that trying to read what she had written." "But she worked very hard at it and didn't like to be told she hadn't written a good chapter. She also didn't like it when the book's editor had her slash many of the names. She had a tremendous memory for names and they were very important to her."[16] In Breckinridge's defense, she was no doubt well aware that without the financial and public support of the numerous people and agencies that helped her through the years, the FNS would not have survived, much less flourished, and she probably wanted to give credit where credit was due.

In the 1950 summer issue of the *Quarterly Bulletin*, Breckinridge reported to readers that she was working on the book "five or six hours a day." "I get through around five thousand words a week, including research and revisions, usually starting my day between four and five A.M. since I work best in the mornings. Thumper (secretary Lucille Knechtly) is handling my correspondence. After noon luncheon, I read my mail and then go out of doors to do things around the place in the open air. At Wendover, we have tea at four P.M. I rarely work after that. Around eight P.M. I fall asleep for eight unbroken hours of sleep before my day begins again."[17] The book's purpose, she explained, was to raise funds for the FNS, with all royalties going direct to the organization. Recognizing it was not a scholarly work, Breckinridge acknowledged that it had no footnotes, no appendix, and no apologies.

That same summer a group of dental students from the University of Louisville came to visit Breckinridge at Wendover. They found her lifestyle at the Big House comfortable, but not pretentious. And they found Breckinridge herself far from the stiff-necked icon some had preconceived. "When she sat down with us," said one of the dental students, "she took out a cigarette, inserted it into a pencil-sized holder about eight inches in length, lit it, and puffed away as we talked. Later, she lifted the cozy off the tea pot and there sat a bottle of wine which was our 'tea' for the afternoon."[18]

As Breckinridge's seventieth birthday approached, the FNS staff went into high gear planning a celebration, one that she had given them permission to hold "as long as it was a little one." It was, however, her first birthday party since her childhood, so in the end no detail was overlooked, despite her modest protests. February 17, 1951, dawned warm and sunny, as though Mother Nature planned to salute Breckinridge as well. More than twenty people — men and women who worked on the FNS property — paraded into her room at precisely eight A.M. to sing "Happy Birthday." Other staff members, close to fifty of them, crowded into the Big House dining room for a noonday meal. On the menu were Breckinridge's favorites: spoon bread with turkey hash, mustard greens, and young green onions. The cook whipped up a vanilla cake from

scratch and carefully pushed seventy candles into the thick creamy icing, decorated with yellow and white roses. Agnes Lewis set arrangements of fresh daf-
fodils about the living room and Scottish nurse Ann MacKinnon "Mac" stood
up at the dinner table and proposed a Gaelic toast: "Lang may your lum reek,"
which translated meant, "Long may your chimney smoke."[19]

The Hyden telephone operator called to say she had so many telegrams
on hand for Breckinridge that she couldn't possibly read them all over the
phone. Could someone come get them? And as the day ended, Breckinridge
was presented with a gift from the entire staff — a four-volume set of books on
Robert E. Lee, with inscriptions from everyone who had contributed to its purchase. Breckinridge spoke briefly, genuinely touched by her staff's attention.
As night fell on her seventh decade, shadows stole across the Middle Fork River
and crept toward the rock-strewn path to the Big House, past the little stone
chapel and the giant beech trees. Unlike the early years, the 1950s would prove
a more stable time for the Frontier Nursing Service, with fewer money and
administrative problems and less staff turnover.

By 1951, the FNS had delivered more than eighty-five hundred patients
since its inception, with more than sixty-five hundred cases delivered *in the
home*. Ten maternal deaths were reported. The result was a gross maternal death
rate of 1.2 per thousand live births, a number that compared with the U.S. rate
of 7.5 per *ten thousand* in 1951. (By contrast, the maternal death rate in 2001
was 1.0 per ten thousand within the U.S.)[20] Nationwide, the postwar economy
was booming and families were increasing their standard of living. A new car
could be had for about two thousand dollars, gasoline was running twenty-
seven cents a gallon, and televisions were becoming more commonplace.
Though World War II had halted sales and public broadcasts, post-war buyers
had purchased more than thirteen million TVs by 1951. President Truman made
his first coast-to-coast broadcast in September of that year, and the *I Love Lucy*
show premiered.

Though the Wendover staff had no TV as yet (Breckinridge could barely
manage to operate a radio much less a new-fangled TV), she would be asked
to come as a guest for a taped segment of *This is Your Life*, an Emmy-winning
documentary series hosted by its producer, Ralph Edwards. It originally aired
in 1952 before a live audience. The format was simple: Edwards surprised his
guest, a celebrity or public figure, with family members, friends, or old acquaintances from their past who made public tributes to the guest from an infamous
"red book" that Edwards used for his mini-biographies. It was really quite an
honor, indicative of Breckinridge's stature on the American landscape by the
1950s. The program's guest roll included famous names and faces from come-
dian Milton Berle to actress Maureen O'Hara who starred alongside John
Wayne, among others. There were even British, Australian, and New Zealand
versions of the show. Yet following the initial shock of being invited, Breckinridge and her staff reconsidered the offer. Assistant FNS director Helen Browne,

in particular, thought it was a bad idea, though it would have certainly boosted FNS public awareness and possibly donations.

Browne corresponded with Ralph Edwards asking him just who they planned to "surprise" Breckinridge with on the show. There was a rumor they would fly in a few of the early FNS British nurses, bringing them to California for the broadcast. "I did try to protect her," said Browne. "What if they brought on Richard Thompson (Breckinridge's second husband) and faced her with *him*?" Few people knew there was rumored infidelity on the part of Thompson while he was married to Breckinridge, and that he had supposedly left her, not the other way around.[21] When the TV show refused to reveal their list of surprise guests, Browne (with Breckinridge's support) wrote back and turned them down. Breckinridge had just been named Kentuckian of the Year by the state's press association and felt that public awareness of the FNS was already high. "But it was a hard thing to do, not going on the show" Browne admitted.[22]

Breckinridge did agree to appear on the *Bob Hope Daytime Show* in 1954 during War Health Day. She was chosen as "woman of the week" representing nurses worldwide who were considered pioneers. Hope found her through the publication of her book, *Wide Neighborhoods*, calling it "as exciting to read as any fiction."[23] Once in print, the book actually received uneven reviews. To her credit, Breckinridge published both positive and negative newspaper reviews in the *Quarterly Bulletin*, contending the comments all "amused" her. After all, she wrote the book for the FNS, not herself she said, and believed that "no one is going to kick an old woman in the face" with crushing criticism. Reviewer critiques ranged from "an honest, eloquent account," to "diffuse, awkward, and overburdened with unimportant minutia."[24] But it certainly had its share of supporters and sold enough copies to warrant a second, and then a third printing. Its first printing run brought the FNS more than two thousand dollars in royalties.

Those who wrote about the FNS, and even a few of its own staff in the early 1950s would begin to refer to the era as a "dull period" for the Frontier Nursing Service, particularly in contrast to its earlier decades of struggle, sacrifice, and the ultimate romanticism of the "heroic, adventurous" nurse-midwives. Such comparisons were relative, of course, and simply a matter of perception. For all intents and purposes, the FNS was still a ground-breaking, historically significant achievement. Through Breckinridge's fundraising efforts (including sales from her book) and her tireless round of speaking engagements (a dozen plus trips in 1952 alone, at the age of seventy) she had managed to raise millions of dollars and devote more than a quarter century of her long life to the Frontier Nursing Service. The next year, 1953, would once again test her mettle along with the stamina of the FNS staff.

23

Fire, Loss and Other Mishaps

No one knows how the blaze began, but it was bad. The call came in at Wendover during a bridge game that the hills behind the hospital and around Beech Fork Center were on fire and they needed all the hands they could find. Ann MacKinnon was the long-time Hyden Hospital superintendent. While her wards filled with new patients requiring standard surgeries, the night sky was lit by flames that came as close as eight hundred feet to the hospital buildings. MacKinnon, who had survived two world wars and numerous crises, was unflappable, going on about her administrative duties while the fires raged nearby.

For over a week in and around FNS property, the air turned acrid with smoke. The nurse-midwives pitched in wherever they could to water horses and cows which were fidgety from the foul air. FNS trustees joined the fire brigade, raking a wide fire ring along the ridge of the mountain behind the hospital and at Beech Fork Center. Brisk winds kept the flames going. There was talk of evacuation, so several of the FNS nurse-midwives packed a suitcase with valuables and boxed up the nursing records, setting them by the door in case they needed tossing in the jeep for safekeeping. Three blows on the horn was a signal that the fire was reaching the nurses' center. One nurse-midwife worried about her horse, Bobbin, wondering if he'd be safe in a fire-encircled pasture. She also had a week-old calf to fret over. If the barn caught on fire, Flossie the cow would be the only animal left to look after her. The school closed and the older children were enlisted to help fight the inferno. By now the entire community was out in full force, raking one huge ring the twelve-mile length of the FNS property at Beech Fork. Finally, it rained and dampened down the smoldering fire.

Hyden in 1953 had a decent highway all the way until the turn-off for Wendover. Then the road became a creek bed. When a new courier arrived in February, she was met by an FNS staff member driving an old Dodge truck. There were now twenty horses at Wendover, a mule, fourteen jeeps, and a station wagon besides the old truck. The new courier was instructed to put her typewriter and radio up on the seat and keep her feet up in case water came through the truck's floorboards. "Why?" she asked. They were on dry land. "Because we have to ford the river," said the driver, revving the engine. Later the courier, relating the event, wrote to her sister: "I do not think any G.I. could have handled any army truck better than this woman did. She just pushed that old truck against the river bed, in we went, and then out again. And we made it with no water in the truck."[1]

Though it was February, with snow dappling the mountaintops, crocuses were in bloom. To the newcomer's surprise, there were not only windows in her room at the Big House, but steam heat and running water. "The little cabins up the hill overlook everything," she said, "and they have a fireplace in every room, but no running water. I believe I am going to be very happy here."[2] What she did not anticipate upon her arrival, was the impending death of a long-time FNS staff member, the unflappable jokester, Gaelic toastmistress, World War I medalist Ann P. MacKinnon, or "Mac." Born in the Scottish Highlands in 1885, Mac was the youngest of twelve children and despite time and distance remained close to most of her siblings throughout her life. Gaelic was her native tongue, the language in which she told her friends at the FNS she tended to think.

She volunteered for World War I at the request of the French Army, one of eight British sisters in the French Flag Nursing Corps. Moved to the front lines, the women were often under fire. When not on the field tending to the wounded, they stayed in clearing station — dugouts, huts, sometimes even a house. Mac was cited for her "remarkable coolness and courage" under fire, receiving the Croix de Guerre, the French medal of honor for exceptional gallantry. Throughout the war, she kept a small tartan-covered book in which she jotted notes or had others sign their messages. It was one of the few personal keepsakes she carried when she came to eastern Kentucky as a Frontier Nurse in 1928. The other thing she brought was a tremendous fear of thunder storms. When working indoors, she would literally duck and hide until the thunderous noise subsided. She explained it was too much like the roar of the great guns.

As superintendent of Hyden Hospital, her administrative skills were considered superior and her ability to roll with the punches one of her best qualities. "She took everything in stride," said Breckinridge. "During one of the many renovations at the hospital, the dust would get so bad she would have to leave her duty station and go wash out the inside of her mouth. But the hospital continued to run with exquisite order."[3] She returned to England in May 1940 along with a dozen other FNS nurse-midwives who felt the need to assist their home countries during the European siege. In England she was made superintendent of a casualty evacuation train, transporting injured men, women, and children from some of the most blitzed areas of the country to hospitals, or treating them on board when necessary. To cheer up her patients, she was known to take up collections for surprise gifts, and once created a garden spot on the train from items she found in a rubbish dump. The hospital train was bombed at one point and Mac sustained a broken back. Breckinridge wrote to her during this time, thanking her for the care she had provided to Breckinridge a decade earlier during her own back injury, and telling her, "I wish there was something I could do for you." She could not mention the bombing in the FNS *Quarterly Bulletin* due to wartime censorship, but Mac's meticulous care of her was something she said she would never forget.[4]

Yet it was Mac's appreciation for the absurd that people remembered most. Every New Year's Eve she arranged for a costume party, telling guests to come dressed as book characters, movie stars, or her theme of the year. The games they played often spilled over into the ward, including Mac's version of "Hide & Seek," in which a nurse, dressed in costume, might pop out from under a patient's bed, carefully choosing wards where no one was *too* ill. Now Mac herself became the patient. As rain was falling that helped douse the forest fires, Mac was hit with a coronary occlusion. She was placed in a hospital bed in the same ward in which she had just worked.

At Wendover, Helen Browne received word of Mac's heart attack by phone and called Breckinridge in Chicago where she was on a fund-raising trip. Betty Lester accompanied Mac to Lexington in the FNS station wagon that also served as an ambulance, then returned to Hyden to take over as superintendent until Mac was back on the job. Mac stayed eight weeks at the Good Samaritan Hospital in Lexington, treated with such care that physicians "tiptoed in and out of her room, peeking into her oxygen tent as though to assure her she was in good hands," according to Breckinridge, who added: "Her own Kentucky mountain crowd never let more than a few days pass without a visit." That included Breckinridge, of course.[5] When the Lexington hospital had done all they could for her, Mac was sent by ambulance back to Hyden where she was placed in her old room at the hospital's nursing quarters. Her friend and colleague, Betty Lester, took over her care, along with running the hospital as superintendent.

Mac was too good a nurse herself, said Breckinridge, to deny her own prognosis. "She knew her chances of pulling through were slim," said Breckinridge.[6] Betty Lester stayed close by her friend, often bending over her to hear Mac whisper names from her childhood. Breckinridge came into her room even when she lay unconscious, speaking softly to her, expressing her appreciation for her years of devotion to the Frontier Nursing Service, as well as to her. "When my glance fell upon her desk," said Breckinridge, "I was humbled anew. For there on the wall two pictures were hung — one of Winston Churchill and one of me."[7] Mac died on February 9, 1953, and was buried in the Wendover cemetery where Bucket was laid to rest four years earlier. It was fitting, said Breckinridge, that she should overlook the river she had crossed so many times during her twenty-five years as a Frontier Service Nurse.

A year later, a new drug room was dedicated to MacKinnon at the Hyden Hospital as a memorial to the late superintendent. More than a hundred fifty people attended the ceremony, including Breckinridge, who noted the room cost twelve hundred dollars to build, with less than a hundred owed due to generous donations. The hospital's Women's Auxiliary baked a total of thirty homemade cakes to serve as refreshments in the nurses' quarters after the dedication. Following Mac's death, Helene Brown and Betty Lester announced they both needed a vacation. They left together on a train headed to New York. Lester went on to England for a three-month visit to her family — the first in eight years. She also planned to attend the International Congress of Midwives in London and return to the States by plane — her first airborne experience.

Brownie headed off to Alberta, Canada, to spend time with friends who were ex-FNS nurse midwives and couriers. Breckinridge took a break too, visiting her sister-in-law in the Virginia Shenandoah Valley, the only holiday she took in 1954. At Wendover, Agnes Lewis was left to put out the word that FNS couriers, secretaries, and non-midwife nurses were needed. In particular, they were short of junior couriers, stenographers, and typists, partly due to the six weeks annual vacation the FNS generously gave its fulltime staff. Nurses were needed for rotation at the outpost centers since many of the original FNS had moved on to the Graduate School program.

Among those left to handle deliveries and family practice was Anna May January. In an FNS Quarterly Bulletin, she recounted one memorable experience: Clouds hovered just above the mountains that cold memorable night. The wind howled and moaned, causing January to toss and turn, she recalled. *What a night to have a race with the stork*, she thought. "I had paid a call on my patient that day and there was no sign of an imminent delivery. So, after listening with one ear cocked till nearly midnight, I decided fate wouldn't send me out on a four-mile trip up the river from Wendover. So I settled down to sleep."[8] About fifteen minutes later she was called to the phone. "I sure hate to git you out on sich a night," said the father, "but I reckon Judy's time has come. You better hurry."[9]

January dressed quickly and grabbed her midwifery bags. A form appeared in the doorway. It was a young student nurse from Hyden Hospital who was staying for the weekend at Wendover. She wanted to come along. "Then get dressed and follow me," said January. They went to the barn and began to saddle up the horses. "We started off by falling into holes and skirting tree limbs. After what seemed an eternity of thrashing about in the rain, the thunder, the lightning, and the potholes, we finally neared the house — only to find that the barn had blown down and bits of it were flying about." They managed to find a standing fence post and hitched their animals. "Rushing into the house," said January, "I was relieved to find Judy, the mother, sitting up in bed rocking back and forth. She greeted me with three words: 'Cow and mule,' which I got between her pains." "Now Judy," the nurse-midwife said, "what is your pain going to tell me about the cow and the mule? I had no idea what she was talking about, and she had not that much longer to go."

The mule and cow were covered by the fallen barn and Judy was worried about losing them. January, trying to distract her, set about preparing for the delivery. "Reassuring her that her husband would take care of the cow and the mule, I assembled my supplies. Very soon, a ten-pound bouncing baby boy arrived. He greeted the night with a lusty yell."[10] But her troubles were not yet over. "She had a partially separated placenta with hemorrhage. I immediately started her poor husband back down the creek to Wendover to relay word to our Medical Director at Hyden Hospital."

Yet January knew that with no phone operating at night between Wendover and Hyden, and the river at high tide, it could take hours before the medical director was reached. "This meant Judy's life depended on me. I did a manual removal of the placenta and with my assistant's help, treated Judy for shock. I shall never forget the poor student nurse trying to get the foot of the double bed up on a chair." The patient slowly began coming out of shock. "By now, I was a little shocky myself," said January, "for my knees were beginning to shake and I felt like I was on paper legs." The patient continued to improve. The husband returned with a message from Brownie saying she would make the trip to Hyden for the doctor and send him up the creek. "With this assurance," recalled January, "I took care of the baby. When I put him in his mother's arms she smiled at me and said 'Hit's a caution how much he looks like John.'" By seven A.M. that morning, with mother, baby, cow, and mule all alive and well, January said she and her student nurse took their leave. "Only the barn," she added, "failed to survive."[11]

A few British nurse-midwives were still finding their way to the Frontier Nursing Service by the mid–1950s. Among them was Primrose Frances Mary Bowling, born in the village of Wellington Heath in Herefordshire in 1928. She would soon distinguish herself not just as an excellent health care professional, but as the only British-born FNS staff to marry a local. Several of her nursing friends had arrived in eastern Kentucky before her, writing home to tell her of the "strange, but interesting region" in which they worked. Like her predecessors, she arrived in New York by way of ship and was met by an American Red Cross representative. "My first impression of America was that the cars were enormous and in colors I had never seen before — pink, yellow, pale blue. The Red Cross worker took me on a whirlwind tour of the city and we went to several eating establishments. I had never seen a hamburger, or eaten one. Then I learned I was going to Kentucky on a bus. I wasn't too keen on that as I thought it would take forever."[12]

She had one other problem. The dear child, as Breckinridge would soon be calling her, had lugged her thirty-five pound sewing machine all the way across the Atlantic and was now trying to get the thing checked, along with her luggage, onto the bus headed for Kentucky. "Carry it as personal luggage," the check-in clerk instructed. "*What?*" Bowling asked. "I can't lug this wretched thing around. It's much too heavy." The clerk shook his head. "Can't be responsible for it; you'll have to take it as personal luggage."[13] So Bowling hauled it onto the bus, rode as far as Philadelphia, changed buses, rode to Pittsburgh, changed buses again, on to Cleveland, Columbus, and Cincinnati, Ohio, transferring the irksome sewing machine at each stopover. "When I finally got to Lexington it was boiling hot and I had on winter clothing because it was cold when I left England."

When she stepped off the bus in Hyden, exhausted from the heat and the struggles with her unwelcome luggage, she said she could not believe her eyes. "All the buildings in town were wooden. And there were no pavements, just wooden walkways. The main road was gravel with lots of potholes. A man stood on the corner with two pistols on his hip. And I thought it must be some poor, eccentric old gentleman with toy guns. But when I asked the courier who met me about him, she said, 'Oh, that's the High Sheriff.' "So those guns are *real?*" Bowling replied, incredulous. "Of course," the courier said, laughing. *Oh my*, thought Bowling. *What kind of place have I come to?* The courier told her to get in the jeep. "We went up another rough road and crossed the river. It was fairly high water and I couldn't swim so I just held my breath till we got to the other side."[14]

Nothing seemed normal to Bowling until they reached Wendover and she was introduced to Breckinridge, who welcomed her into the fold. Bowling would thereafter refer to Breckinridge as "one of the finest women who ever lived in Kentucky." But her first few months on the job were often as rough-edged as the conditions she first encountered, with hard-won lessons for Bowling. "There was a real lack of social life," she said. "In England, young people in the 1950s had very active social lives but there wasn't much to do in eastern Kentucky. So I often went to church. At my first visit, a woman came up and asked if I was "one of them," and I wasn't sure what she meant. Then she asked what kind of church I attended in England so I tried to explain Church of England. After that, most thought I was Roman Catholic. Even the minister preached on Catholics versus Baptists, which I really didn't appreciate."[15]

When Bowling heard a rumor that the minister was telling his congregation people in England "bow to a King and Queen instead of praying to God," she had enough. "I wanted to explain to him that we bow to a king and queen out of respect, nothing else," she said, "but one of the other nurses told me to leave it alone."[16] "Don't ever criticize," was her friend's advice regarding the locals. What troubled Bowling even more was the fatalistic attitude she encountered among some of the mountain people. "There was so much time spent on worrying about the hereafter instead of the here and now, it seemed strange to be wasting time on that."

One family refused much-needed medical help for their infant, telling Bowling that "whatever happens is the Lord's will." "I ended up just praying with them as that is all they would let me do, and the child died. That upset me very much."[17] Sometimes the cultural differences were simply a matter of taste. On a trip to an FNS outpost clinic with an American nurse-midwife, Bowling was asked if she wanted a root beer. "I don't drink beer," she replied, "especially on the job." "It isn't beer," the American nurse said, grinning. "It's soda pop. Here, try it." Bowling took a large swig and immediately spat it out. "That's the most horrible stuff I've ever tasted!" she said, wiping her mouth.[18]

Lost and scared alone on horseback in the hills, moonshine stills, feuding families, strange old grannys with corncob pipes, children with parasites, shots in the dark — she encountered them all during her first year at the FNS, she said. There were times she thought seriously about loading up her sewing machine and heading back to England. And then something happened. "I was transferred to Red Bird Center, a beautiful log cabin that was funded by Mrs. Henry Ford Company. I drove a jeep all the time and I delivered many babies. One day a man came to the clinic I had never seen before, said his name was Johnny. He wanted me to go see about his wife who was having a miscarriage. Could he ride with me in the jeep? I didn't see any of the people he said were going to help carry his wife out, but at least I had my dog with me."[19]

Though wary of the stranger and uncertain of his intentions, Bowling said she allowed him in her jeep. Johnny reached back to pat the dog on the head. "Wouldn't touch him if I were you," Bowling cautioned. "He can be quite vicious sometimes." The dog jumped in Johnny's lap and began to lick his face. "Well," said Bowling, "we finally rounded the bend in the road and met up with all the people who said they would help. When he got to Johnny's house, sure enough, his poor wife was in a terrible condition. We loaded her on a canvas stretcher and carried her to the main road, using the jeep's headlights to guide us."[20] As the woman was being lifted into the jeep for the trip to Hyden Hospital, her husband reached inside his coat pocket. Bowling drew back, not sure of what he was doing. He pulled out a twenty dollar bill and handed it to his wife. "Been saving for just this occasion," he explained. "Give it to the ones who take good care of you."[21]

A few weeks later, Bowling was privy to saving a young mother's baby when the infant presented as a breech birth. In other circumstances, it would have been a hospital delivery. "This was her first child. We were alone, trapped in her cabin in the snow, with no help from anywhere. She delivered a beautiful baby girl, one that turned out to be her only living child, for she had several miscarriages following that birth."[22] Bowling was finally beginning to realize that these strange people with their unfamiliar ways had many things to teach her; and that their kindnesses often knew no bounds. "I went to deliver a child one night and finished up about two A.M. I was dreading the ride back to the nursing center, alone, in the dark, for the FNS Center was isolated, away from other houses. After the baby and the mother were all settled, the grandmother came to me, holding a beautiful blue silk nightgown she had taken from a trunk. 'You are going to stay with us tonight,' she said. And though she was a strange old lady — smoked a corncob pipe and made her own tobacco — I was very relieved that I didn't have to make the drive back. I stayed the night in a big old double bed in the room with the mother and baby."[23]

It was in this same neighborhood that Bowling met her future husband. "It caused quite a stir in the community when I met Bobby and we began dating," Bowling recalled. "I was the first English girl who ever dated a local man, let alone married him."[24] Uncertain how Breckinridge would take the news of the impending nuptials, Bowling was stunned — and grateful — when the Big House at Wendover was offered up for the nuptials. The FNS staff said that Breckinridge had always wanted a wedding to take place at Wendover for it seemed to her the perfect setting to start a new life. In true FNS style, housekeepers and nurses went to work on decorating the place for "Prim" and her groom, completed with wild daisies, cucumber tree blossoms, and flowers from the garden at the large windows in the living room. The deer head over the stone fireplace wore white satin bows around its antlers, and a resourceful kitchen worker covered a clean garbage can with a white feed sack, then filled it with ice for the fruit punch.

The maid of honor had a slight mishap when her jeep ran off the road en route to Wendover, but neither she nor the LP (long-playing) records she brought for the wedding music were any worse for wear. Bowling's only other diversion was that on the morning of the wedding she had to stop getting ready long enough to teach her relief nurse how to milk the cow. Following the ceremony, a wedding breakfast was held at the walnut dining table in the Big House, the scene of numerous sit-downs meals the FNS nurses, staff, and visitors had shared throughout the past three decades. Before leaving on a short honeymoon, Primrose and Robert Bowling were transported to their car by a friend and neighbor wearing a top hat, in his bright green, mule-driven wagon.[25] Ironically — considering Bowling's reluctant initial acceptance of the locals — her new mother-in-law owned "a nice mule," and was "a true mountain woman" who taught her everything from how to grind corn to how to make soap. In the evenings, the newlyweds — with no TV or decent working radio — played card games with Mrs. Bowling. When the couple moved to Hazard in 1956, Bowling found she actually missed the eastern Kentucky country life she had finally grown to understand, appreciate, and now love.

24

Growing Older

By the mid–nineteen fifties it was telephones rousing the Frontier Nurses rather than the hapless fathers traipsing through the woods, knocking on doors, and calling out the standard "Hallo-oo-oo" whenever their wives were "punishing." Furthermore, by 1955 many more deliveries were performed at Hyden Hospital than in mountain cabins. But none of that was any comfort to Betty Lester as a nurse-midwife instructor in the Graduate School. It was near midnight when the phone rang beside her bed at the Haggin Nurses' Quarters where she had her own residence. On the other end of the line was the hospital duty nurse. "Miss Lester? You need to come right away. Your grandbaby is about to be born!"[1]

Considering Lester wasn't even married, this was news indeed. "You mean Ethel has come in?" she asked. After a quarter century inside the Kentucky hills, she was accustomed to locals claiming her as a relative. It was actually quite a compliment, and a far cry from the outsider status she encountered when she first arrived in 1928. Few people would even talk to her then. Ethel was well advanced in her labor as Lester entered the hospital room. "Oh, Miss Lester, I'm so glad you came," she said, grabbing Lester's hand. "Well, I wouldn't miss this for anything. I'll be right here with you."[2]

She recalled a time many years earlier when a baby girl was born from a young mother who explained her first baby had died. "If you'll just take care of me, I know this one will live," the mother said. And the child did live — now a grown woman named Ethel having a baby of her own. That's why Lester was willing to get up in the middle of the night so not to miss this special event. As Lester cleaned, wrapped, and dressed Ethel's new baby boy, several FNS nurses gathered about. "How do you like my grandson?" Lester asked, proudly holding up the child. "Miss Lester, I didn't know you had any children," a nurse-midwife spoke up. "He's mine only in a way," Lester said, laughing. "I delivered his mother more than twenty years ago."[3] She would also follow this child's progress through the years. When the infant she delivered, named Virgil, was eighteen he left for Ohio to take a job. But Lester kept up with the family. One day she learned that Virgil's new wife was pregnant and wanted to have her baby in Hyden. She would be there at the delivery of this child too, her very own "great-grandchild." When asked why she never married throughout her lifetime, her response was, "I've got a very big family. My children are here, and all over the country."[4]

By the mid–1950s, Lester was Social Services director and had her own secretary in addition to a new, challenging set of responsibilities. The department now had a provisional license from the State Child Welfare Division and could legally handle foster home and adoption placements. In addition, medical bills were paid on behalf of indigent families, including a pregnant woman with tuberculosis sent for treatment and delivery of her baby and a child rushed to Lexington for emergency care of an abscess. Corrective devices were purchased for needy families, along with supplements for transportation, food, school tuition, taxes, or other necessary items. Despite the important work she was doing Lester remarked that she often missed her hands-on approach as a nurse-midwife. To her, there was just no substitution for bringing new life into the world, or saving one about to exit. Like many of her colleagues and peers, when forced to leave the hills of Kentucky on business or to visit her family, Lester couldn't wait to return. "I knew that if I didn't get out of the mountains, I'd spend my life there," said a Social Services secretary to Lester, hired for three months during the busy Christmas season. "Agnes Lewis said that is what happened to her. She did not intend to spend her life there. But she fell in love with the place and could not get away."[5]

So too, did the many of the visitors who came and went at Wendover throughout the 1950s. Most arrived with one impression and left with another. "People thought we were totally isolated back in these hills," said FNS secretary Lucille Knechtly. "But the truth is we knew what was going on with current events, for the world often came to us."[6] A young doctor from Nicaragua stopped in and brought a life-sized rag doll that was promptly dubbed Nella, graciously introducing her in his broken English as his "girlfriend." Through the stories he heard of the FNS, he knew that Breckinridge had a keen sense of humor. Two physicians arrived from South Korea during the Korean War. In an effort to make conversation, Breckinridge asked them what they thought of Americans stationed in their country. One bluntly told her, "We wish they'd get out and stay out!" A couple of strapping young football players came to visit two of the Boston couriers and caused a stir when they attended the local square dance held in the Wendover basement. It was a hot summer night and before long the boys were panting and drenched with sweat, much to the amusement of the locals.

Breckinridge was the ultimate hostess to any guest, sometimes to the chagrin of her staff. "She would insist that our guests pile their plates high with food," said Knechtly. "If they didn't, she did it for them. Her favorite comment was, 'There's oceans more [food] in the kitchen'—even if there wasn't."[7]

Nonetheless, the cooks and housekeeping staff remained loyal and devoted to Breckinridge and the Frontier Nursing Service throughout this period. One laundress at Wendover said she washed her son through law school and was amply rewarded for her hard labor when he became a respected attorney in Hyden. This same woman, who seldom missed a day at the Big House, rode her horse, Old Bob, to work. Riding home one winter evening along an icy path, she fell off. Old Bob didn't move, allowing her to grab his leg and pull herself up. Leaning on the animal, she walked the rest of the way home. "Wilson," she said to her husband as she came in, "I think I've done broke my neck. Go for the nurse."[8] At Hyden Hospital, the medical director confirmed that indeed, she had a broken neck. But she would not hear of traveling to Lexington for specialized care. Nor would she stop going to work. She was rigged to a traction device to support her fracture, and within days was back at Wendover doing laundry.

There was always a night watchman on duty on the Big House premises, stationed just beyond the entrance to Pig Alley. Without exception, he would come into the house on cold mornings, build a fire for the women, and have a pot of coffee brewing when Breckinridge came downstairs. Two of the maids, sisters Alabam and Ellen, were notorious jokesters, who lived in a room on the Upper Shelf. One was always trying to catch the other one courting and would hide behind the furniture if a boyfriend showed up. One night when Ellen missed her curfew of eleven P.M., Alabam rigged her bed. When Ellen climbed in the bed collapsed, creating a huge racket. Ellen was so scared of waking everyone up (and Breckinridge discovering she'd missed her curfew) she spent the night frozen in place, headboard up and footboard on the floor. Secretary Lucille Knechtly, known as "Thumper," once missed curfew herself when she got caught in a torrent of rain following a summer dance and a picnic planned for the couriers, secretaries, maids, and neighborhood boys. "I was in charge, more or less," she said. "Just as we reached the picnic spot, it began to rain. The river was low so we waded across, carrying the food, lanterns, records, and a record player. Usually the boys provided live music but this time they wanted to dance, so they left their instruments at home."

As the lively crowd consumed cold hot dogs and marshmallows, the rain grew worse. Someone went to check on the river level. "Thumper," the boy said upon his return, "the only way we can get back now is to swim!" The Middle Fork was raging. "It kept on raining so we kept on dancing," she said. "Our curfew approached and there we were, stranded on the wrong side of the river."[9] The group eventually had to walk a path around the river carrying all their gear, find a cabin, and ask for transport in a boat. Once across the river, they walked the rest of the way to Wendover, arriving well past midnight. "I admonished them to be very quiet," said Knechtly, "as Agnes Lewis had keen ears. The next morning revealed a serene Middle Fork River, flowing innocently below the Big House. Where we were, however, a flash flood had come and gone. So no one believed our tale."[10] "The river," said a long-time FNS nurse-midwife, "is almost a standard by which we live and work. We watch it carefully for we know that when it is high, the creeks we have to travel will be even higher. It can mean walking along rocky slippery paths to reach our patients, and all hope of getting them to the hospital abandoned. In those cases, we do what we can ourselves, for the doctor's help could be hours and hours away."[11]

One such case involved a young boy who had been kicked in the face by a mule and was badly injured. Two of the FNS nurses were having dinner at Wendover when they got the call telling of the accident. Grabbing their gear, they headed for the jeep, and hurried toward their patient. Driving miles through heavy rain, they found their way blocked by dead branches and rubble just short of the where the boy lay injured. "Jeeps are truly remarkable and will go almost anywhere," the nurse said. "But I knew we would have to be airborne before we could get beyond this rubble. We finally had to park it and wade through thick mud to the river bank where a boat was tied." They could see the river was still rising as the heavy rains continued. "Cain't cross here much longer," the boy's father called out. The women climbed into the boat, spanned the river, and walked the remainder of the way, coming upon a small but rickety footbridge. "There were only two flashlights for the four of us, so it made for much stumbling and slipping," said the nurse. "Just as I was about to yell to Nancy to shine the light so I could see to cross the bridge, she crashed through it. It was like a trap door opening. In a split second there was Nancy. And in another second she was gone!"[12]

The women had shared many good laughs through the years during their FNS adventures, but this was no laughing matter. Nancy could have been badly hurt. "Hit held us all this time," the father said, apologizing for the mishap.[13] Nancy scrambled out unharmed and the group moved forward. When they reached their sixteen-year-old patient, Jack, they found his face and forehead badly swollen. He was barely able to speak. His facial tissue was so mangled that bone was visible. Stitches were needed but not possible without further medical attention. The boy had been unconscious for several hours after the accident, possibly had a fractured jaw, and the FNS nurses were wary of moving him due to a possible concussion. "And we knew we could never get him out of the creek," they both agreed.[14]

At the cabin where his family lived, the nurses worked over him, checking his blood pressure and other vital signs. They cleaned and dressed the wound; gave him an anti-tetanus shot; and administered pain medication. Now all they could do was keep him quiet while they monitored his progress, and wait for the weather to break. It was two days before he could be brought to Hyden Hospital, where his wound was checked and his skull X-rayed. The medical director found the boy doing well with no other fractures or injuries, thanks in large part to the skillful work of the FNS nurses. At the hospital, just as the pink dogwoods were beginning to bloom, the first day of the annual surgical clinic was about to begin. For weeks, the staff had prepared for the event, cleaning, ordering supplies, conducting maintenance checks. On April 23, a Monday, the physicians were ready to open the week-long clinic. Suddenly, there was no water. The pumps had stopped. Plumbers were called in from Harlan, thirty-five miles away and worked diligently to get the water flowing again. Then the rods would not budge. There must be sand in the well, they reported — a major disaster for a hospital with a water usage of six thousand gallons a day. FNS executive secretary Agnes Lewis was assigned the task of getting the problem fixed and making arrangements for the hospital to obtain water from other sources. "Friends in Hyden with working wells were always sympathetic and generous when something like this happened," she said. "So they invited the doctors, nurses, and family members into their homes for drinking water, bathing, and cooking purposes."[15]

An FNS Graduate School student collected exotic fish as a hobby and worried that with the water shortage, the latest additions to her aquarium would not survive. Another nurse gave up her scant supply of water to keep the filter working, explaining to the bewildered superintendent that not having the fish around would unsettle the pediatric patients, for when the aquarium was brought into the ward, they were fascinated by "the intriguing little things." Lewis got on the phone for help with assessment, contacting an experienced FNS trustee who left his job at Ford Motor Company on Red Bird River to measure the damage at Hyden. There was almost forty feet of sand in the well, he said, resulting in a cave-in. The sand would have to be bailed out. It was just a matter of how deep to go. At Wendover, Breckinridge had come down with the flu and was recovering in her room. But she told Lewis to keep her informed of every development. As usual, she had her own opinions of what should be done. Her advice was to drill beyond the cave-in and replace whatever was necessary to get the pump working again. It would take nearly a month, a second round of plumbers and drilling, a new rod, pump, motor, and controls to reestablish water at the hospital. In the meantime, the ever-resourceful local community took matters into their own hands. Whenever visitors arrived at the hospital, instead of bringing flowers to a patient, they brought a jug of water.[16]

Things soon settled down to a normal routine. Ruth White was an R.N. who worked the night shift at Hyden Hospital. "I like to work nights," she said. "Our lives are filled with so much noise and busyness; it's good to be quiet and alone."[17] On a calm autumn night in 1957 she was just starting her shift, walking from the nurses quarters a few yards from the hospital. With no moon, the stars blazed high in the sky and below her, the little town of Hyden flashed its own set of lights. The clinic was dark as White entered. Good. That meant an easy night ahead. Narcotics had to be counted, syringes and baby bottles sterilized, sleeping patients checked and monitored. White completed her chores and picked up a baby blanket she was crocheting. Through an open window, she heard a coal truck chugging by on its way to the mines. A baby cried in the children's ward.

Infant Joe was getting a bit restless. Billy was awake and needed a bottle. Eight babies required diapering and delivery to their mothers and dry pads placed in their cribs supplementary feedings prepared for the preemies. In the hospital's entry downstairs a mother called for a nurse. Her young son was sick and having trouble breathing. The child was whisked into an examining room and the doctor on duty called by phone. The boy would be admitted before the night was over. A pre-natal patient wandered into White's ward where she was tending to the babies. "What is it, Bessie?" White said. "Are you all right?" She wondered if she should call the FNS nurse-midwives, though she disliked disturbing them unless the mother appeared close to delivery. "My back hurts," Bessie replied. "And I think I might be getting sick."[18] White, who didn't want to be catching any new babies tonight, knew she would soon be notifying the FNS nurse-midwives.

On the radio, in the news, the Russians launched Sputnik, setting off the space race and changing the balance of the stalemated Cold War between America and Russia. Each country presumed the other was out to annihilate it with nukes. That same year, President Eisenhower ordered troops into Little Rock, Arkansas, to federally enforce school desegregation, setting off riots that would last well into the next decade; and the behemoth, short-lived Edsel was born via the Ford Motor Company, destined to become a commercial flop. A stay-at-home mother named Betty Friedan in Grandview, New York was working on an article in 1957 that would be rejected by major women's magazines because the content might not sit well with traditional, conservative housewives. Angry, Friedan began a manuscript utilizing her researched material and stored it in the china cabinet while she scrubbed the kitchen and tended her children. The book, *The Feminine Mystique*, would not see the light of day until 1963, but when it did, it set off a chain reaction that would revolutionize the way women were perceived in America, and coin the term "feminist." And in Hyden, Kentucky, a new British nurse was getting adjusted to the area after three years as a Queen's Nurse in Canada. Breckinridge was particularly proud of Molly Lee, for she brought a wide range of experience to the FNS, along with her prestigious title (Queen's Nurses demonstrated a high level of commitment to patient-centered practice) and an ability to relate well to the rural population. She also knew horses. Paid one hundred twenty dollars a month for her services, not required to sign a contract, nor wear an FNS hat (she hated hats), Lee would, like most of the FNS nurses, devote a good bit of her life to the Frontier Nursing Service. But in the end, her sacrifices would prove greater and more tragic than all of those who had come before her.

25

The Explosion

Molly Lee came to eastern Kentucky after an English friend and mentor told her about the region. She was hesitant at first, afraid that eastern Kentucky was too populated and "too civilized" for her taste. So she went to British Columbia, Canada, for three years working for the Red Cross in their Outpost Services, living on a farm and riding a bicycle to work. Much of what she did in Canada, she thought, would prepare her for the Frontier Nursing Service. Like Betty Lester, now a thirty-year veteran with the FNS, Lee also thought the idea of having her own horse, dog, and working in a mountainous rural area would be "utopia." That is, until she arrived in Hyden, traveling by train from Saskatchewan, Canada, to Lexington, Kentucky, then by bus to Leslie County where she arrived between Christmas and the New Year holidays. "It was really a dead time of year," she recalled, "not much going on and not many people around. The hills were high and tight, unlike the rolling country I was used to, and no one really took much interest in me except the dog. I don't even remember who met me. But the dog with her seemed glad to see me."[1]

Lee went first to Hyden Hospital where she met a female doctor who was performing a Caesarean section delivery under local anesthetic, a surgical procedure which Lee found "most interesting" coming from her rural outpost. "Then I was assigned to clean a big, old-fashioned metal isolette that was in storage. It looked like a bathtub and was obsolete in most hospitals. But it did keep the babies warm." Within a matter of days, she was told to go to Wendover where she would meet Breckinridge and learn from the couriers how to groom horses. Her first impression of Breckinridge was that she appeared "very down-to-earth" yet in full control of her staff. "She came across like a mother in a household," said Lee. "Most of her time was spent upstairs in her room, but she was still very much the administrator. Yet you had to be part of the "inside crowd," added Lee, in order to receive a daily report from Breckinridge's command post in her bedroom.

Another FNS nurse had vacated her post at Beech Fork Clinic, so Breckinridge directed Lee to the district for her first official assignment. She would be provided with a horse and an FNS uniform, and would work with two other nurse-midwives. As part of her duties, Lee also had to train student nurses enrolled in the Graduate School program. "Beech Fork had the highest number of deliveries of any clinic," Lee said. "Sometimes we'd have six or seven in a three-week period. The students would, of course, want to come out and train during this time."[2] When winter struck hard with temperatures dipping into the single digits, ice and snow covering the ground, Lee said she often felt protective of the girls, whether on horseback or in the FNS jeep — which she barely knew how to drive. "There was one girl in particular, engaged to be married, who came out during a terrible winter storm. We had to drive up the creek bed for a home delivery to the top of the hill where the patient lived. I didn't know much about driving down a precipice, especially in bad weather, so I would stop, get out, walk ahead to look at conditions, and get back in the jeep. I was afraid we would hit something and get thrown. That's why I didn't like carrying people."[3]

Only later did she learn she could put the jeep in its lowest gear, or tap on the brakes to ease her way down a steep decline. She much preferred to travel on horseback, for the animals were shod with protruding nails similar to a mountain climber and with them, she always knew what to expect. "On a horse, you could walk up an icy creek and not fall down. I never had a horse fall with me the entire time." She found she could also ford the swollen river on a horse, not always possible in a motorized vehicle, and that she must learn to read the rivers' many moods so she wouldn't get stranded. "If it was raining, or a sudden storm came up, you had to be careful that when you got out, you could get back in."[4]

Other things surprised her about the region: that despite the poverty which still existed, many people had electricity and washing machines in the 1950s; that unlike the tight English city houses, American homes were seldom infested with human fleas; and that even as late as 1960, patients still paid their medical bills with in-kind goods or services. "It took one woman two-and-a-half years to pay us, and she did it all by bringing us eggs. That's how proud these people were, and how they would work out any way they could to pay their debt."[5] She found too that not every medical condition could be treated by a nurse-midwife, even one as experienced as she was. "I was working with a companion nurse who had gone to the patient's home and she was taking a very long time getting back. So I went to see if anything was wrong. The woman had twins and the placenta was trapped. We had to bring the lady into the hospital to remove the placenta because we had no anesthetic. At Hyden Hospital, Betty Lester gave her dropped ether. A doctor was called from Hazard and he took the placenta, which was very difficult. We had lots of things happen like that."[6]

Breckinridge announced she wanted to see the clinic while Lee was stationed at Beech Fork. Lee recalls the frantic preparations for her visit. "We had to find a three-ply board to put under her bed because of her fractured spine. So we were running around in the attic trying to find this board. The local people really wanted to honor her, so the men went out and shot squirrels so we could cook them for breakfast. But it was always nice when she came to visit."[7] Breckinridge took a moment to speak to the live-in maid at the clinic, a young girl whose father had forbidden her from going to school beyond the eighth grade because he didn't want her riding the bus with boys. The girl was saving her money to return to school on her own and would ultimately complete high school *and* college. It was one of the many cultural differences Lee encountered in Kentucky. Another was a baby's delivery that took place at a home where the family was actively involved in its annual making of molasses.

A craft as old as the hills, producing sorghum from sugar cane was still common in Appalachian in the early 1960s. In simple terms, the cane was cut, stripped of its leaves and tassels, and then placed in orderly heaps near the press. Mules pulled the bar that worked the rollers, crushing the cane stalks. Cane juice (a thin, green sticky fluid) was extracted, collected in a large tub, and strained. The finished product was dipped at the end of the day. It could take up to three days for the grand finale — the stir-off — in which neighbors gathered to celebrate another year's harvest. "We were invited to a taste event at the stir-off," said Lee, "and came at the edge of dark to find the celebrations were almost over. The men had whittled down corn stalks and we dipped them like lollipops into the warm molasses, sucking off their sweetness like kids with a candy apple." Lee says that from an outsider's point of view, it was an experience she would never forget. "In the moonlight, we drove back down the hollow in the open jeep to the echo of 'Come back agin!' And we did, to deliver a baby daughter early the next morning before the sun had topped the hill."[8] Where once upon a time some local younger children thought babies came from the saddlebags of the Frontier nurses, they now suspected the source was FNS jeeps.One little girl whose mother had just given birth at home remarked to her friends the following day: "I know how we get a baby. The next time someone calls the nurses, we'll just go out in the road and stop the jeep. That way, we'll get a baby before they go to the next house."[9]

Lee was also present when Breckinridge celebrated her eightieth birthday in February 17, 1961, at Wendover and when she received word that Breckinridge had won the National League of Nursing's highest award. Reflecting on decades with her beloved Frontier Nursing Service, Breckinridge recalled a day thirty years earlier when a twelve-year-old boy rode his mule to the Big House and said he had brought the nurse-midwives a gift. "We aim to have our baby paid for," the boy announced, presenting the women with two hand-made split bottomed chairs. "Our fee in those days," said Breckinridge, "was five dollars (compared to forty dollars in 1961). The two hand-made chairs were worth five dollars. We would never have asked for anything more in payment because the husband and father had died before the birth of his baby. This boy was now the head of the household. And his gesture was a code of honor in the American pioneer."[10]

Expounding on age differences now that she was eighty and her generation was "going into the wings," Breckinridge said that while no one generation was better than another, she had come to know this younger crowd well because so many of them were serving with her in the FNS. "If anything, the girls of today are a step ahead of my own girlhood. They have much more initiative."[11] What she decried was that in her day, people dreaded debt and did not buy things they wanted until they could pay for them. As a visionary, she could easily have been referring to our current generation. "Americans are in debt up to their eyebrows. This is one of the reasons we have inflation and the failure of a few big financing companies could bring on a crash for millions of people. This represents a complete break with the past. Rare today would be a boy of twelve who took over his father's obligations."[12]

Despite the seriousness of her position, Breckinridge — even at eighty — retained her self-deprecating sense of humor. When a group of local school children commemorated her by pronouncing her a "historical character" in their classroom, she responded by sharing some of their comments in a *Frontier Nursing Service Quarterly Bulletin*. An eleven-year-old sixth grader wrote a paper and titled it: "That Blessed, Old, Grey-Haired Critter Mrs. Mary Breckinridge." The child's essay won a state-sponsored contest for American History Month and Breckinridge told the student she would probably go on to become a historical figure herself.

At the walnut dining table at Wendover, Breckinridge was honored on her special day with her favorite meal and a triple jovial toast by Dr. Rogers Beasley, a well-liked FNS medical director in a long line of FNS administrators. "First, a toast to you as our teacher," he said, holding his glass high. "By your brilliant introduction of the nurse-midwife into the Kentucky Mountains, you have pointed the way for rural maternal care all over the world. You have taught us how to be good neighbors. You have even been willing to teach us how to raise chickens—though I don't think you had many takers on that one. Second, a toast to you as our friend, Mrs. Breckinridge; you have been the most enthusiastic, loyal, and generous of friends. Yes, we *accuse* you of being our friend. And finally, we toast you as the 'Rose of Wendover.' For years you have recorded in your daybook the blooming of the first rose. But for us, you are the rose that has bloomed without fail for eighty years. So here is a toast to you — our teacher, our friend, and our Rose of Wendover."[13]

Breckinridge still worked every day, fed her chickens, pigs, and ducks, and due to her back, was most comfortable when propped by pillows in her bed. Yet she could also be encountered on a given afternoon anywhere from the Wendover barn to the outpatient clinic at Hyden Hospital. Her fulltime staff included twenty-six nurses and nurse-midwives, a medical director, and administrative help. There were five working outpost centers covering twelve districts, plus the Graduate School located at Hyden Hospital. Every six months, the school produced seven new certified midwives. Many of its graduates were now working in places as far flung as South America and the Middle East. An Australian physician, a friend of Breckinridge's, wrote to tell her of his progress with Bush Nursing in the Outback.

The FNS continued to serve the same seven-hundred square mile region in which it began, using its fleet of twenty jeeps and eleven horses, and a mule to work the Wendover garden. Tea was still served every afternoon at four in the living room at the Big House. There, daily problems and new challenges were suspended for at least an hour while Breckinridge sat in her designated overstuffed chair holding court with her staff. Always nearby were the dogs, waiting patiently for their bits of cheese. Couriers served the tea then settled on the cushioned window seat that spanned the length of the double windows, hoping to catch a bit of gossip or worthy news. But things were slowly changing both within and outside the FNS, including the local economy. Once a region with a cash crop of oak and black walnut timber, it was now dependent upon the rise and fall of coal mining that determined employment and unemployment throughout eastern Kentucky. The FNS budgetary expenses ran nearly three hundred thousand dollars a year in 1961. FNS income came from its four thousand subscribers who paid a set amount per year, plus an endowment fund, revenue from the Wendover Post Office, sales of Breckinridge's book *Wide Neighborhoods*, annual grants, the ten dollar hospital fee charged to adults patients (children still received free medical care) and donations from the various FNS committees.

Though still spry, Breckinridge in her eighties was forced to reduce her travel and speaking engagements. Unbeknown to most, her eyesight was failing and she was suffering from a cancer of the bladder that had become invasive. True to form, she was blunt with her physician, whom she referred to by his first name. His daughter had served one summer as an FNS courier. "Ed, I've got some things I have to try and get done. How long do you think I've got? If I could get two more years out of this thing...."[14] He told her he was *hoping* for more than two but he knew her long-term prognosis was bleak. Breckinridge underwent radiation treatment at the University of Kentucky Medical Center that certainly would have, along with her age, zapped her strength. But two years later, she was still going.[15]

Despite her failing health, she rallied for a local parade designed specifically for her that would continue long past her death. It was the first annual Mary Breckinridge Day, sponsored by the Leslie County Development Association. Held on a Saturday in Hyden in 1962, the initial event drew people from all the country. The white-haired Breckinridge, decked out in a FNS uniform complete with tie and insignia, led the parade herself, riding the spirited Doc, one of her favorite horses. At the conclusion of the program, Breckinridge was informed that a park on the Middle Fork of the Kentucky River and the trail behind it had been named in her honor.[16] Molly Lee, Kate Ireland, Betty Lester — now known as "the social worker" — and other FNS staff stepped in to help by attending committee meetings and assisting with the ever-present need for fundraising. More and more often, it was Assistant Director Helen Browne who served as the primary FNS representative, taking Breckinridge's place as public speaker. Lester spoke before a large group at a covered dish supper at the Protestant Episcopal Church in Lexington, showing color slides of the FNS operation and sharing stories from her many years as a nurse-midwife. It was a typical collaborative effort on the part of the FNS staff.

Kate Ireland, head courier, received accolades following her talk and a slide show in Cleveland. One woman wrote to Ireland telling her, "Most of us left feeling we ought to do something for the great work in the Kentucky Mountains."[17] When Breckinridge eventually became too frail to attend even the annual FNS meetings, members came to Wendover instead. One of the Graduate School nurse-midwives, Elsie Maier, recalls Breckinridge during this period. "I found her to be a strong individual still, very much in control of everything within the FNS. Whether you told her anything or not, she always found out and knew what was going on."[18]

When Maier debated over whether or not to leave the FNS in 1964 in order to get married, she went to Breckinridge in confidence and asked her advice. They sat across from each other in the living room of the Big House. "I asked her," said Maier, "if indeed I made this decision not to marry, would she consider having me come back on staff? I can see her sitting in her chair and in her kind voice responding, 'Dear, you always have a home here.' Most of us were single women with families far away. And because of that, she created a family atmosphere and made us feel we were welcome."[19] Though few spoke of what would happen to the Frontier Nursing Service once Breckinridge was gone, no one wanted to see the organization fade away. Important work was still pending. The Kentucky Division of the American Cancer Society awarded a grant to study breast cancer in nursing mothers in 1961 to a Lexington physician who conducted surgical clinics at Hyden Hospital. That field work would take several years.

The topic of birth control was just beginning to gain national attention in the 1960s and attitudes were beginning to change. (It was not until 1965 that a Supreme Court decision legalized birth control for married couples and not until 1967 that family planning was included among services for women on public assistance.)[20] Breckinridge was generally open-minded on most medical topics, but she had never been a strong proponent of birth control in eastern Kentucky for reasons mentioned in her 1930s published essays. (Primarily, she didn't think it would work due to ingrained cultural attitudes. Furthermore, poverty was the biggest problem, she contended, not birth control.) So it was surprising when she agreed to have the FNS participate in one of the first clinical studies of oral contraceptives in humans.

One reason was that she had a close relationship with ob-gyn Dr. John Rock, of the Worchester Foundation, who conducted the trials. His wife was a friend of Breckinridge's from her early days in France and was involved in FNS committee work, along with the couple's daughter. Dr. Rock visited Breckinridge at Wendover to discuss the trials, knowing that the rhythm method and diaphragms were the most common form of birth control for FNS patients. He also knew the FNS had kept meticulous records through the years, which could advance his cause. He and his colleagues were collecting data on the efficiency of Enovid and needed a control group in order to confirm conclusions they had already reached in their own clinic. The group's ultimate goal was to convince the Food and Drug Administration to approve Enovid for marketing through the Sell Corporation. Rock found Breckinridge "broad-minded and a very sociable lady," though she disapproved of his drinking cocktails and refused to join him in a drink at Wendover — a somewhat hypocritical stance considering her nightly sherry. She also found him a complex character, particularly in view of the fact that here was a physician working to promote birth control commercially while he was a practicing Catholic. Regardless, the study at the FNS (and in Puerto Rico) went forward and the Sell Corporation eventually marketed the pill.[21]

While winds of change were definitely blowing through Leslie County by the mid 1960s, some things were destined to remain the same. Molly Lee, the British FNS Queen's Nurse who had spent these past few years in service as a FNS nurse-midwife, invited her sister, Nora, to visit her at Wendover from Devon, England. Nora had never been to America and was excited about the trip. On a warm Friday afternoon in July 1965, the two women were driving the FNS jeep from Wendover to visit a patient who lived about seven miles from Hyden. The jeep hit a bump in the road and suddenly there was a huge explosion. Two men working at the bottom of the hill looked up, saw the shooting flames and billowing smoke. They ran toward it. Lee had severe lacerations on one arm and both legs. Her right foot and ankle were crushed. But it was her sister, Nora, sitting on the passenger side, who had suffered the brunt of the explosion.

Despite her own injuries Lee began giving instructions to the men who had rushed up the hill. "Go phone for a doctor, morphine, and an ambulance!" she shouted. All she could surmise was that they had been hit by an explosive device planted in the road.[22] Medical Director Dr. Rogers Beasley and his nurse dropped what they were doing and headed to the scene. Someone got word to Wendover. Helen Browne and Betty Lester raced to a jeep and drove to the accident site. They would follow the ambulance to Harlan, the largest medical facility nearby. There, Nora learned that she had lost both her legs and the sight in one eye. Molly was less seriously injured, but wanted to remain near her sister. The two women stayed in the hospital for weeks.

The Kentucky State Police, investigating the explosion, determined that a homemade bomb was set as a trap in the road but that neither the sisters nor the Frontier Nursing Service were the intended victims. The sisters were simply in the wrong place at the wrong time. Brownie, now acting FNS director, worried that the press would get word to the Lee family in England before she could. She contacted the British Consul in Cleveland, Ohio, and enlisted their help in reaching the relatives just thirty minutes prior to an announcement by the British Broadcasting Corporation (BBC). It was not the type of press preferred by the Frontier Nursing Service.

Nora Lee returned home to England without her legs, while Molly Lee continued her work in the FNS as a nurse-midwife. "It is deeply distressing to the citizens of Leslie County that not only was one of their nurses hurt, but that a visitor to this country has suffered in such a senseless catastrophe," wrote an administrative staff member in the *FNS Quarterly Bulletin* a few weeks after the explosion.[23] The perpetrators were not caught and only rumors remained about what really happened that July day. Some said it was a Hatfield and McCoy-style family feud. Others said it was moonshine driven. To this day, no clear story has emerged.

In summer 2007, retired from nursing and living in her native town of Devon, England, Molly Lee, at eighty-one, spoke fondly overall about the FNS and her years of service. But she was reluctant to discuss the incident that severely injured her sister. Nora died in October 2003 after suffering a stroke. "She had many complications through the years," said Lee, "but overcame them all with true Christian spirit."[24] Words—and sentiment—despite the tragic incident in Hyden forty-two years earlier—that were spoken like a true Frontier Service Nurse.

26

Death of an Icon

FNS nurse-midwife Anna May January was completing her day's work in the clinic when she spotted a shy young boy clutching a note in his hand. "Mama wants you to come quick," he said in a soft voice. January scanned the note: "I'm sure my time has come. Hurry right along." She asked the courier to get the horse saddled while she changed clothes. Evening shadows settled over the hills and valleys as she wended her way up Sargos Creek. The first snow of the season had dressed the trees in sparkling white and a carpet of white lay below. She had suspected twins at one point but had not heard two fetal heartbeats on her last examination.

Arriving at the home, January rushed in with Timmy, the boy who had come to fetch her. The mother, Martha, was standing in the kitchen and invited her to dinner. "I cooked you a blackberry pie," she said, motioning to the table.[1] January felt things were a little too imminent to sit down to dinner so she politely declined and began to set up her supplies. When her water broke, Martha finally agreed to lie down, settling her young son Timmy by the fire. Within an hour, a baby girl arrived and January called to Timmy. She handed the baby to him and he carefully moved toward the fireplace so he could keep his new sister warm. As January was preparing the mother for post-delivery, another little head appeared. "Timmy," January called. "Put Samantha down and come get this one!" "Where am I gonna put her — on the hearth?" he said. Samantha was placed in her mother's arms just after baby Samuel, all three pounds of him, arrived. With mother and twins doing well, January took Timmy by the hand and sat down at the dining room where they each had a healthy slice of homemade blackberry pie.[2]

What January never shared with her patients was the horseback accident that nearly took her life a few years earlier while on duty. Her horse had plunged into soft mud, slid over an embankment, and tossed her onto the ground. The pommel of the saddle flew off and hit her in the abdomen, causing internal injuries. Because she was at an isolated outpost district miles from help, it was hours before she could be reached. She was taken by ambulance to Lexington where surgery was performed, a transfusion given, and new antibiotic administered to prevent peritonitis. "The gallant Anna May's life was saved," reported Breckinridge following the incident. "And she rides again."[3]

The Frontier Nurses continued their far-flung duties as late as 1965, even as horses began their decline of service within the FNS; even as the federal government began to poke around in the Appalachian hills and valleys; even as a new generation wrought changes to the forty-year-old organization; and even as Mary Breckinridge and her courageous, spirited, sacrificial, and innovative life drew to a close. Breckinridge was just as adamantly opposed to government interference in her work in 1963 as she was in 1923 when plans for the FNS were at the embryonic stage. No one knew her position on government assistance better than Dr. Louis Hellman, who pioneered the establishment of midwifery instruction at Kings College in New York. He also served on President Kennedy's national Panel on Mental Retardation, was enamored of the Kennedy family, and a Breckinridge acquaintance.

During one of the FNS fundraising talks that he attended, he questioned Breckinridge's statistics regarding infant and maternal mortality rates, believing they might have been filtered to support the organization's fund-raising goals. In time, he would change his mind, especially after getting to know Breckinridge and recognizing the inherent integrity of the program. "I think, despite the poverty in the region, very damn few people died," he admitted. "I think her figures were probably right."[4] In the spring of 1963, he came to Wendover and got into a philosophical disagreement with the "peppery" Breckinridge about government aid, whom he added could be resistant to change and "extremely difficult about innovative ideas," such as computerizing the FNS data or publicizing the FNS through national media channels. He also found that she had tunnel vision regarding the FNS, as though midwifery existed only at Wendover, Kentucky. When he suggested she utilize government funds in the development of the FNS, he really struck a nerve, surmising that she probably didn't appreciate this fifty-two year-old "youngster" coming in and telling her what to do. "She was very much opposed to government participation in private endeavors, saying 'no way, we will raise our *own* money in order to remain independent.' She also made no bones about telling me, 'I don't like that president and I don't like your attitude.'"

Hellman said in the end, Breckinridge was someone he never expected to get along with, but he did. Along the way, he gained a grudging respect for the Frontier Nursing Service in general and Breckinridge in particular. "She made a significant contribution to midwifery against what was probably a fair amount of opposition," he concluded. "She was a reactionary in many ways who liked to do things by herself." Women like Breckinridge and her FNS nurse-midwives were "admirable sorts," he concluded, "special people with courage."[5] Typifying the core philosophy of the Frontier Nursing Service during this era was Betty Lester, who, by 1964, had spent thirty-six years with the FNS. She was now birthing the babies of babies she had delivered in her first few years. Her varied posts within the agency included midwifery supervisor, Hyden Hospital superintendent, outpost district nurse-midwife, and director of Social Services. Her life's work had affected literally hundreds of people. British-born, she returned to England during the war, but now called Hyden, Kentucky, her home, and the Frontier Nursing Service her family. To reward her service and dedication, the State of Kentucky commissioned Betty Lester a Colonel on July 23, 1964. In a letter addressed to the "Honorable Betty Lester," Governor Edward T. Breathitt stated: "I know the high esteem in which you are held by the people of the mountains, and I am confident you will continue to serve them faithfully and devotedly. May you enjoy this new title."[6]

That same year, the Frontier Graduate School of Midwifery, which now had its own six-bedroom cottage complete with heat, electricity, plumbing, and maid service near Hyden Hospital, reported that students were admitted twice a year on scholarships at a cost of eight hundred dollars for the six-month course, plus a stipend of twenty-five dollars a month to each student. The FNS medical director provided regular lectures at the midwives quarters and travel throughout the thousand-square mile region was conducted primarily by jeep. Among the students was Martha Lady, who spent time as a nurse missionary in Rhodesia prior to entering the six-month nurse-midwife course at the FNS. She found herself intrigued by the similarities she found working in Africa and in eastern Kentucky, particularly women's attitudes toward childbirth. "To many of the women, having a baby was not considered a big deal," she explained. "I think it was their basic oneness with nature, the sense of 'I was born to have children so let's get down to work and have a baby.' Life in Africa was basic, too, not complicated with a lot of trappings, and the same was true in Kentucky."

Lady said she met Breckinridge a couple of times during her training, noting that she was becoming more physically frail. "Yet, even when she was in her room upstairs, her presence could still be felt," said Lady. "You knew she was there and in command and I was impressed with that fact."[7] In theory, Breckinridge, as director, and her staff were the consultants to the faculty of the School of Midwifery. But in reality, Breckinridge, eighty-four years old, was conducting little of the actual day-to-day operations of the FNS. In fact, Breckinridge had been in declining health for quite some time, spending more of her time upstairs at Wendover propped in bed. It had been rumored for years that her eyesight was failing, fueled by her weakened condition and the constant use of a cane to get around the familiar terrain at Wendover.

Her longtime secretary Agnes Lewis recalled an incident a full decade earlier at an annual meeting in Lexington when Breckinridge apparently failed to recognize her own FNS staff member after she walked up to her at the meeting. Breckinridge extended a hand and said "Nice to meet you" to her head courier. "She finally told us both at the conference that her oculist informed her she was losing her middle vision," recounted Lewis. "She said faces were out of focus and that she didn't want to worry us, but that was the reason she didn't recognize the courier. Then we all laughed about it as the word went round that Mrs. Breckinridge didn't know her own staff when they were not dressed in blue jeans."[8] Her fading health was a topic seldom mentioned again, for Breckinridge did not want pity from her staff or loss of confidence among the public. Just as bad, she had to give up reading, one of her favorite pastimes. When it got to the point that she could not read even typed memos the FNS staff prepared, she requested they produce their memos using a black felt tip pen so she could make out the words.

Following her radiation treatment for bladder cancer in 1963, she had little energy for even feeding her beloved chickens and geese. According to her physician, Dr. Edward H. Ray, she overcame that initial cancer but now had leukemia. On days when she was unable to come downstairs, the night watchman fixed her coffee and brought it to her, then lit the coal in her open fireplace. Every morning, her assistant, Helen Browne, and secretary, Agnes Lewis, came to her room to deliver reports. Many of her staff recalled that even though she was physically ill, her mental faculties remained clear and sharp. When well-wishers dropped by to visit, Breckinridge welcomed them to her bedside, at times sharing or reminiscing in uncharacteristic fashion. Mary Stewart was an old friend and former junior courier for the FNS who came to Breckinridge after learning of her most recent illness. "As a courier, we never could have talked this way," she said. "But now I was an older woman and we were just two friends who had both been through some similar times. And I think when you know the end is

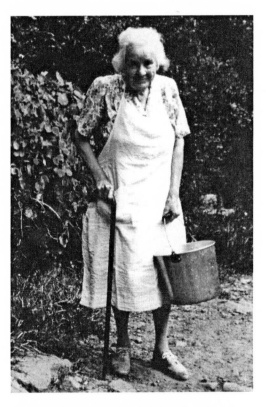

Mary Breckinridge in her eighties, founder of the Frontier Nursing Service. The best part of her day, she said, was feeding her beloved chickens, ducks, and geese on the Wendover property, headquarters of the FNS, and her home for forty years. This photograph was taken a short time before her death in 1965. (courtesy Frontier Nursing Service, Inc.).

near there is a tendency to open up a little more. We shared tragedies in our families, had both lost our parents, and had both been through a divorce. I recall she was sitting in a chair that day and I had on my coat because the room was chilly."[9]

Breckinridge admitted that being a divorced woman in the 1920s was considered "a major catastrophe" within her family and one that took more out of her than she liked to admit. She also spoke of losing her two children as something a person never gets over. But the conversation then veered into the general rather than specific, leaving Stewart with a lasting, insightful impression of Breckinridge. "Though she had a lot of good friends and was a gracious, warm person, I believe there was always a part of her that she kept to herself. And she never let anyone into that part."[10] Agnes Lewis was among the few people privy to her employer's vulnerabilities. Unlike much of the staff, Lewis knew about the important role Breckinridge's spiritual advisor, Sister Adeline, played throughout Breckinridge's life. And she knew that in Breckinridge's last remaining days, she often spoke aloud to Breckie, startling the night watchman who entered her room to light the coal fire. Not only did Breckinridge entrust Lewis with destroying her private papers and other items that she feared would be exploited after her death, it was Lewis she turned to in an effort to disperse her personal belongings among the staff.

The secretary was having a difficult time, however, accepting that Breckinridge would not be around much longer and an even more difficult time imagining anyone but Breckinridge living in the room at the end of the hall. "She tried so hard to get me to say things that things in her room would go to certain people, and which one of us would stay in her room. I didn't want to tell her, but not one of us wanted to take over that bedroom."[11] Assistant Director Helen Browne sidestepped the issue by telling Breckinridge she might someday use it as an office. "It will be a good place to think in," Browne said diplomatically. It was one of many times she saw herself playing devil's advocate, a position not very comfortable for the immediate staff who—unlike Browne—did not fall in line with whatever Breckinridge wanted. "Agnes was raised in the FNS era when everybody did exactly what Mrs. Breckinridge said," explained Browne, "and she [Breckinridge] could make you feel like a worm if you didn't do it."[12]

Browne, Lewis and FNS nurse-midwife Anna May January were close by when Breckinridge learned that her favorite nephew, John, had been killed in Vietnam. She did not support the war, believing that the U.S. should have learned from the French who had entered the country before the Americans. The death of yet another young person important to Breckinridge rocked her to the core. Browne said later it was the only time she ever saw Breckinridge lose her faith. "It nearly destroyed her," said Browne. "It was the third major loss in her life after her young husband and her children. I was very worried about her because she was almost hysterical. She wouldn't talk to anyone, wouldn't eat. Anna May would literally sit with her in her room for hours at a time because we couldn't leave her alone."

Breckinridge would gaze at her nephew's pictures, pointing and speaking to the photos. Finally, in desperation, Browne called the doctor for a sedative, though Breckinridge rarely took drugs. "It hit her pretty quickly and fifteen minutes later she was sound asleep. The next morning when I went to her room, boy did she take it out on me!" "You put me to sleep last night and I should have stayed awake and helped John get over to the other side," Breckinridge railed.[13] For the next two days, she wouldn't speak to Browne. "On the third morning I went back up to her room and she said, 'Brownie, I want to tell you something.' I realized then she was coming around." "What did you do after you told me John had died?" Breckinridge asked. "Well, Mrs. Breckinridge," said Browne, somewhat taken back, "I went to the chapel and commended his soul to God's care." "Ah, that's what I should have done," she replied. "But I couldn't." "That cooked it," recalled Browne. "I knew then she was all right."[14]

Browne reminded her they belonged to the same Episcopal faith. In turn, Breckinridge confessed there were times the church didn't mean that much to her. (She also once said during a barely averted financial crisis that "God is niggardly. He will give you just want you need, but never any more.")[15] It was during these last few days of her life that those closest to her began to see Breckinridge in all of her multi-faceted complexity. Browne believed that Breckinridge, due to her position of leadership within the FNS, was "desperate" for real friends. According to Browne, Breckinridge looked up at her one day and implored, "Brownie, you *do* love me, don't you?" Her response was, "Mrs. Breckinridge, I have a tremendous admiration for what you've done."[16] "I'd never permit myself to say I loved her," Browne explained. "I was afraid to because she could use that against you."[17] It was an answer that perhaps said more about Helen Browne, destined to take over the Frontier Nursing Service, than it did about Breckinridge.

Margaret Gage arrived at Wendover just a short time before Breckinridge passed away. She first met Breckinridge during a slide show presentation in the 1920s and became interested in the FNS organization. Now long-time friends, the two socially connected women maintained a correspondence through the years. Gage had planned a trip to the Big House in the summer of 1965 but when Breckinridge wrote and asked her to please come earlier, she agreed. "I think she had a psychic sense," said Gage. "And how marvelous that I was able to go when I did, for I would never have seen her again."[18] Gage arrived on May 14 and found Breckinridge upstairs in bed, physically fragile but "alert." They drank a glass of sherry together and Breckinridge told her to come see her again in the morning as she wanted Gage's input on articles scheduled in an upcoming issue of the FNS *Quarterly Bulletin.* "So the next morning I went to her room and we had a nice visit. I read through what she was working on.

She made excellent suggestions throughout the text. She was still just as bright as a tack."[19]

Looking forward to an extended visit, Gage said she was sitting in the Big House living room that evening with Brownie, Agnes, and FNS medical director Dr. W.B. Rogers Beasley, who had stopped in for dinner. "We heard her ring the buzzer from her room," recalled Gage, "and Brownie went up to see about her. She told Brownie she wasn't feeling all that well."[20] A few minutes later Breckinridge managed to get out of bed and come downstairs. "I'm so tired," she told the group gathered in her living room. "Can anyone give me something to make me sleep?" She had refused supper that night and her staff knew something was wrong. Dr. Beasley advised them to keep her quiet and calm, and just watch her, as there was little else they could do. Betty Lester volunteered to sit with her during the night. Sometime during the evening Browne entered the room and noticed that the side of Breckinridge's face was drooping. As usual, Breckinridge was propped upright in bed. Browne approached the bed, tipping over a lamp. "Brownie, what are you doing?" Breckinridge mumbled. "Oh, sorry, I knocked something over. Would you like to lie down and turn over?"[21]

Breckinridge allowed the two nurses to shift her body into a more comfortable position and she drifted off back to sleep. That was the last time she spoke to anyone. Later that morning, Sunday, May 16, 1965, half a dozen or so of the staff met in Breckinridge's room, aware that this remarkable woman's time was finally coming to a close. Besides Brownie, there was Margaret Gage, Agnes Lewis, Betty Lester, and FNS secretary Lucille Hodges. British FNS nurse-midwife Anne Cundle was one of several who actually nursed Breckinridge.

As the day wore on, others came to the bedroom door and quietly paid their respects. Lewis, in particular, was having a hard time. Brownie contended that "it would have killed Agnes if Mrs. Breckinridge's death had been difficult."[22] "I felt that Sister Adeline, her spiritual advisor, was with her too," said Gage. "She died very peacefully, very quietly; just stopped breathing. It was really quite beautiful and the right kind of passing for her."[23] No pomp and circumstance — just the way the eighty-four-year-old Breckinridge would have wanted it. In their final act of devotion to their founder, the Frontier Nursing Service staff began the process of making funeral arrangements — no small feat in view of the public attention that would surely follow the death of Mary Breckinridge.

Browne didn't want the funeral home coming in and "snatching" the body away, as she put it, so the staff decided to allow Breckinridge to remain in her room the first few hours. Phone calls were made, a long list of telegrams prepared. The Board of Governors and the City of Hyden chairman were notified. Prepared for a slew of publicity, Browne contacted the *Lexington-Herald* and requested they put the news on the Associated Press wire services. Along with the statewide Kentucky newspapers, *The New York Times* and the *Washington*

Post ran a biographical feature on Breckinridge and her lifelong contribution to public health nursing. The *Courier-Journal* referred to her as the "Angel of the Frontier, and the most illustrious Kentucky woman of all time, certainly of her own time."[24] Letters and telegrams arrived from as far away as Troon, Scotland, and Sydney, Australia. Locally, the outpouring of gratitude, sentiment, respect, and admiration was immediate and almost overwhelming.

To accommodate the crowd expected at the funeral, and to allow Leslie County residents to see Mrs. Breckinridge one last time, the FNS staff agreed to have her body dressed in her FNS uniform, and the casket remain open at the funeral home in Hyden. She would be interred at the family plot in Lexington. The service was held in the auditorium at the local high school, the same site where Breckinridge had attended the Mary Breckinridge Day Festival, the same spot where she had looked over the crowd and viewed the numerous faces of babies safely delivered by the FNS nurse-midwives throughout its many decades. Many of the attendees were now adults with children of their own. "All those pretty young things," she called the FNS babies.[25] At her service, the casket was covered in wild honeysuckle and mountain laurel. Though her favorite flower was a yellow rose, Breckinridge made it clear that she didn't want people spending money on flowers for her funeral. Instead, she left instructions to give a charitable donation to the poor.

Since someone had to man the FNS headquarters at Wendover, Kate Ireland offered to stay behind and therefore missed the service. Following the funeral, several people recalled their fondest memories of Breckinridge. One nurse recounted that when Breckinridge stopped by to view her clinic she noticed the place was lacking in aesthetics. "It's not pretty like an English garden," Breckinridge remarked bluntly. "Plant some flowers." "But I don't know how," the nurse replied. "Then *learn*," said Breckinridge.[26] Lucille "Thumper" Knechtly, who became Breckinridge's secretary in 1943, said that whenever her boss' diction became too wordy, she would turn to Knechtly and say "Thumper, help me. I have verbal diarrhea!"[27] And many talked of Breckinridge's penchant for getting her staff to follow her instruction, despite the fact it was a bad idea.

Courier Jean Hollins often drove Breckinridge to Lexington. Though Breckinridge could not operate a vehicle herself, she nonetheless would direct Hollins' up and down the numerous one-way streets throughout the city. "Even when Mrs. Breckinridge instructed her to turn the wrong way — she didn't argue, she just went," said Knechtly. "She said it was easier than arguing and if the cops caught them, she knew Mrs. Breckinridge could talk her way out of it."[28] But most of all, those who remembered her spoke of her integrity, her strong work ethic, her keen intelligence, her love of animals and children, her surprising sense of fun (at square dances she could do a mean hoedown), the confidence she inspired in others, and her unflagging generous spirit. FNS blacksmith Leonard Howard said she had a heart "as big as a truck."[29]

Della Gay grew up on a mountain farm near Hyden, grinding corn, making molasses, stringing beans. She remembers granny midwives who delivered the babies of young women like herself in the 1920s and how difficult it was to reach a doctor. Her first three labors were long and dangerous and she "liked to have died" she said. There was no doctor available to attend to her with the first baby, a time when her labor came to a sudden stop. "The granny woman came and just did the best she could," Gay said. "After the baby was finally born, I was sick for about a month. I couldn't stand up."[30] When the FNS began coming into the area in the 1930s Gay says a nurse-midwife showed up at her house one day in Jack's Creek. "One morning at daylight I looked out the window and I see'd her getting off from the horse. She come in with some medicine and doctored my young'un. That's how good they tended to you. And all they used to charge was a dollar a year. When they delivered the baby it was just five dollars. They would bring bundles of clothes, big bundles, and you could get one of them for five dollars, all the clothes the baby had to have. Can you imagine that?"[31] As for Breckinridge, Gay said, "I've never know'd nobody being like her. When she was getting old, she come over here to the center one day and a woman got sick trying to have a baby. The other nurses were all gone. I heard she delivered that baby before the nurses got back. I wish she could be a living today." (There was no documented case of Breckinridge conducting a delivery during her tenure in the FNS, particularly in her latter years.)[32]

Gay was not alone in wishing immortality on the charismatic, unforgettable Mary Breckinridge. A stalwart admirer of the FNS and Breckinridge, FNS employee Hobert Cornett was one of many who grieved for the mistress of the Big House long after she was gone. "I don't see why a person like her can't live forever," he said.[33] Of the Frontier Nursing Service staff, veteran secretary Lucille Knechtly summed up why so many women were willing to offer so many years of their life for what was considered modest pay and few benefits, other than the sheer romanticism inherent in the work. Part of it was the inspirational pull from Breckinridge —"that little woman with the big identity"— who was, throughout its first forty years, the heart and soul of the FNS. Another reason was the type of women the organization attracted. "Those of us from the 'outside' were here because each in our own way wanted to serve," said Knechtly. "We believed in ourselves, as human beings put on earth for something besides material gain."[34]

She said what she received in return was more satisfying than gold — words and sentiments echoed through the years by the majority of the nurse-midwives who worked for the Frontier Nursing Service. Many spoke of the deep friendships and camaraderie they encountered not only among themselves, but within the tight-knit communities where they tended the sick, aided the poor, and served as nurse, teacher, and friend.

When asked what becoming an honorary Kentucky Colonel really meant to her in July 1978, British-born nurse-midwife Betty Lester—who had despaired fifty years earlier that the locals would never accept her, thought for a moment and replied: "Well, you get a special invitation to the Kentucky Derby each May, and to the derby parties. It's quite important! But the *nicest* thing ever said to me was that I was not a 'foreign lady.' I was one of their own."[35]

Epilogue

In the decade following the death of Mary Breckinridge, the Frontier Nursing Service underwent a major, and some say inevitable, evolution. Medicare and Medicaid made their way into the Kentucky Mountains as well as other complicated government programs that were part of the War on Poverty. The subsidized help came with a price. At one point in the mid-seventies, the FNS was forced to file a lawsuit against the federal government for failure to reimburse them in Medicare funds. As a result, in addition to new forms of media — TV and eventually the Internet — attitudes began to change toward the FNS. There was greater exposure to new ideas and outside influences. "I think people watching TV medical shows in the 1970s suddenly thought they weren't getting everything in medical services that people in New York got," said Nancy Damman, a one-time junior courier. "They wanted these TV-type doctors to help them instead of the nurses."[1]

Getting in and out of Hyden, Kentucky, was boosted with the completion of the Daniel Boone and Hal Rogers Parkways, which meant a driver could get from Hyden to Lexington in about two and a half hours, the same amount of time that it once took to get to London from Hyden, only thirty-five miles away. There was internal bickering that served only to weaken the aging organization and a new Advisory Board was set up to counter what many thought were rubber-stamp requests Breckinridge had submitted to the FNS Boards in the past. Wendover, as a nursing center, along with several of the outpost centers, closed due to lack of funds, and the organization became centralized versus the decentralized structure Breckinridge had so successfully set in place. While the FNS nurse-midwives were once an integral part of the community, nursing and the medical profession in general became more of an institutional entity. New drugs, new procedures, more specialized care, and concurrent liability issues all served to change the face of rural health care. Higher fee structures were put into place to offset skyrocketing health care costs and many local residents found they were ill prepared for the reality of modern day medical costs. No longer could they pay their bills in chickens, labor, or eggs. "Treatments became much more sophisticated after 1965," said Ohio-born Kate Ireland, former head courier of the FNS. "Nurses could no longer do as Anna May January once did —'honey, you just got a bad throat.' Those days were gone. Now you had to know what type of bad throat so you would know what type of medicine to prescribe."[2]

Of the Frontier Nursing Service staff through 1965, very few are still alive today. Director Helen E. Browne stayed on through controversy and internal changes for eleven years until her retirement in 1975. She believed that all nurse-midwives should speak with a single voice and thus worked to merge the FNS-based American Association of Midwives with the American College of Nurse-Midwifery. It became the American College of Nurse-Midwives. She received numerous awards for her work, including Commander of the Most Excellent Order of the British Empire in 1976 and had the honor of being greeted by the Queen Mother at Buckingham Palace. Browne was living in Milford, Pennsylvania, when she died at home on January 20, 1987.

Agnes Lewis, FNS executive secretary, stayed on at Wendover for two years after Breckinridge's death. She had given nearly thirty-seven years to the FNS organization without a break in service other than one nine-month period due to family illness. It was an impressive show of loyalty for someone who thought the FNS was located in Lexington when she took the job; who grew "physically ill" at the first sight of Hyden; and who regularly submitted her resignations to Breckinridge because she feared she could not please her. Breckinridge, in turn, regularly ignored them. After her retirement, Lewis moved to Maryville, Tennessee, to live with her sister. She spent her last years in a nursing home in Maryville and died on Valentine's Day, 2000 — two months shy of her one hundredth birthday.

British nurse-midwife and Social Services director Betty Lester, who never returned to her family in England, retired in 1971. She was often spotted driving a Volkswagen around Hyden as she dodged the huge coal trucks on the narrow mountain roads. Whenever she stopped in at Wendover, she noted, in her soft English voice that it was "lonely without the horses." When President Nixon came to visit the Republican stronghold of Leslie County in 1978 Lester had her picture made alongside him. It held a prominent place in the mobile home where she lived at the foot of Hyden Hospital. Lester remained active and well-respected within the community until the day she died.

Kate Ireland, who came to the FNS as a junior courier in 1951, then the outspoken board chairperson of the FNS, returned to Tallahassee, Florida. Like Breckinridge, Ireland was born into a prominent family. After her stay at the FNS she returned to manage the nine-thousand acre plantation purchased by her father, complete with pheasants and hunting dogs, where she continued to live as of 2007. Feisty as ever at eighty-plus, she is a three-time cancer survivor and an activist in exemplary land stewardship through her favorite cause, Tall Timbers. Her Frontier Nursing Service legacy includes a stint as honorary chairman of the FNS Foundation. There is a healthcare facility in Manchester, Kentucky, that bears her name. There is also a Kate Ireland Drive in Hyden on which the Mary Breckinridge Home Health Agency sits and the FNS Rural Healthcare Centers.

Molly Lee, well into her eighties, returned to England and lives in Devon. By 1975, home deliveries by the FNS had decreased from about 80 percent to 11 percent, mostly due to better accessible medical facilities and the fact that these type deliveries were not covered by insurance. In addition, childbirth, once seen as a natural, normal event, was now a full-fledged medical procedure requiring hospitalization. When the eighty bed, not-for-profit Mary Breckinridge Hospital was completed in 1975, serving as a critical access facility for Leslie County, FNS director Helen Browne said the construction cost was "almost as frightening as the high cost of independence. But if we have inherited enough of Mrs. Breckinridge's faith, we shall have our new hospital."[3]

Betty Lester in Hyden, Kentucky, sometime during the 1970s. Retired in her seventies as an FNS nurse-midwife, she never returned to England to live. Instead, she made her home at the foot of Hyden Hospital and became a beloved member of the small community. "They were my family," she said (courtesy Frontier Nursing Service, Inc.).

With a few exceptions, the standing structures at Wendover have stayed remarkably close to their original state. The little chapel in which Breckinridge held evensong ceremonies and Sunday services was torn down after her death. Some thought it should have been left standing. The barn and nursing quarters became a gift shop. The Garden House was renovated into an administrative building. The Upper Shelf sits vacant in much the same condition as when FNS nurse-midwives held parties there. Today, Frontier Nursing Service, Inc., is the parent holding company for Mary Breckinridge Healthcare, Inc., and Frontier Nursing Healthcare, Inc., which includes six rural healthcare clinics. Fully accredited, the Frontier School of Midwifery and Family Nursing offers distance learning for all fifty states, seven foreign countries, and includes a community-based nurse practitioner program.

As of 2007, the Frontier School of Midwifery and Family Nursing (renamed from Frontier Nursing School) has graduated nurse-midwives from every U.S. state and Puerto Rico, training almost one-fourth of the more than six thousand certified American nurse-midwives currently practicing within the profession. The FNS Courier Program continues as a twelve-week internship for adults eighteen and older. They shadow the medical staff observing healthcare in a rural setting and volunteer on projects from Hospice to the Rape Crisis Center. Beech Fork Clinic, also known as the Jessie Draper Memorial Nursing Center, built in 1926, was restored to its original state in 2003. A new clinic was completed in 1981 to fulfill the needs of a growing community. Its focus today is disease prevention and health promotion. A computerized sign at the clinic lists the cost of a pregnancy test at sixteen dollars. New patients ages twelve and older are charged a hundred forty dollars for a complete work-up. But unlike most medical clinics throughout the country, there is no reference to payment due upon receipt of services.

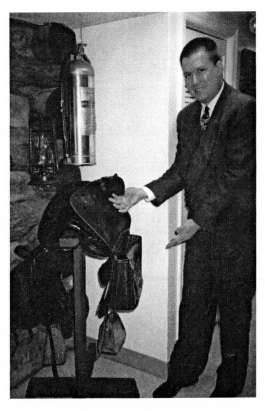

FNS development coordinator Michael J. Claussen showing visitors an authentic FNS saddlebag used by the nurse-midwives. Fully stocked bags could weigh up to forty pounds each (photograph by Marie Bartlett, courtesy Frontier Nursing Service, Inc.).

Within the modern-day Frontier Nursing Service, some things remain the same. Children remain a large part of the patient load and working families still struggle to pay their medical bills on minimum wages. "We had a woman with asthma who needed medications but had no money to pay for them," said a contemporary Frontier Nurse Practitioner (FNP). "I did what any good Frontier provider has always done ... improvise, scrounge, and make do."[4] More important, what also hasn't changed is the strong sense of community support.

When a family lost everything due to a fire in 2006, neighbors got together and donated baby and household items.

The Mary Breckinridge Day and Festival Parade remains an annual community event the first week of October. The FNS *Quarterly Bulletin* is still published, continuing its list of "urgent needs" in its closing pages. The Leslie County newspaper, *Thousandsticks News*, features current headlines that reflect contemporary times: "Mobile Meth Lab Explodes," and "Drug Testing May Begin This Year in Schools." But readers are also apt to see a story on "How the Banana Split," or "Jim's Father Come Back from the Dead," for locals still love a good story, both the hearing and the telling.

Wendover was designated as a National Historic Site and turned into a bed and breakfast in 1991 and as of 2007 had accommodated more than twenty-five hundred guests throughout its long history. The house retains much of its original charm, with many of the furnishings used by the FNS staff still in place. Breckinridge's books line the shelves in the living room; the stone fireplace harbors her photos and keepsakes; the dark wood banisters still gleam. Her room has the same simplistic elegance. From the bedroom window, there is a view of the grounds, the rustic outbuildings, and in the distance, the soothing sound and perpetual flow of the Middle Fork River. There is no swinging bridge now but the moody river still rages through periodic "tides." Though chickens, pigs, ducks, and geese no longer roam Pig Alley, it continues to serve as the entrance to the rustic Big House, evoking the strong sense of a former time and place.

At times, a maintenance worker will follow the trail that leads along the rock-strewn path to the Big House and swears he sees Breckinridge in the window. Footsteps have been heard in the upstairs rooms, or a door mysteriously opened, as though the Frontier Nursing Staff has returned to resume their duties. Whatever spirits remain, if any, are surely benign; Breckinridge would have it no other way. Perhaps she is there making sure that all is right with the place; perhaps "Aggie" or "Brownie" or Betty Lester are still looking after those who once came seeking medical attention. Or perhaps they are *all* looking out for those still to come that might — just might — need their help.

Chapter Notes

Chapter 1

1. Nellie Asher interview by Dale Deaton (hereinafter DD) 08/27/80, Frontier Nursing Service Oral History Project, Louie B. Nunn Center for Oral History, University of Kentucky Libraries (hereinafter cited as FNSOHP)
2. *Ibid.*
3. *Ibid.*
4. *Ibid.*
5. Mary Breckinridge and J.C. Breckinridge, *Midwifery in the Kentucky Mountains, An Investigation*, p. 23
6. *Ibid.*, p. 12
7. *Ibid.*, p. 13

Chapter 2

1. Mary Breckinridge, *Wide Neighborhoods: A Story of the Frontier Nursing Service* (Lexington: University Press of Kentucky, 1952).
2. "A Frontier Nurse Speaks Out," *Lexington-Herald*, August 11, 1940.
3. Breckinridge, *Wide Neighborhoods*, p. 1, 2.
4. Laura E. Ettinger, *Nurse Midwifery: Birth of a New American Profession* (Columbus: Ohio State University Press, 2006), p. 16–20.
5. Breckinridge, *Wide Neighborhoods*, p. 3–6.
6. *Ibid.*, p. 20, 52.
7. *Ibid.*, p. 35.
8. Hazel Corbin interview, by Carol Crowe-Carraco, 04/30/79, FNSOHP.

9. Lucille Knechtley interview, by DD, 07/09/79, FNSOHP.
10. Breckinridge, *Wide Neighborhoods*, p. 49.
11. *Ibid.*, p. 51.
12. *Ibid.*, p. 57.
13. *Ibid.*, p. 58.
14. Ruth Eichor interview, by DD, 07/16/79, FNSOHP.
15. Florence McLaughlin and Mary McLaughlin interview, by DD, 07/16/79, FNSOHP.
16. Emily E. Saugman interview, by DD, 03/09/79, FNSOHP.
17. Ruth Eichor interview, by DD, 07/16/79, FNSOHP.
18. Catherine T. Arpee interview, by Linda Green, 12/02/78, FNSOHP.
19. Zaydee Dejong Harris interview, by DD, 06/14/79, FNSOHP.
20. Beatrice Williams interview, by Anne Campbell, 01/26/79, FNSOHP.
21. Breckinridge, *Wide Neighborhoods*, p. 109.
22. *Journal of Midwifery & Women's Health*, no. 48, (2003): 86–95.

Chapter 3

1. Ettinger, *Nurse-Midwifery: Birth of a New American Profession*, p. 39.
2. FNS *Quarterly Bulletin* 1, 1926, p. 5.
3. FNS *Quarterly Bulletin*, Vol. 1, p. 7–8.

4. *Ibid.*, p. 11.
5. Betty Lester interview, by Jonathan Fried, 03/03/78, FNSOHP.
6. Breckinridge, *Midwifery in the Kentucky Mountains*, p. 2.
7. *Ibid.*, p. 2–4.
8. *Ibid.*, p. 4–6.
9. Jean Tolk interview, by DD, 11/01/78, FNSOHP.
10. Breckinridge, *Midwifery in the Kentucky Mountains*, p. 25.
11. *Ibid.*, p. 11–12.
12. *Ibid.*, p. 11–12.
13. *Ibid.*, p. 13.
14. M. Stobbe, "U.S. Maternal Deaths on the Rise," *www.medscape.com*.
15. Harvard Public Health Now, *www.hsph.harvard.edu* 12/18/04.
16. Mary Breckinridge, "Nurse on Horseback," *Woman's Journal*, February 1928.
17. Correspondence between Dr. Veech and Mary Breckinridge, October-November 1923.
18. Breckinridge, *Midwifery in the Kentucky Mountains*, p. 27.
19. FNS *Quarterly Bulletin* 1, October 1925, p. 4.
20. *Southern Mountain Life & Work*, October 1926, p. 8–9.
21. Edna Rockstroh interview, by Betty Lester, 09/22/77, FNSOHP.
22. *Ibid.*
23. *New York Times*, "Prim-

itive America on Screen," undated, 1926.

24. Ettinger, *Nurse-Midwifery*, p. 51.

25. Correspondence from
Mary Breckinridge to Elizabeth Brice, September 23, 1926.

Chapter 4

1. Betty Lester interview,
by DD, 07/27/78, FNSOHP.

2. *Ibid.*

3. *Ibid.*

4. *Ibid.*

5. Betty Lester interview,
by Jonathan Fried, 03/03/78,
FNSOHP.

6. FNS *Quarterly Bulletin*
24, 1949, p. 2–4.

7. *Ibid.*

8. Edna Rockstroh inter-
view, by DD, 12/01/79, FN-
SOHP.

9. Written account by
Betty Lester provided to FNS,
undated letter.

10. Betty Lester interview,
by DD, 07/27/78, FNSOHP.

11. *Ibid.*

12. *Ibid.*

13. *Southern Mountain Life
& Work*, October 26, p. 9.

14. J. Hopp, *Babies in Her
Saddlebags* (Nampa, ID: Pacific
Press, 1986).

15. Interview with Betty
Lester on film produced by Appalshop, Inc. Whitesburg, Kentucky.

16. *Ibid.*

17. Betty Lester interview,
by DD, 07/27/78, FNSOHP

18. Mary　　Breckinridge,
"Nurse-Midwife — A Pioneer"
(reprint), *American Journal of
Public Health*, November 1927,
p. 1147–1151.

19. *Ibid.*, p. 1147–1151.

20. E. Poole, *Nurses on
Horseback* (New York: Macmillan, 1932).

21. *Ibid.*, p. 38.

22. Hopp, *Babies in Her
Saddlebags*, p. 11–12.

23. Carlyle Carter inter-
view, by Linda Green, 01/20/79,
FNSOHP.

24. Agnes Lewis interview,
by DD, 01/05/79, FNSOHP.

25. Breckinridge,　　*Wide
Neighborhoods*, p. 196.

26. FNS *Quarterly Bulletin*
20, Autumn 1944, p. 28–34.

27. Agnes Lewis interview,
by DD, 01/05/79, FNSOHP.

28. Hopp, *Babies in Her
Saddlebags*, p. 12–13.

29. *Ibid.*, p. 13.

30. Betty Lester interview,
by DD, 07/27/78, FNSOHP.

31. Hopp, *Babies in Her
Saddlebags*, p. 14–16.

Chapter 5

1. FNS *Quarterly Bulletin*
19, p. 3.

2. Walter Morgan inter-
view, by Sadie Stidman,
04/11/79, FNSOHP.

3. Breckinridge,　　*Wide
Neighborhoods*, p. 174.

4. *Southern Mountain Life
& Work*, October 1926, p. 9.

5. Jessie Shepherd inter-
view, by Linda Green, 08/22/78,
FNSOHP.

6. Breckinridge,　　*Wide
Neighborhoods*, p. 190.

7. FNS *Quarterly Bulletin*
19, Winter 1944, p. 3.

8. Breckinridge, "Nurse
on Horseback," *Woman's Journal*, February 1928.

9. Breckinridge,　　*Wide
Neighborhoods*, p. 198.

10. Breckinridge,　　"The
Nurse Midwife — A Pioneer,"
*American Journal of Public
Health*, November 1927, p.
1150.

11. Breckinridge, *Wide Neighborhoods*, p. 231.

12. *Ibid.*, p. 232.

13. *Ibid.*

14. *Southern Mountain Life
& Work: Mothers & Babies in
Leslie Co.*, October 1926, p. 10.

15. Mary Lewis Biggerstaff
interview, by DD, 02/12/79,
FNSOHP.

16. *Courier-Journal*, Louisville, Kentucky, July 8, 1928.

17. Interview with Martha
Prewitt Breckinridge, by Carol
Crowe-Carraco, 3/30/79, FN-
SOHP.

18. *Ibid.*

19. *Ibid.*

20. *Ibid.*

21. *Ibid.*

Chapter 6

1. Breckinridge, *Wide Neighborhoods*, p. 229–230.

2. Hopp, *Babies in her Saddlebags*, p. 37.

3. Poole, *Nurses on Horseback*, p. 121.

4. Breckinridge, *Wide Neighborhoods*, p. 241.

5. FNS *Quarterly Bulletin*
16, no. 3 (Winter 1941), reprint.

6. Lucille Knechtly, *Where
Else But Here?* (Pippa Passes,
Kentucky: Pippa Valley Print-
ing, 1989), p. 24.

7. Interview with Corbin
Pennington, by Sadie Stidham,
March 18, 1979, FNSOHP.

8. Hopp, *Babies in Her
Saddlebags*, p. 48–50.

9. Interview with Jean
Tolk, by DD, November 1,
1978, FNSOHP.

10. *Ibid.*

11. *Ibid.*

12. *www.cdc.gov.*

13. Interview on film with
Betty Lester, Appalshop, Inc.
1984.

14. *Ibid.*

15. FNS *Quarterly Bulletin*,
undated volume, 1926, p. 8.

16. *Ibid.*, p. 8–16.

17. Interview with Betty
Lester, by DD, July 27, 1978,
FNSOHP.

18. Interview with Betty
Lester, by DD, August 3, 1978,
FNSOHP.

19. Interview with Marvin
Breckinridge Patterson, by
DD, May 13, 1978, FNSOHP.

20. www.Midwiferytoday.
com.

21. Interview with Sadie &
Juder Stidham, by DD, De-
cember 1, 1978, FNSOHP.

22. Hopp, *Babies in Her
Saddlebags*, p. 27–28.

23. *Ibid.*, p. 26.

24. *Lexington-Herald*, May
30, 1934.

25. *Ibid.*

Chapter 7

1. Interview with Roe
Davidson, by DD, July 20,
1978, FNSOHP.

2. Interview with Grace
Reeder, by Carol Crowe-

Carraco, January 25, 1979, FN-SOHP.

3. E. Poole, *Nurses on Horseback* (New York: Macmillan, 1932), p. 26.

4. M. Breckinridge, *Cornbread Line*, reprinted from *The Survey*, 1930, p. 2.

5. Poole, *Nurses on Horseback*, p. 24.

6. *Ibid.*, p. 25.

7. Breckinridge, *Wide Neighborhoods*, p. 343.

8. FNS Campaign correspondence, New York committee chairman, October 1931.

9. Poole, *Nurses on Horseback*, p. 48.

10. *Ibid.*, p. 50.

11. *Ibid.*, p. 44; Wikipedia, Rockefeller-hookworm.

12. Breckinridge, *Wide Neighborhoods*, p. 267.

13. Interview with Agnes Lewis, by DD, January 5, 1979, FNSOHP.

14. *Ibid.*

15. *Ibid.*

16. *Ibid.*

17. *Ibid.*

18. *Ibid.*

19. Interview with Martha Prewitt Breckinridge, by Carol Crowe-Carraco, March 30, 1979, FNSOHP.

20. *Ibid.*

21. *Ibid.*

22. Interview with Agnes Lewis, by DD.

23. *Ibid.*

24. *Ibid.*

25. *Ibid.*

26. *Ibid.*

27. *Ibid.*

28. *Ibid.*

29. Interview with Margaret Gage, by Marion and W.B. Rogers Beasley, October 16, 1978, FNSOHP.

30. FNS *Quarterly Bulletin*, undated volume, p. 34–36.

31. *Ibid.*

32. Poole, *Nurses on Horseback*, p. 29–30.

33. *Ibid.*, p. 90–91.

34. *Ibid.*, p. 90–97.

35. Interview with Zaydee Dejong Harris, by DD, June 14, 1979, FNSOHP.

36. Poole, *Nurses on Horseback*, p. 97.

37. *Ibid.*, p. 101.

38. *Ibid.*

39. *Ibid.*

Chapter 8

1. Interview with Agnes Lewis, by DD, January 5, 1979, FNSOHP.

2. *Ibid.*

3. Interview with Phoebe Hawkins and Mary Martin, by Anne Campbell, May 23, 1979, FNSOHP.

4. Interview with Zaydee Dejong Harris, by DD, June 14, 1979.

5. Mary Breckinridge correspondence dated December 8, 1931.

6. Interview with Agnes Lewis, by DD, January 5, 1979, FNSOHP.

7. Interview with Alden Gay, by Linda Green, September 1, 1978, FNSOHP.

8. *Ibid.*

9. E. Poole, *Nurses on Horseback*, p. 32–33.

10. *Ibid.*

11. *Ibid.*, p. 34–36.

12. Interview with Agnes Lewis, by DD, January 5, 1979, FNSOHP.

13. Correspondence to FNS donors dated December 8, 1931.

14. "Brother Can You Spare A Dime?" *Washington Post National Weekly*, October 25, 1999.

15. "Open Letter from Mary Breckinridge," FNS *Quarterly Bulletin*, undated volume.

Chapter 9

1. E. Poole, *Nurses on Horseback*, p. 52.

2. *Ibid.*, p. 86.

3. J. Hopp, *Babies in Her Saddlebags*, p. 30–31.

4. Interview with Dorothy Caldwell, by Marian Barrett, January 18, 1979, FNSOHP.

5. Hopp, *Babies in Her Saddlebags*, p. 47.

6. *Ibid.*, p. 38.

7. *Ibid.*, p. 17–18.

8. *Ibid.*, p. 17–19.

9. Interview with Betty Lester, by DD, July 27, 1978, FNSOHP.

10. *Ibid.*

11. J. Hopp, *Babies in Her Saddlebags*, p. 20.

12. *Ibid.*, p. 20–22.

13. Interview with Betty Lester, by DD, July 27, 1978, FNSOHP.

Chapter 10

1. Interview with Anne Winslow, by Anne Campbell, September 25, 1979, FNSOHP.

2. FNS *Quarterly Bulletin* 28, Winter 1953.

3. L. Knechtly, *Where Else But Here?*, p. 31.

4. Interview with Primrose Bowling, by Charles Bowling, December 10, 1985.

5. FNS *Quarterly Bulletin* 30, p. 30.

6. Interview with Leonard Howard, by DD, July 9, 1979, FNSOHP.

7. M. Breckinridge, "An Adventure In Midwifery," Harmon Foundation Quarterly Award, 1928.

8. L. Knechtly, *Where Else But Here?*, p. 17.

9. FNS *Quarterly Bulletin* 30, p. 21–22.

10. L. Knechtly, *Where Else But Here?*, p. 13.

11. Interview with Agnes Lewis, by DD, January 5, 1979, FNSOHP.

12. L. Knechtly, *Where Else But Here?*, p. 23.

13. *Ibid.*, p. 23–24.

14. Interview with Margaret Gage, by Marion and W.B. Rogers Beasley, October 16, 1978, FNSOHP.

15. L. Knechtly, *Where Else But Here?*, p. 3, 25.

16. *Ibid.*, p. 5.

17. *Ibid.*, p. 8–9.

18. *Ibid.*

19. FNS *Quarterly Bulletin* 29, p. 21–22.

Chapter 11

1. Correspondence from Louis Dublin to Mary Breckinridge, May 22, 1935.

2. FNS *Quarterly Bulletin*, undated volume, p. 17.

3. *Good Housekeeping Magazine*, June 1932, p. 6.

4. *Ibid.*
5. Mary Willeford, FNS *Quarterly Bulletin*, 1932, reprint.
6. E. Poole, *Nurses on Horseback*, p. 163.
7. *Good Housekeeping Magazine*, June 1932, p. 2.

Chapter 12

1. Interview with Agnes Lewis, by DD, January 5, 1979, FNSOHP.
2. *Ibid.*
3. *Ibid.*
4. *Ibid.*
5. M. Breckinridge, *Wide Neighborhoods*, p. 282.
6. *Ibid.*, p. 218.
7. Historical Statistics of U.S. Department of Commerce Census Bureau, 1975.
8. M. Breckinridge, "Is Birth Control the Answer?" *Harper's Monthly Magazine*, 1931.
9. *Ibid.*
10. *Ibid.*
11. Laura E. Ettinger, *Nurse Midwifery: Birth of a New American Profession* (Columbus: Ohio State University Press, 2006), p. 143.
12. Interview with Roger Egeberg, by DD, April 27, 1979, FNSOHP.
13. *Ibid.*
14. *Ibid.*
15. FNS *Quarterly Bulletin* 38, p. 17–19.
16. *American Journal of Nursing* 38, no. 11 (November 1938), reprint.
17. "Letters From Our Frontier Hospital," by a staff nurse, *Frontier Nursing at War*, April 1943.
18. M. Breckinridge, "The Frontier Nursing Service," reprinted from *The Centurian*, October 1939.
19. FNS *Quarterly Bulletin*, undated volume.
20. FNS booklet, *You're Wanted on Cutshin*, 1939.
21. M. Breckinridge, *Wide Neighborhoods*, p. 323.
22. M. Breckinridge, "The Rural Family and its Mother," *The Mother*, April 1944, in Frontier Nursing Service Collection, Southern Appalachian Archives, Berea College.
23. *Ibid.*

Chapter 13

1. Interview with Betty Lester, by Jonathan Fried, March 3, 1978, FNSOHP.
2. Interview with Betty Lester, by DD, July 27, 1978, FNSOHP.
3. *Ibid.*
4. M. Breckinridge, "A Frontier Nurse Speaks Out," *Lexington Herald*, August 11, 1940.
5. M. Breckinridge, "Childbirth & War," FNS *Quarterly Bulletin* 18, Autumn 1942, reprint.
6. *Ibid.*, p. 7.
7. Correspondence from Betty Lester to FNS staff, Easter, 1941.
8. Interview with Betty Lester, by DD, July 27, 1978, FNSOHP.
9. *Ibid.*
10. J. Hopp, *Babies in Her Saddlebags*, p. 52–53.
11. *Ibid.*, p. 53.
12. FNS *Quarterly Bulletin* 16, Winter 1941.
13. Correspondence (compiled) from Frontier Nursing in War letters, FNS *Quarterly Bulletins*, 1943.
14. M. Breckinridge, "The Mother," Reprinted from *American Journal of Public Health*, November 1927.

Chapter 14

1. Interview with Agnes Lewis, by DD, January 5, 1979, FNSOHP.
2. *Ibid.*
3. *Ibid.*
4. *Ibid.*
5. *Ibid.*
6. *Ibid.*
7. *Ibid.*
8. *Ibid.*
9. *Ibid.*
10. Interview with Lucille Knechtly, by DD, July 9, 1979, FNSOHP.
11. *Ibid.*
12. *Ibid.*

13. L. Knechtly, *Where Else But Here?*, p. 44–45.
14. Interview with Lucille Knechtly, by DD, July 9, 1979.
15. FNS *Quarterly Bulletin* 19, Summer 1943.
16. FNS *Quarterly Bulletin* 19, Winter 1944, p. 35.
17. FNS *Quarterly Bulletin* 19, Summer 1943, p. 17–18.
18. *Ibid.*
19. *Ibid.*
20. *Ibid.*, p. 19.

Chapter 15

1. FNS *Quarterly Bulletin* 19, Winter 1944, p. 30–32.
2. *Ibid.*, p. 30.
3. *Ibid.*
4. *Ibid.*, p. 85–86.
5. *Ibid.*, p. 89.
6. FNS *Quarterly Bulletin* 21, Spring 1946, no p. number.
7. *Ibid.*
8. *Ibid.*, p. 55.
9. Interview with Lucille Knechtly, by DD, July 9, 1979, FNSOHP.
10. J. Hopp, *Babies in Her Saddlebags*, p. 56.
11. Interview with Betty Lester, by DD, July 27, 1978, FNSOHP.
12. *Ibid.*
13. FNS *Quarterly Bulletin* 21, Spring 1946.
14. *Ibid.*
15. *Ibid.*
16. *Ibid.*
17. Florence Samson, RN, "Water," FNS *Quarterly Bulletin* 21, Spring 1946.
18. *Ibid.*
19. FNS *Quarterly Bulletin* 21, Spring 1946.
20. *Ibid.*
21. *Ibid.*
22. *Ibid.*, p. 40–42.
23. *Ibid.*
24. FNS *Quarterly Bulletin* 21, Spring 1946.
25. *Ibid.*
26. *Ibid.*, p. 7–8.
27. *Ibid.*
28. *Ibid.*

Chapter 16

1. Diagram presented to Mary Breckinridge by Ellen Wadsworth, February 17, 1941.

2. Interview with Mary Wilson Neel, by Anne Campbell, December 1, 1979, FNSOHP.

3. L. Knechtly, *Where Else But Here?*, p. 27.

4. Interview with Catherine Towbridge Arpee, by Linda Green, December 2, 1978, FNSOHP.

5. *Ibid.*

6. *Ibid.*

7. *Ibid.*

8. L. Knechtly, *Where Else But Here?*, p. 29.

9. M. Breckinridge, *Wide Neighborhoods*, p. 72.

10. Interview with Brooke Alexander, by Anne Campbell, September 25, 1979, FNSOHP.

11. *Ibid.*

12. Interview with James Parton, by Anne Campbell, May 25, 1979, FNSOHP.

13. *Ibid.*

14. *Ibid.*

15. *Ibid.*

16. *Ibid.*

17. Interview with Mary Wilson Neel, by Anne Campbell, December 1, 1979.

18. Interview with Mardi B. Perry and Susan Putnam, by Anne Campbell, January 25, 1979, FNSOHP.

19. *Ibid.*

20. Interview with Fredericka Holdship, by DD, March 25, 1979, FNSOHP.

21. Interview with Mary Wilson Neel, by Anne Campbell, December 1, 1979, FNSOHP.

22. *Ibid.*

23. *Ibid.*

24. *Ibid.*

25. *Ibid.*

26. Interview with Allyn J. Shepherd, by Marian Barrett, January 18, 1979, FNSOHP.

27. Interview with Mary Wilson Neel, by Anne Campbell, December 1, 1979, FNSOHP.

28. *Ibid.*

29. *Ibid.*

30. Interview with Marianne Harper, by Linda Green, April 9, 1979.

31. Interview with Mary Wilson Neel, by Anne Campbell, December 1, 1979, FNSOHP.

32. Interview with Mardi B. Perry and Susan M. Putnam, by Anne Campbell, January 25, 1979, FNSOHP.

33. Interview with Mary Wilson Neel, by Anne Campbell, December 1, 1979, FNSOHP.

34. M. Breckinridge, *Wide Neighborhoods*, p. 276.

Chapter 17

1. Interview with Dorothy Caldwell, by Marian Barrett, January 18, 1979, FNSOHP.

2. Interview with Nancy Damman, by DD, no date provided, FNSOHP.

3. Interview with Dorothy Caldwell, by Marian Barrett, January 18, 1979, FNSOHP.

4. *Ibid.*

5. FNS *Quarterly Bulletin* 20, Winter 1945, p. 11–13.

6. *Ibid.*, p. 11.

7. *Ibid.*

8. *Ibid.*, p. 11–13.

9. *Ibid.*

10. *Ibid.*

11. *Ibid.*

12. *Ibid.*

13. *Ibid.*, p. 4–11.

14. *Ibid.*

15. *Ibid.*

16. *Ibid.*

17. *Ibid.*

18. *Ibid.*

19. Interview with Mary Stewart, by Marian Barrett, January 15, 1980, FNSOHP.

20. *Ibid.*

21. *Ibid.*

22. *Ibid.*

23. *Ibid.*

24. M. Breckinridge, *Wide Neighborhoods*, p. 341

Chapter 18

1. FNS *Quarterly Bulletin* 21, Summer 1945, p. 62.

2. L. Knechtly, *Where Else But Here?*, p. 29.

3. *Ibid.*, p. 28.

4. B. Lester, "Operation Louise," FNS *Quarterly Bulletin* 28, Summer 1952, p. 17–21.

5. *The Road*, produced by Vision Associations, 1967.

6. FNS *Quarterly Bulletin* 21, Winter 1946, p. 8.

7. *Ibid.*, p. 8–10.

8. *Ibid.*

9. *Ibid.*

10. FNS *Quarterly Bulletin* 21, Summer 1945, p. 18–20.

11. FNS *Quarterly Bulletin* 20, Spring 1945, p. 5.

12. *Ibid.*

13. *Ibid.*, p. 5–8.

14. *Ibid.*, p. 2.

15. FNS *Quarterly Bulletin* 21, Summer 1945, p. 27.

16. *Ibid.*, p. 21–25.

17. *Ibid.*

18. *Ibid.*

19. *Ibid.*, p. 25.

Chapter 19

1. FNS *Quarterly Bulletin* 21, Winter 1946, p. 15.

2. *History of Social Work 1905–1940*, Massachusetts General Hospital Website.

3. FNS *Quarterly Bulletin* 23, Spring 1948, p. 28.

4. FNS *Quarterly Bulletin* 22, Winter 1947, pgs 10–11.

5. *Ibid.*

6. *Ibid.*, p. 11, 63.

7. *Ibid.*

8. M. Breckinridge, *Wide Neighborhoods*, p. 329.

9. FNS *Quarterly Bulletin* 23, Summer 1947, p. 51.

10. M. Breckinridge, *Wide Neighborhoods*, p. 320.

11. FNS *Quarterly Bulletin* 23, Summer 1947, p. 4.

12. *Ibid.*, p. 6.

13. *Ibid.*, p. 4.

14. *Ibid.*, p. 17–34.

15. *Ibid.*

16. *Ibid.*

17. FNS *Quarterly Bulletin* 22, Winter 1947, p. 4.

18. FNS *Quarterly Bulletin* 23, Spring 1948, p. 42–43.

19. *Ibid.*, p. 44.

20. FNS *Quarterly Bulletin* 22, Winter 1947, p. 26.

21. FNS *Quarterly Bulletin* 24, Winter 1949, p. 3.

22. *Ibid.*

23. FNS *Quarterly Bulletin* 23, Autumn 1947, p. 9.

Chapter 20

1. FNS *Quarterly Bulletin* 23, Autumn 1947, p. 48.
2. FNS *Quarterly Bulletin* 24, Summer 1948, no page number.
3. FNS *Quarterly Bulletin* 22, Spring 1947, p. 58–59.
4. *Ibid.*
5. *Ibid.*
6. FNS *Quarterly Bulletin* 24, Winter 1949, p. 46.
7. M. Breckinridge, *Wide Neighborhoods*, p. 321.
8. L. Ettinger, *Nurse-Midwifery: Birth of a New American Profession*, p. 33, 36, 46.
9. M. Breckinridge, *Wide Neighborhoods*, p. 322.
10. Interview with Elizabeth Lansing, by Anne Campbell, June 6, 1980, FNSOHP.
11. *Ibid.*
12. *Ibid.*
13. *Ibid.*
14. M. Breckinridge, *Wide Neighborhoods*, p. 333.
15. *Ibid.*
16. *Ibid.*

Chapter 21

1. FNS *Quarterly Bulletin* 25, Autumn 1949, p. 14.
2. Interview with Kate Ireland, by DD, November 1, 1979, FNSOHP.
3. *Ibid.*
4. *Ibid.*
5. L. Knechtly, *Where Else But Here?* p. 30.
6. FNS *Quarterly Bulletin* 29, Autumn 1953, p. 5–7.
7. *Ibid.*
8. L. Ettinger, *Nurse-Midwifery: Birth of a New American Profession*, p. 53.
9. *Courier-Journal*, Louisville, Kentucky, May 31, 1950.
10. *Ibid.*
11. FNS *Quarterly Bulletin* 25, Winter 1950, p. 44.
12. *Ibid.*
13. Alliance for Improvement of Maternity Services (AIMS), *www.aimsusa.org*.
14. History of Midwifery, *www.mnmidwife.org*.
15. L. Ettinger, *Nurse-Midwifery: Birth of a New American Profession*, p. 140.

16. M. Breckinridge, "Figures That Are Facts," no primary source or date provided.
17. FNS *Quarterly Bulletin* 25, Winter 1950, p. 5–7.
18. *Ibid.*
19. *Ibid.*
20. *Ibid.*
21. FNS *Quarterly Bulletin* 26, Spring 1950, p. 3–14.
22. *Ibid.*
23. *Ibid.*
24. *Ibid.*
25. *Ibid.*
26. *Ibid.*
27. *Ibid.*

Chapter 22

1. M. Breckinridge, *Wide Neighborhoods*, p. 328.
2. Interview with Helen E. Browne, by Carol Crowe-Carraco, March 26, 1979, FNSOHP.
3. *Ibid.*
4. *Ibid.*
5. *Ibid.*
6. *Ibid.*
7. *Ibid.*
8. *Ibid.*
9. *Ibid.*
10. *Ibid.*
11. *Ibid.*
12. *Ibid.*
13. *Ibid.*
14. *Ibid.*
15. *Ibid.*
16. *Ibid.*
17. FNS *Quarterly Bulletin* 26, Summer 1950.
18. "Dentistry & the FNS," *Ibid.*
19. FNS *Quarterly Bulletin* 26, Summer 1950.
20. National Center for Health Statistics.
21. Interview with Helen E. Browne, by Carol Crowe-Carraco, March 26, 1979, FNSOHP.
22. *Ibid.*
23. FNS *Quarterly Bulletin* 29, Spring 1954.
24. FNS *Quarterly Bulletin* 28, Summer 1952.

Chapter 23

1. FNS *Quarterly Bulletin* 28, Spring 1953.
2. *Ibid.*

3. FNS *Quarterly Bulletin* 28, Winter 1953, p. 8–9.
4. *Ibid.*
5. *Ibid.*, p. 11.
6. *Ibid.*, pgs 9–11.
7. *Ibid.*
8. FNS *Quarterly Bulletin* 30, Winter 1955, pgs 7–9.
9. *Ibid.*
10. *Ibid.*
11. *Ibid.*
12. Interview with Primrose Bowling, by Charles Bowling, December 10, 1985, FNSOHP.
13. *Ibid.*
14. *Ibid.*
15. *Ibid.*
16. *Ibid.*
17. *Ibid.*
18. *Ibid.*
19. *Ibid.*
20. *Ibid.*
21. *Ibid.*
22. *Ibid.*
23. *Ibid.*
24. *Ibid.*
25. FNS *Quarterly Bulletin* 29, Summer 1953, p. 58.

Chapter 24

1. J. Hopp, *Babies in Her Saddlebags*, p. 70–71.
2. *Ibid.*
3. *Ibid.*, p. 70–71.
4. *Ibid.*
5. Interview with Carolyn Booth Gregory, by Linda Green, March 31, 1979, FNSOHP.
6. L. Knechtly, *Where Else But Here?*, p. 54.
7. *Ibid.*, p. 56.
8. *Ibid.*, p. 62.
9. *Ibid.*, p. 64–65.
10. *Ibid.*
11. FNS *Quarterly Bulletin* 30, Spring 1955, p. 3.
12. FNS *Quarterly Bulletin* 26, Spring 1956, p. 11–14.
13. *Ibid.*
14. *Ibid.*
15. *Ibid.*
16. *Ibid.*
17. FNS *Quarterly Bulletin*, Autumn 1957.
18. *Ibid.*

Chapter 25

1. Interview with Molly Lee, by Carol Crowe-Carraco, February 6, 1979, FNSOHP
2. *Ibid.*

3. *Ibid.*
4. *Ibid.*
5. *Ibid.*
6. *Ibid.*
7. *Ibid.*
8. FNS *Quarterly Bulletin* 37, Spring 1962, p. 11–13.
9. *Ibid.*, p. 25.
10. FNS *Quarterly Bulletin* 36, Summer 1960, p. 21.
11. *Ibid.*
12. *Ibid.*
13. FNS — *80 Years of Service Mary Breckinridge* — The Rose of Wendover, ProQuest Information.
14. Interview with Dr. Edward Ray and Louise Ray, by DD, December 7, 1978, FNSOHP.
15. *Ibid.*
16. *Courier-Journal*, Louisville, Kentucky, September 22, 1962.
17. FNS *Quarterly Bulletin* 37, Spring 1962, p. 29.
18. Interview with Elsie Maier, by DD, December 5, 1978, FNSOHP.
19. *Ibid.*
20. www.imr.bsd.uchicago.edu.
21. Interview with Dr. John Rock, by DD, June 15, 1979, FNSOHP.
22. FNS *Quarterly Bulletin* 41, Summer 1965, p. 49–50.
23. *Ibid.*
24. Phone interview with Molly Lee, conducted August 17, 2007.

Chapter 26

1. FNS *Quarterly Bulletin* 37, Winter 1962, p. 1–4.

2. *Ibid.*
3. M. Breckinridge, *Wide Neighborhoods*, p. 299.
4. Interview with Dr. Louis Hellman, by Anne Campbell, November 29, 1979, FNSOHP.
5. *Ibid.*
6. FNS *Quarterly Bulletin* 40, Summer 1964, p. 41.
7. Interview with Martha Lady, by DD, August 4, 1978, FNSOHP.
8. Interview with Agnes Lewis, by DD, January 5, 1979, FNSOHP.
9. Interview with Mary Stewart, by Marian Barrett, January 15, 1980, FNSOHP.
10. *Ibid.*
11. Interview with Agnes Lewis, by DD, January 5, 1979, FNSOHP.
12. Interview with Helen E. Browne, by Carol Crowe-Carraco, March 26, 1979, FNSOHP.
13. Interview with Helen E. Browne, by DD, March 27, 1979, FNSOHP.
14. *Ibid.*
15. *Ibid.*
16. *Ibid.*
17. *Ibid.*
18. Interview with Margaret Gage, by Marian and W.B. Rogers Beasley, October 16, 1978, FNSOHP.
19. *Ibid.*
20. *Ibid.*
21. Interview with Helen E. Browne, by DD, March 27, 1979, FNSOHP.
22. *Ibid.*
23. Interview with Margaret Gage, by Marion and

W.B. Rogers Beasley, October 16, 1978, FNSOHP.
24. *Courier-Journal*, Louisville, Kentucky, May 17, 1965.
25. L. Knechtly, *Where Else But Here?*, p. 82.
26. Interview with Georgia Ledford, by Carol Crowe-Carraco, August 17, 1978, FNSOHP.
27. L. Knechtly, *Where Else But Here?*, p. 78.
28. *Ibid.*
29. Interview with Leonard Howard, by DD, July 9, 1979, FNSOHP.
30. Interview with Della Gay, by Linda Green, September 8, 1978, FNSOHP.
31. *Ibid.*
32. *Ibid.*
33. L. Knechtly, *Where Else But Here?*, p. 83.
34. *Ibid.*, p. 86.
35. J. Hopp, *Babies in Her Saddlebags*, p. 78.

Epilogue

1. Interview with Nancy Damman, by DD, no date provided, FNSOHP.
2. Interview with Kate Ireland, by DD, November 1, 1979, FNSOHP.
3. FNS *Quarterly Bulletin* 41, Winter 1966.
4. FNS online, ProQuest Information and Learning Company, Spring 2006.

Bibliography

One of the best sources I had access to, thanks to the University of Kentucky, Berea College, and Frontier Nursing Service, Inc., was a comprehensive FNS Oral History Collection. Spanning 1900 to 1985, this documented account of the FNS contained one hundred ninety-two interviews with nurse-midwives, couriers, administrative staff, and residents of Leslie County who recalled, sometimes in great detail, their associations with the FNS and Mary Breckinridge. Initiated in 1978, the project was conducted under the supervision of Dale Deaton. Principal interviewers were Deaton, Anne Campbell, and Carol Crowe-Carraco. This project provided an in-depth look at the FNS from the people directly involved. I also visited the FNS site in Wendover, Kentucky, on three occasions, and toured the Hyden Hospital and the Beech Fork Clinic. At the Big House, I was privy to resources that ranged from photo collections to films, books, and correspondence. Simply being on the grounds and in the actual home of Mary Breckinridge and the FNS brought the history of the organization to life. In addition, I traveled to Tallahassee, Florida, where I interviewed Kate Ireland, FNS head courier, and Anne Cundle, British FNS nurse-midwife; talked by phone with FNS nurse-midwife Molly Lee in England about her years at the FNS, and Dr. Richard A. Carter in Nashville, Tennessee, who answered my medical questions. I also contacted Dr. Joyce Hopp, Ph.D., in California, who wrote a book on FNS nurse-midwife Betty Lester, and corresponded frequently with Michael Claussen, FNS Wendover development coordinator, for follow-up questions. At the University of Kentucky and Berea College I found, through the helpful staff, the FNS Special Collection of FNS materials that provided rich insights into the day-to-day operation of the FNS. Among the materials housed were more than a hundred issues of the FNS *Quarterly Bulletin*, from its first issue in 1925 to the current year, and several articles produced by Mary Breckinridge as part of her fund-raising efforts.

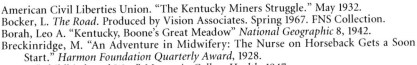

American Civil Liberties Union. "The Kentucky Miners Struggle." May 1932.
Bocker, L. *The Road.* Produced by Vision Associates. Spring 1967. FNS Collection.
Borah, Leo A. "Kentucky, Boone's Great Meadow" *National Geographic* 8, 1942.
Breckinridge, M. "An Adventure in Midwifery: The Nurse on Horseback Gets a Soon Start." *Harmon Foundation Quarterly Award*, 1928.
_____. "Childbirth and War." *Mountain College Health*, 1947.
_____. "The Cornbread Line." *The Survey*, 1930.

_____. "A Frontier Nurse Speaks Out." *Federal Union, Inc.*, 1940 (originally appeared in *Lexington Herald-Ledger* on August 11, 1940).

_____. "The Frontier Nursing Service." *Centurian*, October 1939.

_____. "Is Birth Control the Answer?" *Harper's Monthly Magazine*, 1931.

_____. "The Nurse-Midwife — A Pioneer." *American Journal of Public Health* 17, no. 11 (November 1927).

_____. "The Nurse on Horseback." *The Woman's Journal*, February 1928.

_____. "The Rural Family and Its Mother." *The Mother*, April 1944.

_____. *Wide Neighborhoods: A Story of the Frontier Nursing Service*. Lexington: University of Kentucky Press, 1952.

Breckinridge, Mary Marvin. "The Forgotten Frontier." 1928. FNS Collection.

Breckinridge, Mary, and J. C. Breckinridge. *Midwifery in the Kentucky Mountains: An Investigation*. 1923.

"Brother, Can You Spare a Dime?" *Washington Post National Weekly*. October 25, 1999.

Buck, Dorothy. "The First Nursing Service." *Mountain Life and Work*, January 1934.

Casey, Baretta R., et al. "Rural Kentucky's Physician Shortage." *UK Center for Rural Health*, September 2005.

Courier-Journal. "Nursing Service Marks Its 25th Year." May 31, 1950.

Creason, J. "Hossback to Jeep." *Courier-Journal Magazine*, June 11, 1961.

Dorland's Illustrated Medical Dictionary. 29th ed. Philadelphia: W.B. Saunders, 2000.

Ettinger, L. *Nurse-Midwifery: Birth of a New American Profession*. Columbus: Ohio State University Press, 2006.

FNS pictorial. *"Reflections of Our Past & Present, FNS Celebrating 80 Years: A Collection of Photos from the FNS."*

Godby, Allan, and Dorothy Godby. "Dentistry and the FNS." Summer 1950. Excerpt provided by ProQuest Information & Learning Co.

Hopp, J. *Babies In Her Saddlebags*. Nampa, ID: Pacific Press Publishing Association, 1986.

Knechtly, L. *Where Else But Here?* Pippa Passes, KY: Pippa Valley Printing, 1989.

Lansing, E. *Rider on the Mountains*. New York: Thomas Crowell, 1949.

Lester, B. Written account from Lester to the FNS of her arrival in Hyden. 1928. FNS Collection.

Lexington-Herald. "Reports on Work Done by FNS Given at Annual Meeting." May 30, 1934.

National Center for Health Statistics, 2001.

New York Times. "Nurse on Horseback Rides the Lonely Kentucky Trails." January 18, 1931.

Poole, E. The Nurse on Horseback." *Good Housekeeping Magazine*, June 1932.

_____. *Nurses on Horseback*. New York: Macmillan, 1932.

Prewitt, M. "Mothers and Babies in Leslie County." *Southern Mountain Life and Work*, October 1926.

Summers, V. "Saddle-Bag and Log Cabin Technique." *American Journal of Nursing* 38, no. 11 (November 1938).

Trout, A. "Nurse and Angel of the Frontier Dies." *Courier-Journal*, May 17, 1965.

"The Year That Changed America." *U.S. News & World Report*. August 20, 2007.

Web Sites

www.answers.com/Cumberland-plateau
www.answers.com/topic/banking
www.agpix.com
www.bluegrassgrotto.org/ (Floyd Collins)
www.cb.com/women (in American history)
www.CenterforNursingAdvocacy.org
www.city-data.com/Hyden-KY
www.geocities.com (1920s & 1930s)
www.kclibrary.nhmccd.edu (American Cultural History 1920–29
www.kernel.uky.edu (1920s)

www.leslie.K12.KY.us/LCHS
www.MassGeneralHospital.org "History of Social Work"
www.medicine.net/com
www.medscape.com/nurse-midwifery in U.S.
www.midwiferytoday.com
www.publicschoolreview.com
www.wikipedia.org/Alpha_Omicron_Pi
www.wikipedia.org/Appalachian (Mountains)

www.wikipedia.org/Great (Depression in the United States)

www.wikipedia.org/Louis_Brandis

www.wikipedia.org/This_Is_Your_Life

www.wikipedia.org/Queen's (Nursing Institute)

www.wikipedia.org/World (War II and V-I Flying Bomb)

www.willrogers.org

Index

Numbers in *bold italics* indicate pages with photographs.